Handbook of
Drug Therapy
Monitoring

Handbook of Drug Therapy Monitoring

Charles H. Brown, M.S., R.Ph.

Associate Professor of Clinical Pharmacy
Purdue University
School of Pharmacy and Pharmacal Sciences
West Lafayette, Indiana

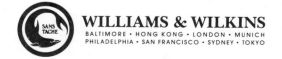

WILLIAMS & WILKINS

BALTIMORE · HONG KONG · LONDON · MUNICH
PHILADELPHIA · SAN FRANCISCO · SYDNEY · TOKYO

Editor: John P. Butler
Associate Editor: Linda Napora
Project Editor: Eden Delcher
Designer: Bets Ltd.
Illustration Planner: Lorraine Wrzosek
Production Coordinator: Charles E. Zeller

Accurate indications, adverse reactions, and dosage schedules for drugs are
provided in this book, but it is possible that they may change. The reader is urged
to review the package information data of the manufacturers of the medications
mentioned.

Printed in the United States of America

Library of Congress Cataloging in Publication Data

Brown, Charles H.
   Handbook of drug therapy monitoring.

   Includes index.
     1. Chemotherapy—Evaluation.   2. Patient monitoring.   I. Title.   [DNLM:
1. Drug Therapy.   2. Monitoring, Physiologic.   WB 330 B877h]
RM263.B77   1989   615.5'8   89-5500
ISBN 0-683-01091-3

                                        90   91   92
                        3   4   5   6   7   8   9   10

To my wife Betty,
and my son Mark,
whose devoted love, support, and encouragement
have been invaluable.

C.H.B.

Preface

The purpose of this textbook is to assist senior pharmacy students (B.S. or Pharm. D) and practicing pharmacists in developing clinical drug therapy monitoring skills. Drug therapy monitoring is becoming an essential activity for pharmacists in community and hospital pharmacy settings. The reasons for this role change for pharmacists include the growing complexity of multiple drug therapy and the evolution of clinical pharmacy practice. Today, pharmacists are becoming more involved in providing drug information and education, conducting drug utilization reviews and patient care audits, detecting and reporting adverse drug reactions, and conducting clinical drug studies and investigational drug trials. The *Handbook of Drug Therapy Monitoring* presents a comprehensive, practical, systematic approach to the how's and why's of drug therapy monitoring.

The process of drug therapy monitoring involves collecting various patient data along with drug and disease monitoring parameters to determine: (1) the appropriateness of therapy and specific drug choice, drug dose, drug dosage form, route of administration and duration of therapy for the patient and the disease/ disorder; (2) a patient's beneficial or adverse response to drug therapy; (3) that appropriate serum drug levels are achieved for the particular patient; and (4) whenever needed, recommended dosage adjustments to assure that therapeutically effective serum drug levels are achieved and toxic serum drug levels are avoided.

The processes of effectively assessing drug therapy and performing follow-up patient monitoring are often complex in nature and take time and clinical experience to develop and refine. One of the most difficult tasks a pharmacist has in performing drug therapy monitoring is in developing an effective and efficient approach or plan. To assist the pharmacist in developing such an approach, this book reviews the contents of a typical medical chart by utilizing Jane Doe's simulated patient case. The format of this book allows the pharmacist to extract essential patient data from the medical chart and guides him/her in developing a formal patient case write-up of Jane Doe. By utilizing the problem-oriented medical record and guided design approaches presented in this text, the pharmacist progresses through an extensive review and evaluation of Jane Doe, her medical problems and their drug therapies. Other simulated patient case exercises, with varying degrees of difficulty, are also included to provide the student with opportunities to refine their clinical skills, develop problem identification and problem solving skills, and perform drug therapy monitoring. Following each simulated patient case exercise is a suggested answer sheet for the student to check his/her responses. By working through these exercises, the pharmacist has an opportunity to develop an effective, efficient approach to drug therapy monitoring.

CHARLES H. BROWN, M.S., R.Ph.

Contents

Introduction

The increased potency and complexity of modern drugs, along with patients' varied responses to drug therapy, present health care professionals with the monumental problem of adequately overseeing patients' pharmaceutical needs. A solution that has proven both cost-efficient and clinically effective is the utilization of clinically trained pharmacists to: act as drug therapy consultants and to perform general drug therapy monitoring; provide drug information and education; participate in drug utilization review and patient care audits; detect and report adverse drug reactions; conduct clinical drug studies; and monitor investigational drug studies (1–24).

The process of monitoring drug therapy involves more than just the assessment and management of a patient's drug therapy. For the purpose of this text, the term drug therapy monitoring is defined as utilizing patient-, drug- and disease-monitoring parameters to determine: (1) appropriateness of drug choice, drug dose, drug dosage form, route of administration, and duration of therapy for the patient and disease/disorder; (2) a patient's beneficial or adverse response to drug therapy; (3) serum drug levels and, whenever needed, recommend dosage adjustments to assure that therapeutically effective serum drug levels are achieved and that toxic serum drug levels are avoided; and (4) that serum drug levels are appropriate for the particular patient being evaluated to either cure or control the disease/disorder. Prior to entering clinical pharmacy practice, the pharmacist needs to have developed competency in pathophysiology, therapeutics, interpersonal relationships, and communication skills, as well as possessing a sympathetic and caring attitude for the patient. All of those elements are necessary for the clinical pharmacist to better communicate with the patient and other health professionals.

■ Goals of Monitoring Drug Therapy

The primary goals of having a clinically trained health care professional assess and monitor a patient's drug therapy should be to: (1) assure appropriate, rational drug therapy is utilized to achieve the desired therapeutic objective; (2) maximize the drug's beneficial effects and prevent or minimize the drug's undesirable effects; and (3) help reduce the cost of medical care for patients. These goals may be achieved when the clinical pharmacist identifies existing or potential medication problems and either initiates problem-solving measures or recommends them to appropriate health care professionals. Problem-solving measures are those which help to improve the efficiency of drug therapy or decrease the risk of adverse drug effects in patients.

However, to accomplish these goals fully, the pharmacist will need to develop his or her clinical skills so that he or she feels comfortable in a clinical setting and is self-confident and resourceful. It is very important that the pharmacist develop a rational plan for approaching both routine and complicated aspects of drug therapy. The clinical pharmacist should remember that monitoring drug therapy is an ongoing process, and it must be re-evaluated at regular intervals to keep up with patient progress and drug therapy modifications.

■ Need for Drug Therapy Monitoring By Pharmacists

As a result of acute and multiple chronic diseases, short- and long-term drug therapy becomes an integral part of the total medical care most patients receive. It is not uncommon to find patients residing in their homes, hospitals or nursing homes who receive more than eight different medications daily, with some receiving as many as 20 drugs each day (25–28). Since the elderly take more medication per patient than any other segment of our population, these patients may require closer drug therapy monitoring than younger adults. This situation may be further complicated because some patients, especially the elderly, may exhibit a modified drug response resulting primarily from altered pharmacodynamic and pharmacokinetic effects. A modified drug response may occur in patients as a result of altered patterns of absorption, distribution, metabolism, and excretion or elimination of drugs. These alterations are due, in part, to physiological and pathological changes in patients as a result of aging. Examples of such physiologic changes as a result of aging include: (1) decreased hepatic and renal function; (2) alteration in body lean muscle mass and fat composition; (3) alteration in blood flow to vital organs, especially kidneys and liver; and (4) decreased protein (albumin) binding of drugs (27–35).

The reduced ability of some patients to handle drugs often leads to altered and unexpected drug responses even when only one medication is used. When multiple drugs are taken concurrently, abnormal drug responses are even more difficult to explain or predict. As one might expect, the incidence of adverse drug reactions (ADRs) increases dramatically with increasing age and increasing or multiple drug use (36–38). Studies have reported that the incidence of ADRs for elderly patients ranges from 24 to 67 percent as compared with about 11 percent in younger adults 31–40 years old. Drugs most often reported as causing ADRs in patients include: (1) diuretics; (2) antihypertensives; (3) antiparkinson agents; (4) psychotropic agents; and (5) cardiac drugs, especially digoxin (37–38). A clear relationship between increasing age and the incidence of ADRs has been demonstrated for the benzodiazepine derivatives, such as chlordiazepoxide, diazepam, flurazepam, and nitrazepam (38–42).

■ Necessary Skills for the Clinical Pharmacist

There are several areas in which the clinical pharmacist needs to develop skills to accomplish fully the goals of drug therapy monitoring:

Interpersonal Relationships

The clinical pharmacist must learn to understand and appreciate the role of other health care professionals (e.g., physicians, nurses, therapists, etc.). He/she must also be able to interact with and function as a member of the health care team. Sound drug therapy is largely based upon the cooperative efforts of each team member. Whenever possible, the clinical pharmacist should accompany the physician on medical rounds. Some drug-related problems could be avoided if the pharmacist could directly assess the appropriateness of prescribed medication as well as provide drug information to assist the physician. In addition, the pharmacist could present his/her findings resulting from monitoring the physician's patients and make requests for laboratory tests or other necessary measures. Interactions with nurses and various therapists may arise when they have a specific question about the mechanism of action of a certain medication a patient is taking. They may also want to know if the side effects of a specific medication include a change in the patient's behavior, mental alertness, activity level, etc. Only when physicians, nurses, therapists, and the clinical pharmacist have developed a cooperative professional relationship can the full potential and expertise of each health care professional be realized to enhance the quality of patient care in any institution.

Communication Skills

The clinical pharmacist must be able to communicate his/her recommendations and findings to the physician or other health professional in a clear and concise manner. He/she must use a team approach, respecting others' expertise while displaying confidence in his or her own.

Empathy

The clinical pharmacist must possess a deep sense of shared responsibility to patients for the medical care they receive. Empathy will be immediately discerned by the patient. It will facilitate the taking of the patient's drug history and develop patient confidence in the professional care being provided.

Clinical Skills

To monitor drug therapy efficiently and effectively, the pharmacist will first need to become familiar with specific aspects of common diseases and their appropriate drug therapy. These aspects include: (a) disease etiology; (b) disease signs and symptoms; (c) pathophysiology; (d) criteria for diagnosis; (e) clinical laboratory tests; (f) applied therapeutics; and (g) pharmacokinetics. In addition, the clinical pharmacist must also learn to cope with many emotional and psychological factors involved in working closely with patients who may be critically ill and never fully recover from their disease(s).

A pharmacist who has been clinically trained to: (1) relate drug therapy to specific diseases or disorders; (2) review drug doses and administration; (3) monitor patient response to drug therapy and drug side effects; and (4) provide information on rational drug use and appropriate drug dosages can have a positive impact on the quality of patient care in an institutional environment. Numerous studies have shown that when pharmacists routinely performed drug therapy monitoring on patients in long-term care facilities (LTCFs) and hospitals, the average number of medications consumed by patients significantly decreased. Due to this decrease, patients experienced fewer ADRs and realized a substantial reduction in medication costs. The amount of didactic and clinical training that the pharmacist receives makes him/her the most capable and highly trained professional to identify drug-related problems through regular monitoring of patients' drug therapy (1–5).

Drug Therapy Monitoring System

It is imperative that the clinical pharmacist develop a rational plan for approaching monitoring routine and complicated aspects of drug therapy. Monitoring drug therapy is an ongoing process because acute or chronic changes in a patient's condition often dictates therapy modifications (7–9). While there is no perfect drug therapy monitoring system or model available which can be easily adopted by all individuals, this self-instructional approach to drug therapy monitoring presents some basic guidelines for an organized monitoring system. These guidelines provide a step by step, standardized, organized, and accountable system of drug therapy monitoring. The approach is basic yet comprehensive and will help improve the pharmacist's understanding of patients' medical charts and the clinical skills and knowledge needed to monitor drug therapy accurately. In addition, it enables the pharmacist to function and communicate with other health care professionals in a team approach to improve patient care. Drug therapy monitoring in the context of institutionalized patients is more effective and easier for the pharmacist to perform since there is a more complete data base for these patients. However, it is hoped that many of the same monitoring processes presented here can be adapted for monitoring the drug therapy of non-institutionalized or home-bound patients.

■ Learning Objectives

The learning objectives listed below follow a sequential order in the learning process for monitoring drug therapy. Upon completion of this self-instructional course on drug therapy monitoring, the student/pharmacist should be able to:

1.   State the purpose and goals for monitoring a patient's drug therapy.
2.   List sources of patient information that should be examined in monitoring drug therapy.
3.   List specific patient information that should be extracted from a patient's medical record.
4.   List the steps involved in drug therapy monitoring.

5. Classify potential problems under each of the following categories that should be considered in drug therapy monitoring:
   a. drug related
   b. disease-management related
   c. administration
   d. physical status of patient
6. Identify factors that correlate with a high incidence of adverse drug reactions.
7. List drug categories responsible for causing most adverse reactions.
8. Identify clinical laboratory tests that should be performed periodically when patients are taking medication.
9. Identify indications for requesting serum drug levels.
10. Identify monitoring criteria and additional parameters used to determine the appropriateness of therapies for common illnesses.
11. Describe formal methods of communication with physicians about findings of drug therapy assessment and the process of documenting those findings in the medical chart.

■ References

1. Kidder SW. The cost benefit of drug reviews in long-term care facilities. *Today's Nursing Home* May 1982.
2. Kidder SW. Saving cost, quality and people. *Am Pharm* 1978; 18:18.
3. Kidder SW. Skilled nursing facilities—a clinical opportunity for pharmacists. *AJHP* 1977; 34:751–753.
4. Parker RD. The SNF: a unique opportunity for consultant pharmacist service. *Hosp Form* 1977; 12:693–695.
5. Kuwahara J, Kane RL. The role of the clinical pharmacist on a nursing home care team. *DICP* 1976; 10:268–271.
6. American Society of Consultant Pharmacists, *Standards of Practice for Consultant Pharmacists*. Bulletin, American Society of Consultant Pharmacists, Arlington, VA, 1977.
7. Cheung A, Kayne R. An application of clinical pharmacy services in extended care facilities. *CA Pharm* 1975; 23:22–25, 28, 43.
8. Brown CH. A systematic approach to drug regimen review. *Contemporary Writings on Long Term Care Pharmacy*, Vol 2, American Society of Consultant Pharmacists, Arlington, VA, 1980.
9. Sam MJ, Cheung A, *et al*. A systematic approach to drug therapy monitoring. *Hosp Pharm* 1977; 12:155–161.
10. Vancura EJ, Martilla JK; Monitoring drug therapy: An applied approach. *Comtemp Pharm Pract* 1981; 4:238–245.
11. Herfindal ET, Bernstein LR, Kishi DT. Effect of clinical pharmacy services on prescribing on an orthopedic unit. *Am J Hosp Pharm* 1983; 40:1945–1951.
12. Rich DS, Mahoney CD, Jeffrey LP, Pezzullo JC. Evaluation of a computerized digoxin pharmacokinetic consultation service. *Hosp Pharm* 1981; 16:23–27.
13. Abramowitz PW, Ludwig DJ, Mansur JM, Nold EG. Controlling moxalactam and cefotaxime use with a target drug program. *Hosp Pharm* 1983; 18:416–420.
14. Alexander MR, Alexander B, Mustion AL, Spector R, Wright CB. Therapeutic use of albumin: 2. *JAMA* 1982; 247:831–834.

15. Bukle WS, Lucarotti RL, Matzke GR. Documenting the influence of clinical pharmacists. *Am J Hosp Pharm* 1982; 39:481–482.

16. Knapp DA, Knapp DE, Michocki RJ, Speedie MK, Jankel CA. Drug prescribing and hospital cost containment. *Top Hosp Pharm Manage* 1982; Nov:7–14.

17. Slaughter RL, Schneider PJ, Visconti JA. Appropriateness of the use of serum digoxin and digitoxin assays. *Am J Hosp Pharm* 1978; 35:1376–1379.

18. Elenbaas RM, Payne VW, Bauman JL. Influence of clinical pharmacist consultations on the use of drug blood level tests. *Am J Hosp Pharm* 1980; 37:61–64.

19. Dick ML, Winship HW III, Wood GC. A cost effectiveness comparison of a pharmacist using three methods for identifying possible drug related problems. *Drug Intell Clin Pharm* 1975; 9:257–262.

20. Kelly KL, Covinsky JO, Fendler K, Bauman JL. The impact of clinical pharmacist activity on intravenous fluid and medication administration. *Drug Intell Clin Pharm* 1980; 14:516–520.

21. Schondelmeyer SW. Strategy to effect change in pharmacy practice. *Am J Hosp Pharm* 1982; 39:2137–2142.

22. Monson R, Bond CA, Schuna A. Role of the clinical pharmacist in improving drug therapy: clinical pharmacists in outpatient therapy. *Arch Intern Med* 1981; 4:1441–1444.

23. Nelson AA, Beno CE, Davis RE. Task and cost analysis of integrated clinical pharmacy services in private family practice centers. *J Fam Pract* 1983; 16:111–116.

24. Pathak DS, Nold EG. Cost-effectiveness of clinical pharmaceutical services: a follow-up report. *Am J Hosp Pharm* 1979; 36:1527–1529.

25. Lamy PP. *Prescribing for the Elderly*, Publishing Sciences Group, Littleton, MA, 1980; 53–54.

26. Office of Long-Term Care, Long-Term Care Facility Improvement Campaign, Monograph No. 2. Physician's Drug Prescribing Patterns in Skilled Nursing Facilities (DHEW Pub. No. 75–50059), Rockville, MD, 1976, p. 23.

27. Brown CH, DeSimone EM. Use of PRN medication in skilled nursing facilities. *Contemp Pharm Pract* 1980; 3(4):209–215.

28. Brown CH. Automatic stop-order policy for PRN medication in skilled nursing facilities. *Contemp Pharm Pract* 1981; 4(2):59–63.

29. Triggs EJ, Nation RL et al. Pharmacokinetics in the elderly. *Eur J Clin Pharmacol* 1975; 8:55.

30. Triggs EJ, Nation RL. Pharmacokinetics in the aged: A Review. *J Pharmacokinet Biopharm* 1975; 3:387.

31. Crooks J, O'Malley K, Stevenson IH. Pharmacokinetics in the elderly. *Clin Pharmacokinet* 1976; 1:280.

32. Lamy PP, Vestal RE. Drug prescribing for the elderly. *Hosp Pract* 1976; 11:111.

33. Hollister LE. Prescribing drugs for the elderly. *Geriatrics* 1977; 32(8):71.

34. Richey DP, Bender AD. Pharmacokinetic consequences of aging. *Annu Rev Pharmacol Toxicol* 1977; 17:49.

35. Vestal RE. Drug use in the elderly: A review of problems and special considerations. *Drugs* 1978; 16:358.

36. Greenblatt DJ, et al. Drug dispositon in old age. *N Engl J Med* 1982; 306:1081–1088.

37. Steel K, German PM, Crescenzi C, Anderson J. Iatrogenic illness on a general medical service at a university hospital. *N Engl J Hosp Pharm* 1981; 304:638–642.

38. Miller RR. Drug Surveillance utilizing epidemiologic methods: a report from the Boston collaborative drug surveillance program. *Am J Hosp Pharm* 1973; 30:584–592.

39. Hurwitz N. Predisposing factors in adverse reactions to drugs. *Br Med J* 1969; 1531.

40. Williamson J, Chopin JM. Adverse reactions to prescribed drugs in the elderly: a multicentre investigation. *Age Aging* 1980; 9(2):73.

41. Boston University Medical Center. Clinical depression of the central nervous system due to diazepam and chlordiazepoxide in relation to cigarette smoking and age: a report from the Boston collaborative drug surveillance program. *N Engl J Med* 1973; 288:277–280.

42. Greenblatt DJ, Allen MD, Shader, RI. Toxicity of high-dose flurazepam in the elderly. *Clin Pharmacol Ther* 1977; 21:355–361.

43. Greenblatt DJ, Allen MD. Toxicity of nitrazepam in the elderly: a report from the Boston collaboraive drug surveillance program. *Br J Clin Pharmacol* 1978; 5:407–413.

Chapter 1
Components of the Patient's Medical Chart

While reading through this chapter, the pharmacist will become familiar with many different types of patient information contained in various parts of a typical medical chart. The medical chart is a source of information about a patient's past and present medical status. It is the data bank which provides the basis for the health care professional's review and assessment of drug therapy.

To obtain sufficient pertinent patient data for drug therapy monitoring on institutionalized patients, the clinical pharmacist needs to examine the patient's medical record. Although a patient medication history may have been obtained by a nurse or physician upon admission, the pharmacist should also attempt to verify the accuracy of the chart's past medication record as well as to determine if the patient has any medication allergies or hypersensitivities. Patient information is collected and written in the patient's medical chart by various healthcare professionals (e.g., physicians, nurses, therapists, dietician) who interact with the patient. Once a person is institutionalized, a complete record of everything that happens to the patient on a daily basis is recorded in various sections of a patient's medical record. Examining all patient information in the medical record helps the clinical pharmacist monitor and assess the patient's drug therapy and response to drug therapy.

It is important to remember that not all medical charts or sections of a chart will be complete for a given patient. As a patient's medical chart increases in size, some sections may be thinned-out and filed either in a folder in a file cabinet at the nurses' station or in the medical records department. At times, it may be necessary to review the filed chart or "old chart" to find essential patient information from the current or a previous admission. Also, the organizational sequence of a chart will vary greatly from one health care facility to another. With this in mind, the most common sections of a sample medical chart for a patient

(Ms. Jane Doe) will be reviewed along with a brief description of the types of patient information usually recorded in each section. The various sections will be discussed in order of their usual appearance in a typical medical chart. It is important to remember that, in most sections of the medical chart, the most current patient information appears on the beginning sheets and the oldest data appear on the last sheets or toward the end of the section.

■ Admission Record

This section is usually the first division of a medical chart, and it provides general demographic, economic, and medical information on the patient at the time of admission to the health care facility. In some instances, these data are not recorded elsewhere in the patient's medical chart. Information included on the admission sheet section is usually gathered by an admission secretary or director; the admission medical assessment record is usually completed by a nurse and other health care professionals. With continuous monitoring of the patient's drug regimen and medical status, the pharmacist can easily determine if the patient has progressed or regressed since the date of admission. Specific patient information the clinical pharmacist should review that is usually recorded in the admission record includes:

1. General patient information (e.g., patient name, age, date of birth, sex, race, religion, date of admission, medical records number or patient number, admission or visit number, insurance number);
2. Attending physician(s);
3. Admitting diagnosis (primary and/or secondary diagnoses);
4. Patient's drug allergies and/or drug sensitivities;
5. Nurse's assessment (vital signs, review of systems, etc.);
6. Dietician's assessment;
7. Physical therapy assessment;
8. Occupational therapy assessment;
9. Speech therapy assessment;
10. Social worker's assessment and discharge plan.

Before going on to the next section of Jane Doe's medical chart, read through the following pages of her facility Admission Record example and locate the previously mentioned patient information. At times, medical abbreviations or terminology are used in this section by various healthcare professionals to conserve time and space. If the reader is not familiar with the meaning of a specific medical term or abbreviation, he or she should refer to Chapter 6 (Medical Terminology) for its meaning. Knowing the meaning of each term will enhance the reader's understanding of this section.

FIGURES 1.1-1.5   ADMISSION RECORD

			PRIOR ADM. DATE	MEDICAL RECORD NO. 04227

PATIENT ACCOUNT NO. 04227	ADMISSION DATE 7-29	TIME 1:15 pm	EDP NO.	SOC. SEC. NO. 309 01 6670	ROOM & BED 148 A	ACC	SERVICE

PATIENT NAME Doe, Jane Q.	PATIENT ADDRESS 102 Brown Street Lafayette, Indiana	CITY	STATE ZIP 47904

PHONE 479-7766	BIRTH DATE 12-04-95	AGE 89	SEX F	M/S M	RACE W	RELIGION P	PARISH/CHURCH Church of Christ	NF

P A T I E N T

SM	CLS	FC	SACRAMENT TO THE SICK	ADM. BY CHB

EMPLOYER Retired	EMPLOYER ADDRESS	CITY	STATE ZIP

NEAREST RELATIVE Elizabeth Rumble	NEAREST RELATIVE ADDRESS 1014 Brown Street Lafayette, Indiana 47904

RELATIONSHIP Daughter	N R PHONE 479-3606	N R EMPLOYER Acme, Inc.	PHONE 425-1155	EXT. 299

EMERGENCY RELATIVE Joseph Delane	REL S	EMERGENCY RELATIVE ADDRESS 1018 Brown Street	CITY Lafayette, Indiana 47904	STATE ZIP

EMERGENCY RELATIVE PHONE 479-6438	COMMENTS

GUARANTOR NAME Medicare Part A	GUARANTOR ADDRESS	CITY	STATE ZIP

INSURANCE COMPANY NAME, ADDRESS, CODE, POLICY NUMBER, POLICYHOLDER NAME

I N S U R A N C E

1ST	SS 309-01-6670
2ND	
3RD	
4TH	

ADMITTING DIAGNOSIS 1 Rt. Shoulder Fx Humeral Head	ADMITTING DIAGNOSIS 2 CHF with pleural effusions, ASHD

M E D

ADMITTING PHYSICIAN B. Casey, M.D.	ATTENDING PHYSICIAN J. J. Omar, M.D.	SURGEON

REFERRING PHYSICIAN	DISCHARGE DATE & TIME

Allergies: NKA

ADMISSION

Patient Admission Instruction:
- ☑ Introduction to Roommate & Staff
- ☑ Smoking
- ☑ Belongings Identified
- ☑ Call Light
- ☑ Regulations
- ☑ Valuables/Money Home
- ☑ Laundry
- ☑ Visiting Hours

Hearing No problems c̄ hearing

Hearing Aid ☐ Yes ☒ No

Vision Wear glasses all the time

Glasses ☒ Yes ☐ No

Cognitive Function
Alert – but forgetful

Dentures ☒ Upper ☒ Lower ☐ Partial
in mouth

Bowel Habits
BM yesterday 7-28
goes about q o d

Eating Habits
poor appetite

Sleeping Habits (energy patterns)
OK – has no problems getting
to sleep or staying asleep

Bladder Habits foley Cath
patent c̄ dark clear urine

Pacemaker ☐ Yes ☒ No

Smoker ☐ Yes ☒ No

Height 5' 3"

Weight 108 lb/49 kg

Blood Pressure 110/70

Temperature 98⁶ (o)

Pulse AP 82

Respiration 20

Other —

Indicate skin condition, lesions, bruises, amputations, scars

purple area
sling
yellow
red-purple area
both knees edematous warm
pink 1/4 cm open
purple yellow area

Condition prior to this illness:
Lived c̄ son, could do own care + house work.
Fell 7-16, went St. E. Hospital was there prior to
this adm.

Patient's Name (Last, First, MI)	Attending Physician	Room Number	Patient Number
Doe, Jane	J. J. Omar	148A	4227

ADMISSION ASSESSMENT

Review Body Systems — EENT, Respiratory, Circulatory, Gastrointestinal, Urinary, Neurological, Musculoskeletal.

Eyes – sclera white, wears glasses all the time

Nose – no discharge   Throat – clear, no redness noted

Ears – hearing OK, no discharge noted

Resp – non-labored, no coughing or chest pain

Circ – AP 86 reg. Skin – pale, warm + very dry. Turgor – poor

Gastro – appetite poor, no c/o indigestion, N,V., has BM QOD
abd. soft flat c̄ good bowell sounds

Urinary – foley cath, patent c̄ dark yellow urine. No c/o
discomfort

Neuro – alert, forgetful, no weakness

Musculoskeletal – no stiffness, deformities, both knees
edematous + warm. Moves ↑+↓ extremities well
poor standing balance, gait unsteady.

Skin – poor turgor, coccyx pink c̄ 1/4 cm open area. Many purple/
yellow area on ® side.

Speech – clear, speaks when spoken to, fast to respond

Describe Functional Status: Eating, Elimination, Mobility, Dressing, and Grooming.

Eating – appetite poor, needs assist c̄ set up
may need to be fed because of ® arm sling + poor appetite

Elimination – foley cath patent, dark yellow urine, BM QOD

Mobility – moves all extremities, may need assist c̄
repositioning + turning. Standing balance poor
gait unsteady

Dress ⎤
Grooming ⎦ care per staff

SOCIAL ASSESSMENT

Name	Relationship	Lives Near	Visits/Writes
Elizabeth Ramble	Daughter	City	✓
Joe Delone	Son	City	✓
Ruby Beak	Daughter	Peoria, IL	✓

Family Attitude to Admission

Supportive

Prior Living Arrangements

In own home c̄ son

Educational Background

H.S. graduate

Hobbies

Cards, reading

Likes/Dislikes (Pers. Emotional, Social)

watching sports

Who Planned Admission

Pt. + family

Friends

None close

Social Activities/Organizational Memberships

Church of Christ

Occupation (Past/Present)

Homemaker

Expectations/Motivations to Discharge, including Medically Related Social & Emotional needs.

Mrs. Doe is an 89 year old, very pleasant lady who lived at home with her son prior to fall on 7-16. Her daughter lives in the other side of the two-family dwelling. She was born in Carroll County and lived in the area all her life. She had five brothers and said she enjoyed playing all kinds of sports with them. She has been a widow ten years and has three children. Her husband died of a heart attack and she still misses him. Upon discharge, she plans to return home.

Source of Information **Patient**   Interviewed By **Barbara Homes**   Date **7/30**

Patient's Name (Last, First, MI)	Attending Physician	Room Number	Patient Number
Doe, Jane	J. J. Omar	148A	4227

Page 3

ASSESSMENT – DIETARY, ACTIVITY, OTHER

Date	Dept. Name	← Comments	← Signature/Title
7/30	Speech	Speech Th NA at this time	D. Mills,
7/30	O.T.	pt. would benefit from O.T.	M. Cox, O.T.R.
7/30	Dietary	Pt. is alert but forgetful. She has order for 1 gm. na diet. Hx of CHF & ASHD. Denies chewing/swallowing diff., allergies or bowel problems. Can feed self c̄ assist. Likes most foods. Meds. incl. Lasix + Lanoxin. Hgb 11.4, BS 166, Ht. 5'3", Wt. 108# IBW 112-136#. Wt. Hx unknown. Continue to monitor + encourage intake. C. Atter, RDT	
7/30	ACT	Patient is an 89 year old c̄ MD orders of non-exertive activities of choice. No alcohol bev. She was a homemaker, moves all extremities well/poor standing balance/slightly HOH + wears glasses. Her hobbies are reading/sports/music/ PLAN: Have patient attend group Act. 2x wk. will increase ad lib. D. Mills, AD	
7/30	P.T.	No PT at this time per MD order. M. Michael, RPT	

■ History and Physical (H & P) Examination

The medical history section of the chart helps document any past medical problems the patient has encountered and provides background on his or her present medical status. Information included in this division is usually gathered by the patient's attending physician, emergency room physician, consulting physician, or a surgeon or radiologist. In some instances, there may be H & Ps from several physicians who have seen the patient. (See Fig. 1.7, radiology consultation.) The history and physical examination section profiles the patient's medical condition at the time of admission. Ideally, it should contain a description of all medical problems the patient is presently experiencing and the physician's impression or diagnosis of each medical problem and a plan for their treatment. When the patient is admitted to the facility directly from his or her home, the physician may handwrite this information into the chart or dictate the H & P for a secretary to type and put into the chart. However, if the patient was admitted directly from another health care facility, a typed, dictated copy of the patient's medical discharge summary and transfer records is usually included. Patient information presented in this H & P examination section usually includes:

1. Current chief complaint(s);
2. History of present illness;
3. Past medical history;
4. Drug allergies/drug sensitivities;
5. Family history and social history;
6. Physical examination (e.g., vital signs, review of systems);
7. Physician's impression(s) of what is wrong with the patient, including admitting diagnosis and a care plan for hospitalization/institutionalization.

Before going on to the next section of Jane Doe's medical chart, review and read through the following pages of her H & P and locate the previously mentioned patient information. At times, laboratory tests (often written as abbreviations) may be included in the patient write-up. If the reader is not familiar with the meaning of a specific laboratory test, he or she should refer to Chapter 4 (Clinical Laboratory Diagnostic Tests) for its meaning. Becoming more familiar with each laboratory test mentioned will enhance the reader's understanding of this section.

FIGURE 1.6   **HISTORY AND PHYSICAL EXAMINATION**

EMERGENCY ROOM RECORD

Last Name	First Name	Attending Physician	Hosp. No.	Admission Date
Doe	Jane	C. A. John, M.D.	11 21 12	7-29

cc: J.J. Omar, M.D.
    B. Casey, M.D.

C.C.: Total body pain.

ONSET & COURSE OF P.I.: This 89 year old white female fell off a step at home and was noted by the ambulance crew as having pain in her right humerus. The patient however had grunting respirations, and had a respiratory rate of 52/min. Because of this physical finding, the patient had an electrocardiogram as well as a chest x-ray. The chest x-ray revealed a fracture of the right humerus with the head being dislocated. It also revealed a pleural effusion and a consolidated area in the anterior segment of the left lower lobe. An electrocardiogram revealed a left bundle branch block with some PVC's. The chest x-ray also showed cardiomegaly. The patient had a CBC which showed a 10,800 white count and only 11.4 grams of hemoglobin. The rest of the CBC was within normal limits. The patient's creatinine was 1.1. Her BUN was 27 and her electrolytes within normal limits. Electrolytes were drawn because the patient gave a history of taking 1 mg. of Bumex per day. The patient's blood sugar was 166 at approximately 9 o'clock in the evening after having eaten at 15 till 5:00. The patient was demanding water to drink and her breath smelled slightly fruity and for this reason was suspected she had diabetes mellitus. Despite the very small clues that were altered by the patient as to her history, a complete physical was done. It was noted the patient had a circumferential ring just above her knees where she held her stocking and was also noted she had osteoarthritic deformities of both knees. Although the patient was complaining of some pain in the hip area, neither leg was foreshortened and the patient did seem to have a good rotary motion of both hip sockets and it was thought that clinically there was no fractured hip.

The patient had marked swelling of the ankles and the patient had decreased hearing acuity and the tympanic membrane could not be visualized well bilaterally because of cerumen. The pupils were pinpoint and as they constricted with light, it was difficult to do a clear funduscopic examination. The patient was edentulous. The heart beat was noted to be regular on physical examination but no cardiomegaly or murmurs could be detected. Examination of the breasts revealed no masses and examination of the adbomen was within normal limits. No organomegaly or tenderness or fluid was elicited. Further examination of the extremities showed the patient to have a bruised abraded area over the lateral aspect of the left elbow and a small skin tear on paper thin skin on the right elbow. The patient complained bitterly of pain when the right arm was attempted to be rotated in the socket.

FINAL DIAGNOSIS: 1] Cardiomegaly with pleural effusion and left bundle branch block with frequent premature ventricular contractions.

                          2] Fracture dislocation of the head of the humerus on the right side.

                          3] Diabetes mellitus.

C. A. John MD

lag D 7 / 30   2:47   Dictated by: C.A. John, M.D.
      T 7 / 30   12:10

FIGURE 1.7   RADIOLOGY CONSULTATION

RADIOLOGY CONSULTATION

Last Name	First Name	Attending Physician	Hosp No.	Admission Date
Doe	Jane	C. A. Johns, M.D.	11 21 16	7-29

DATE OF CONSULTATION: 7-29

CONSULTING PHYSICIAN: B. Casey, M.D.

H.P.I.:   This 89 year old female apparently fell at her home during the night and injured her right shoulder. She denies having been unconscious. She was seen in the emergency room where she was complaining of pain in the area of the right shoulder. X-rays of the right shoulder reveal a fracture dislocation of the right humeral head with the humeral head lying anterior and inferior to the glenoid with the proximal end of the distal humeral shaft in the area of the glenoid. Circulation and sensation of the right upper extremity appears to be normal. Her X-rays of the chest reveal a left pleural effusion. She also has a history of diabetes mellitus with cardiomegaly and her EKG reveals a left bundle branch block with PVC's. She was placed into a velcro shoulder immobilizer and admitted for further evaluation.

PHYSICAL EXAMINATION

GENERAL: She appears to be alert and oriented. She denies having been unconscious.

The right arm is in a shoulder immobilizer. There is moderate tenderness around the area of the right shoulder. Circulation and sensation of the right upper extremity appears to be quite good. She does have decreased breath sounds in the left pleural base as compared to the right.

X-rays of the right shoulder reveal a fracture dislocation of the right humeral head with the head lying anterior and inferior to the glenoid with the proximal humeral shaft fragment lying in the area of the glenoid.

My impression is: 1.   This lady has a fracture dislocation of the right humeral head.
2.   Cardiomegaly.
3.   Left pleural effusion.
4.   Left bundle branch block with PVC's.
5.   Diabetes mellitus.

In view of this, the patient's age, and other medical problems, I would not recommend a surgical reduction and internal fixation of her fracture dislocation of the right humeral head. I would however recommend that she be treated with a velcro shoulder immobilizer and then go for early motion. I did explain to her that her shoulder motion would never be normal again. She appears to understand what I was saying and agrees with this type of treatment.

Thank you for the opportunity of seeing this patient. I will follow her with you.

Ben Casey, MD

Dictated by: Ben Casey, M.D.

lag   D   7 / 30   7:06
       T   7 / 30   10:35

■ Physician's Orders And Progress Notes

The first portion of this section of the chart focuses on physician's orders and contains a specific listing of such information as current medications, treatments, laboratory tests, therapies, diet, and level of activity prescribed by the patient's physician(s). In time, each component of these orders may be discontinued or altered in response to changes in the patient's condition. If the patient remains in the facility for an extended period of time (e.g., several weeks or months), this section will contain a chronological (from oldest to the most current) listing of all medication orders. The listing of physician's orders will normally be updated or rewritten on a regular basis (e.g., weekly or monthly).

In some facilities, such health care professionals as clinical pharmacists and/or nurse practitioners may write orders for medication, laboratory tests, or other instructions following consultation with the patient's attending physician. However, for legal purposes, these orders (handwritten orders or copies of telephone orders) are generally countersigned by the physician during his or her next visit to the facility. Orders for medication should include the medication's name (generic or trade name), strength, dose, dosage interval, duration of treatment, and route of administration. Medication that is intended to be used only when needed (i.e., prn) includes all of the above information plus an indication of its appropriate use.

Patient information outlined in the physician's orders segment of the chart usually includes:

1. Routine medication orders;
2. PRN medication orders;
3. Orders for taking vital signs, monitoring fluid intake and/or urine output;
4. Orders for treatments (e.g., topical ointments/creams, bladder irrigation);
5. Orders for therapies (e.g., physical, occupational, speech);
6. Orders for level of activity (e.g., complete bed rest, up as tolerated);
7. Orders for clinical laboratory tests (e.g., chemistry profile, serum electrolytes, complete blood count);
8. Special diet order (e.g., 1500 kcal, 2 g sodium, American Diabetes Association [ADA]);
9. Orders for approved bedside medication or other health items;
10. Orders to discontinue or change anything previously ordered (e.g., medication, therapy, laboratory test, treatment, activity);
11. Order for alcohol consumption;
12. Order for generic drug substitution;
13. Standing orders (e.g., acetaminophen 10 gr/orally every 4–6 hr prn pain or temperature more than 100°F).

The second portion of this section of a patient's medical chart is the physician's progress notes. These patient progress notations are made when the physician makes periodic visits to the facility to review the patient's response to drug therapy and changes in the patient's overall medical status. The content and extent of these notes may vary from a few words to a very thorough and organized documentation of the presentation of a given medical problem and an approach or plan for its solution. Some physicians may utilize the problem-oriented medical record (POMR) and write these notes in the subjective, objective, assessment, and plans (SOAP) format. Information presented in the physician's progress notes section of the chart usually includes:

1. Patient's subjective complaints of acute or chronic problems;
2. Physician's objective evaluation of the patient's medical status (e.g., laboratory tests, vital signs);
3. Physician's assessment of the patient's overall medical status;
4. Physician's plans to help correct or improve the patient's condition and therapeutic goals;
5. Requests for consultations (e.g., medical specialist, therapists [occupational, physical, speech], clinical pharmacist, nurse specialist).

In many instances, the goals of drug therapy for a particular medical problem or disease is to make the patient as comfortable as possible and to cure or relieve the problem. However, a cure for every medical disorder or disease is not always possible or realistic. In some cases, the goals of drug therapy may be to improve the patient's quality of life, to maintain or stabilize the patient's present medical status, or to prevent further progression of the disease. For example, the therapeutic goal for an acute infectious disease is to cure that disease. For such chronic diseases as diabetes or congestive heart failure, the goals of therapy would be to halt the progress of the disease and reduce or alleviate its clinical manifestations by returning body functions to as close to normal as possible. Better understanding of the physician's therapeutic goals for each patient helps the clinical pharmacist monitor the patient's progress to assure that the proper course of drug therapy is followed.

Before going on to the next section of Jane Doe's medical chart, read through the following pages of her Physician's Orders and Progress Notes and locate the previously mentioned patient information.

FIGURES 1.8-1.11 **PHYSICIAN ORDERS AND PROGRESS NOTES**

PHYSICIANS' INTERIM / TELEPHONE ORDERS
PHYSICIAN — PLEASE SIGN, DATE AND RETURN WITHIN 48 HOURS*

LAST NAME	FIRST NAME	ATTENDING PHYSICIAN	DATE	PATIENT NUMBER	ROOM NO.	CENTER NAME

SIGNATURE OF NURSE RECEIVING ORDER	TIME ☐ A M ☐ P M	SIGNATURE OF NURSE NOTING ORDER	DATE	SIGNATURE OF PHYSICIAN *	DATE

3

ORIGINAL

PHYSICIANS' INTERIM / TELEPHONE ORDERS
PHYSICIAN — PLEASE SIGN, DATE AND RETURN WITHIN 48 HOURS*

LAST NAME	FIRST NAME	ATTENDING PHYSICIAN	DATE	PATIENT NUMBER	ROOM NO	CENTER NAME
Doe,	Jane	J. Omar	7/30	4227	148A	

1. 2-4 g nat diet

SIGNATURE OF NURSE RECEIVING ORDER	TIME	SIGNATURE OF NURSE NOTING ORDER	DATE	SIGNATURE OF PHYSICIAN *	DATE
E. Edison	4:00 ☐ A M ☐ P M	C. Person	7/30	J.J. Omar, MD	7/31

2

ORIGINAL

PHYSICIANS' INTERIM / TELEPHONE ORDERS
PHYSICIAN — PLEASE SIGN, DATE AND RETURN WITHIN 48 HOURS*

LAST NAME	FIRST NAME	ATTENDING PHYSICIAN	DATE	PATIENT NUMBER	ROOM NO	CENTER NAME
Doe,	Jane	J.J. Omar	7/30	4227	148A	

1. No therapy evaluation at present time
2. B&O supp. as ordered X14 days, then DK

SIGNATURE OF NURSE RECEIVING ORDER	TIME	SIGNATURE OF NURSE NOTING ORDER	DATE	SIGNATURE OF PHYSICIAN *	DATE
E. Eller	12:00 ☐ A M ☐ P M	M. Anderson	7/30	B. Casey, MD	7/31

1 PHYSICIANS' INTERIM / TELEPHONE ORDERS

ORIGINAL

Date	Interim Orders	D/C	Progress Notes
8/1	Lanoxin 0.125 mg god J.J. Omar, M.D.		8/1 Dig. level ↑ at 2.6, will ↓ dose to 0.125. Abdominal aneurism Pt. very confused & disoriented. Vomited some & left pleural effusion. J.J. Omar, M.D.
8/3	Ran Digoxin level @ 4 PM BS R₄ Slow K tab ↑ BID po S₁ K⁺ level on 8-6-85 J.J. Omar MD		8/3 S₁. K⁺ ↓ at 2.9 Pt. not eating well. Will R₄ K⁺ suppl. J.J. Omar, M.D.
8/4	Ran 2 Hr PPBS J.J. Omar, M.D.		8/4 S₁. Digoxin 1.9 now - OK but still high. J.J. Omar MD
8/6	R₄ IV D₅W at 100 ml/hr × 48 hrs. J.J. Omar, MD		8/7 S₁. K⁺ WNL now at 4.2 Abd. soft Will leave IV out & try to ↑ oral feedings & fluid intake. J.J. Omar MD
8/7	Urge oral fluids & oral intake. J.J. Omar MD		

Patient's Name (Last, First, MI)	Attending Physician	Room Number	Patient Number
Doe, Jane	J. J. Omar	148A	4227

Side 2

Rehab Potential ☐ Good ☑ Fair ☐ Poor ☐ Maintenance

Goals:

☐ Unless Checked Generic Substitution Allowed

ORDER DATE	C		Therapy Evaluation - Admission	☐ Speech Therapy ☐ YES ☑ NO

Therapy Evaluation - Admission ☐ Speech Therapy ☐ YES ☑ NO
☐ Occupational Therapy ☐ Y ☑ N (See Therapy Orders & Report for
☐ Physical Therapy ☐ Y ☑ N further orders)

ORDER DATE	C	Orders
7/29	✓	Lanoxin 0.125 mg po ī tab d
	✓	Septra-DS po ī tab BID
	✓	Lasix 40 mg po ī tab d
	✓	B+O rect. supp ī prn bladder spasm × 14 d
	✓	Tylenol 325 mg po īī tabs q 3 hr prn pain
	✓	I fleet enema prn constipation
	✓	Haley's MO 30 ml prn constipation (if no results, use Fleets enema)
7/31	✓	Restoril 15 mg po ī cap q hs prn sleep (MRX1)
	✓	Tigan 2 ml IM q 4 hrs prn nausea

Activity Program Orders
Patient may participate as follows:
☐ No Restrictions
☐ All activities except outings
☐ Only non-exertive activites
☐ Bedside activities only
☐ Reality Orientation

☐ Remotivation
☐ Hair Permanent
☐ Alcoholic Beverages   No
Patient may leave building?
☐ If attended
☐ Unattended
☐ May not leave building

Restrictions

Does patient know diagnosis?   Safety Devices ☐ No ☑ Yes
☑ Yes ☐ No   Give type & reason:
Patient able to receive mail?
☑ Yes ☐ No   posey
If no, Physician must document reason.

Diet: 1 g Na+ diet
      no alcohol

Other Orders:
Change urinary catheter q 6 wk. and prn
Sling for right arm
Posey while up
Up in chair with assistance 1 hr. TID to tolerance
IPPD (no repeat)

Above Orders Noted By   C. Barley, R.N.   Date 7/31

Nurse's Review/Signature & Date
7/31
C. Barley, RN

PHYSICIAN NAME
J. J. Omar
PHYSICIAN PHONE
475-1177

Physician must sign after reviewing above
J. J. Omar, M.D.
Physician's Signature & Date

These Orders Are For The Mo./Yr.
July 19

DIAGNOSIS Fx ® Humeral Head, DM, LBBB-PVC's,   ALLERGIES
Left pleural effusion   NKA

Patient's Name (Last, First, M)	Attending Physician	Room Number	Patient Number
DOE, JANE	J. J. OMAR	148A	4227

PHYSICIAN'S ORDERS

Date	Interim Orders	D/C	Progress Notes
7/29	Adm. Orders : 1. Sling for Rt. arm 2. Up in chair c̄ asst. 1 hr. TID to tolerance (easy while up) 3. PFD (no repeat) 4. Change urin. Catheter q 6 whr. + prn 5. No alcoholic bev. 6. Chest X-ray 7. Chem. Profile 8. UA, C+S 9. CBC 10. Thyroid profile 11. Lasix 40mg po. d 12. Lanoxin 0.125mg po. d 13. Tylenol 5gr. ii tabs po. q 3 hrs. prn pain or ↑ temp 14. Haley's MO 30ml prn constipation (if no results use fleets enema) 15. Fleets enema prn constipation 16. 1g Na⁺ diet c̄ Salt sub. 17. B+O supp ī rect. prn bladder spasm J.J. Omar, MD		7-29 C/o of some pain in Rt. arm chest cong. noted P- ✓ xray + labs J. J. Omar MD
7/31	1. Sr. Digoxin level 2. Sr. electrolytes 3. Restoril 15mg hs po MRX1 prn sleep 4. Septra -DS ī po BID X10d J J Omar, MD		7-31 S- C/o nausea, not eating well arm pain, bladder spasm O- ✓ 12⁹/60, P80, R16 3⁺ Bacteria in urine ↑WBC, BUN 27 (↑) ↓RBC A- prob. UTI, X-ray shows pleural effusion P- TX c̄ ATB, when C+S return Re sleep ✓ Digoxin level later J J Omar

Patient's Name (Last, First, MI)	Attending Physician	Room Number	Patient Number
Doe, Jane	J. J. Omar	148 A	4327

Side 2

■ Universal Progress Notes or Nurse's Notes

These progress notes usually provide the most current comments or observations made by nurses, therapists, pharmacists, dieticians, and other professional staff members. Various health care professionals will report on such things as the patient's progress, response to drug therapy, activities, mental attitude, general feelings, activity, eating habits, and sleeping status. These recorded observations will reflect the overall feelings or status of the patient on a day-to-day basis. Information presented in the universal progress notes or nurse's notes section of the chart usually includes:

1. Vital signs (e.g., temperature, apical pulse, respirations, and blood pressure);
2. Nurse's assessment and daily observations of the patient's status;
3. Onset of additional acute medical conditions or exacerbation of a chronic medical condition;
4. Patient response to drug therapy;
5. Current weight;
6. Documentation of prn medication administered to the patient;
7. Patient's refusal to take medications;
8. Signs and symptoms of adverse drug reactions, drug toxicity, or allergic reactions;
9. Social involvement with visitors, residents, and staff;
10. Documentation of the pharmacist's drug therapy assessment and monitoring findings (in some facilities, may be written in the Physician Progress note section of the medical chart or on a separate page);
11. Urinary catheter changes, patency of urethral catheter, physical appearance of urine;
12. Patient complaints;
13. Notes by therapists (e.g., physical therapy, occupational therapy, speech therapy);
14. Notes by dietician on eating habits, diet, weight changes;
15. Notes by activities director;
16. Notes from social services.

Before going on to the next section of Jane Doe's medical chart, read through the following pages of her Universal Progress Notes or Nurse's Notes example and locate the previously mentioned patient information.

FIGURES 1.12-1.19   UNIVERSAL PROGRESS NOTES OR NURSE'S NOTES

Date	Time	Department (Nursing, P.T., etc.)	Prob. No.	Progress Note / Signature/Title
8/9	3⁴⁵ PM	Nsg.		Called Dr. Omar office regarding pt's poor food intake and skin dryness. Message left. ———————— W Lynch RN
8/9	5³⁰ P	Nsg.		Up in chair for meal. 75% @ supper. Alert + oriented. Vaseline lotion to skin for dry skin. Foley draining. Complaining of pain ® arm. Skin warm and dry. ———————— W Lynch RN
8/9	4⁴⁵ P	Nsg.		Late entry. Dr. Omar phoned in order. W Lynch RN

Patient's Name (Last, First, MI)	Attending Physician	Room Number	Patient Number
Doe, Jane	J. J. Omar	148A	4227

INTERDISCIPLINARY PROGRESS NOTES

Date	Time	Department (Nursing, P.T., etc.)	Prob. No.	◄ Progress Note | ◄ Signature/Title
				dressing applied. —————— R. Goodson RN
8/7	12:15 A	NSG		#22 Angio inserted top of ⓛ hand. IV infusing well. No sign of redness or swelling. Good blood return noted. — R. Goodson RN
8/7	1:30 A	Nsg		Pt. still awake even p̄ Restoril 15 mg was repeated @ 12:30/A. Yelling for "Elizabeth." Hands are restrained to prevent pt. pulling out I.V. IV infusing well. No sign of infiltration L. Nichols RN
8/7	2:45 A	NSG.		PT. PULLED I.V. OUT. UNABLE TO RESTART. WILL CONTACT DOCTOR IN AM. PRESSURE D APPLIED TO OLD SITE TOP OF ⓛ HAND. S. McCoy RN
8/7	6:30 A	Nsg.		I.V. out. Pt taking fluids. Became agitated per report of nurse when I.V. reinserted. Called Dr. Oman + orders rec'd. —— L. Nichols RN
8/7	6:45 A	Nsg.		Called Jones Drugs' pharmacist Jack Phillips and ordered Valium for pt. —— L. Nichols RN
8/7	9:45 Am	Nsg.		K+ report of 4.2 called to Dr. Oman; no new orders. —— S. Wills RN
8/7	10:15 Am	Nsg.		Dr. Oman here. Examined pt. Progress note written. —— S. Wills RN
8/7	6p	nsg		Family here - Pt. took all liquid on supper tray. —— C. Mead RN
8/8	2:30 p	NSG.		16 F 5 cc Catheter pulled out by patient. No bleeding from meatus. Same size catheter anchored c̄ difficulty. —— W. Lynch RN

Patient's Name (Last, First, MI)	Attending Physician	Room Number	Patient Number
Doe, Jane	J. J. Oman	148A	4227

INTERDISCIPLINARY PROGRESS NOTES

Date	Time	Department (Nursing, P.T., etc.)	Prob. No.	◄ Progress Note / ◄ Signature/Title
8/5	1¹⁵ pm	Nsg.		Called Dr. Omar office regarding lab reports called on 8/3 and skin breakdown on sacral area. — P. Thomas RN
8/5	1⁴⁵ pm	Nsg.		Dr. Omar office called orders. — P. Thomas RN
8/6	6¹⁵ A	Nsg.		Lab here and drew blood for K+ A. Goodson RN
8/6	1⁵⁰ P	Nsg.		Called Dr. Omar office regarding pt's nausea and only intake of 10% breakfast and lunch. — K. Miller RN
8/6	2¹⁰ P	Nsg.		Rec'd orders from Dr. Omar office — K. Miller RN
8/6	3¹⁵ P	Nsg.		IV started per L forearm c̄ 22 G angio c̄ good blood return. Secured c̄ Opsite & tape. — M. Evans RN
8/6	3³⁰ P	Nsg.		Pt. has poor skin turgor. Questionable understanding of IV in L arm. — M. Evans RN
8/6	3⁴⁵ P	Nsg.		Order Rec'd. for IV-D5W x 2 days (48 hr.) M Evans RN
8/6	5 PM	Nsg.		IV infusing well. No swelling @ site. Good blood return. Family here. — C. Mead RN
8/6	7 PM	Nsg.		Family c̄ pt. Assisted her c̄ dinner. Ate 90% of meal. — C. Mead RN
8/6	9 PM	Nsg.		IV continues to infuse well. Site not swollen. Good blood return. — L. Nichols RN
8/6	11 PM	Nsg.		No swelling or infiltration @ IV site. — L. Nichols RN
8/6	11³⁰ P	NSG		Pt. pulled IV out. Pt agitated, picking @ sheets. No redness @ old IV site. Pressure

Patient's Name (Last, First, MI)	Attending Physician	Room Number	Patient Number
Doe, Jane	J. J. Omar	148 A	4227

INTERDISCIPLINARY PROGRESS NOTES

Date	Time	Department (Nursing. P.T., etc.)	Prob. No.	◄ Progress Note ❘ ◄ Signature/Title
				and K serum levels. Left message. ————— K. Miller RN
8/1	930 AM	Nsg.		Dr. Omar here, examined pt. Orders re- ceived. ————— K. Miller RN
8/1	940 P	Nsg.		Confused & disoriented. Granddaughter was here for supper. Pt. seemed to know her and had a nice conversation c̄ her. Pt. very confused after she left. Yelling. Thinks she's in her own home with in- truders. ————— L. Nichols RN
8/1	10 PM P	Nsg.		Quieter earlier but has now started to climb over side rails. Restrained in bed per orders. ————— L. Nichols RN
8/2	2 00 A	NSD.		Pt. awake and very agitated. Removed chest restraint and turned self around in bed c̄ head @ foot of bed. Yelling loudly. Alert but very confused. Medicated c̄ Restoril @ 135 A ———— A. Goodson RN
8/2	3 00 AM	NSD.		Lab here and drew blood for chloride, K+ and NA. ———— A. Goodson RN
8/2	915 A	Nsg.		K+ level 2.9. Lytes & dig. level reports called to Dr. Omar. Orders recd. —— B Davis RN
8/3	315 A	Nsg.		Kept off of back while in bed. Has been alert today. C/o mouth feeling dry. Takes fluids well. Does not eat solid foods well. Up in chair c̄ restraint for 1 hr. @ a time. B Davis RN

Patient's Name (Last, First, MI)	Attending Physician	Room Number	Patient Number
Doe, Jane	J. J. Omar	148A	4227

INTERDISCIPLINARY PROGRESS NOTES

Date	Time	Department (Nursing, P.T., etc.)	Prob. No.	Progress Note / Signature/Title
7-31-	3¹⁵ A	Nsg.		Pt. awake and very confused. Pt. thinks she is @ home and can't find her "things." Has awakened frequently since 2³⁰ A. States "I can't sleep." — A. Davidson RN
7/31	8¹⁵ AM	NSG.		PATIENT CARE CONFERENCE: GOAL TO HEAL LEG ULCER. REHAB POTENTIAL GOOD. R. Mathews RN
7/31	10³⁰ am	Nsg.		Pt. c/o nausea. Called Dr. Omar office. Vomited white phlegm. — R. Mathews RN
7/31	2¹⁰ pm	Nsg.		Dr. Omar office called. Order for Tigan rec'd. — J. Michael RN
7/31	6¹⁵ P	NSG		Nausea & small emesis of undigested food. Tigan 2 cc given IM. Also very confused this PM — B. White RN
7/31	8 P	NSG		No more emesis or c/o nausea. Family here and concerned about pt. being confused. Dr. Omar notified and will return call. — B White RN
7/31	8³⁰ P	NSG		Dr. Omar called and gave order for Restoril 15 mg @ h.s. and may repeat x 1 prn for sleep. B White RN
8/1	6⁵⁰ A	Nsg.		Pt. slept better during the night. No yelling. No further vomiting noted. — B. Jones RN
8/1	9¹⁰ AM	Nsg.		Called Dr. Omar office regarding pt. c/o nausea, exhibiting confusion with hallucinations of seeing men in her room. Concerned over chemical imbalance that could be present with Lanoxin/Lasix in her Digoxin level

Patient's Name (Last, First, MI)	Attending Physician	Room Number	Patient Number
Doe, Jane	J. J. Omar	148 A	4227

INTERDISCIPLINARY PROGRESS NOTES

Date	Time	Department (Nursing, P.T., etc.)	Prob. No.	◄ Progress Note ◄ Signature/Title
7/30	4⁵ pm	Rheum.		Drug Regimen Reviewed — Pt. has a DX of DM ō any TX. Rec. getting orders for monthly FBS and Sr. electrolytes every three months. May need K⁺ suppl. Monitor digoxin TX. C/Brown, Rheum.
7/30	5p	late entry NSG		DR. OMAR OFFICE RETURNED CALL — ORDERS RECEIVED. ———————————— E. Edison RN
7-30	740 P	ACT		ICP Review: Res. moves extremities well / Poor balance / Confused @ X's / Slightly HOH Glasses / Res. will be encouraged to attend Grp. Act. Therapy. — Donna Smythe RN
7/30	11p	Nsg.		Appears alert, oriented as to TPPE. Foley cath patent — drng. clear amber urine, Transfers c̄ ÷ assist. Walks c̄ ÷ — ÷÷ assist to BR (per request) for BM — tried to have BM x3 this shift but unable. Checked for impaction — no stool felt in rectum. Apologizes for staff having to help her. ↑ in chair abt. 55 hr. during supper. c/o nausea — returned to bed p̄ eating only few bites supper. ® arm in sling at all times — painful when moved. T 97 P 96 R 18 BP 174/100 ———— C Parson RN
7-31	1⁴⁵ A	Nsg.		Pt. sleeping. No c/o pain @ this time. Alert. Skin intact. Turns c̄ assist. Foley cath patent + draining amber urine. 146/80 - 98 - 86 - 20 ———— A. Goodson RN —

Patient's Name (Last, First, MI)	Attending Physician	Room Number	Patient Number
Doe, Jane	J. J. Omar	148A	4227

INTERDISCIPLINARY PROGRESS NOTES

Date	Time	Department (Nursing, P.T., etc.)	Prob. No.	Progress Note / Signature/Title
7/30	10³⁰A	nsg		Dr. Omar office notified of need for ancillary orders and clarification on diet and B+O Supp. Dr. Casey office called for Therapy orders. Both Doctors are to return calls. ———— N. Andrews RN
7/30	12N	nsg		Dr. Casey returned call and stated "pt not ready for Therapy evaluations at this time. ———— N. Andrews RN
7/30	2⁰⁰P	nsg.		Alert and oriented. B/P 132/76 – 97.6° – 78 – 20. Fed self brkf in room. Ate 50% for brkf but refused lunch. Pain med x 1 for painful arm. Took meds 5 diff. Joked about how big her pills were. Foley cath patent. Pleasant + co-operative ———— C Smithson LPN
7-30	3⁰⁰P	Dietary		Wt 108# IBW 112-136# 1 gm Na diet. Have requested 2-4 gm Na diet or 2 gm Na diet. Appetite poor 10-35%. Needs assist c̄ meals + encouraged. Hx CHF; ASHD; poss. DM mellitus. Meds include Lanoxin + Lasix Hgb 11.4 FBS 166 BP ¹¹⁰/₇₀. Obtain new diet order. Monitor + encourage intake. ———— Sally Stein FSM
7-30	3P	Nsg.		Medication error occurred @ 9 P.M. 7/29 C Parsons RN

Patient's Name (Last, First, MI)	Attending Physician	Room Number	Patient Number
Doe, Jane	J. J. Omar	148 A	4227

INTERDISCIPLINARY PROGRESS NOTES

Date	Time	Department (Nursing, P.T., etc.)	Prob. No.	◄ Progress Note / ◄ Signature/Title
7/29	1$\frac{50}{P}$	Nsg		89 yr. old female admitted to room 148 A via cart per ambulance c̄ family. Alert & oriented to person and place. BP 110/70 P 82 R 20. Answers questions c̄ no problems. (R) arm in sling. (R) arm purple, no edema noted in hand. R pulse 82. No c/o discomforts. Coccyx pink open area 1/4 cm. no drainage. (L) elbow area 1/4 cm opened c̄ yellow drainage op-site intact — J Williams LPN
7/29	5p	nsg.		Family here. Alert & oriented. Pt. arm in sling – warm to touch. Up in w/c for supper. Appetite poor – 10%. Family requests patient to be posied when up in chair. If any problem keeping in bed, they request her to be posied. Some pain in right arm. Refused pain med. TPR 97⁴-84-18 · BP 144/80 J Phelps Rn
7/30	6 A	Nsg.		Pt. has not slept this shift. (R) arm in sling – arm & fingers pink in color and warm to touch. Voices no complaints of pain – alert – cont of B+B T 96.5 BP 120/60 - 84-16 —— BJones R N

Patient's Name (Last, First, MI)	Attending Physician	Room Number	Patient Number
Doe, Jane	J. J. Omar	148A	4227

INTERDISCIPLINARY PROGRESS NOTES

■ Laboratory Tests

The laboratory test section contains copies of a patient's special tests and clinical laboratory reports. These reports are important because they accurately record a patient's medical status at the time the test was conducted and may also reveal evidence of past and/or present medical disorders. Some laboratory tests are very time consuming to run and it may take several hours, days, or weeks for the test to be completed. When the test results are returned from the laboratory to the nursing unit, they will be filed in the laboratory section of the patient's chart. An abnormal laboratory value may be marked "L" for low or "H" for high. Other laboratories may indicate an abnormal value on the report by placing an asterisk (*) following the laboratory value. In some instances, a double asterisk (**) following an abnormal laboratory value indicates a grossly abnormal laboratory value that may be life threatening to the patient. Frequently, the laboratory personnel will report this value directly to the physician by telephone or in person for immediate attention. If a particular laboratory test has been ordered and the results are not in the appropriate chart section, the laboratory test may be one that takes an unusually long period of time to run, or the copy of the laboratory test results may be lost. If it is determined that the copy of the laboratory test is lost, the laboratory should be contacted as quickly as possible to get another copy of the laboratory test results. Some laboratory tests require collecting specimens (e.g., blood or urine) from the patient at a specific time; specimens must be properly stored until the test is conducted. For example, for some test results to be most meaningful, the serum drug level (SDL) must be a peak level and/or trough level, whereas other drugs may require a postdistribution SDL. The laboratory test must also be run on the specimen as quickly as possible so that the specimen does not undergo any chemical or biochemical reactions or contamination.

Information in the laboratory test section usually includes:

1. Results of current laboratory tests or previous reports from another hospital or long term care facility (e.g., complete blood count, fasting blood sugar, blood chemistry profile, serum electrolytes, blood urea nitrogen, serum creatinine, urinalysis, culture and sensitivity report, prothrombin time, partial thromboplastin time);

2. Serum drug levels (e.g., digoxin, phenytoin, theophylline, phenobarbital, tobramycin, procainamide);

3. X-rays, CAT scans, ECG/EKG, EEG, and related tests;

4. Times when laboratory specimens were collected and when laboratory tests were run.

Before going on to the next section of Jane Doe's medical chart, the reader should take some time and read through the following pages of her Laboratory Test examples to gain a conceptual understanding of the various laboratory tests and to locate the previously mentioned patient information. To gain a better understanding of the types of tests typically run on patients, several different clinical laboratory tests are illustrated in this section. If the reader is not familiar with a specific laboratory test, he or she should refer to Chapter 4 (Clinical

Laboratory Diagnostic Tests) to learn more about a specific test. Chapter 4 provides a brief description of several common clinical laboratory tests, their normal laboratory test values, and some interpretations of their test results that could be considered when their values are either elevated or decreased from accepted normal limits.

FIGURES 1.20-1.26   LABORATORY TESTS

```
RUN:  AUG 3                    CLINICAL LABORATORY                    PAGE 1
      7:17 PM

DOE, JANE  0652159  89  F

0818:0462S  RESULTED RECV:  ·8/3    4:35 PM  COLL:  8/3     4:00 PM

   ORDERED:  GLUCOSE, 4:00 PM

GLUCOSE, 4:00 PM - 145 MG/DL

--------------------------------------------------------------------------------
RUN:  AUG 4                    CLINICAL LABORATORY                    PAGE 1
      3:40 PM

DOE, JANE  0652159  89  F

0818:0410S  RESULTED RECV:  8/4    2:12 PM COLL:  8/4     2:00 PM

   ORDERED:  GLUCOSE,2 HR.PP

GLUCOSE,2 HR.PP = 229* MG/DL (50-120)

--------------------------------------------------------------------------------
RUN:  AUG 6                    CLINICAL LABORATORY                    PAGE 1
      10:02 AM

DOE, JANE  065219  89  F

0806:0139S  RESULTED RECV:  8/6    8:28 AM  COLL:  8/6     6:10 AM
   ORDERED:  POTASSIUM

POTASSIUM = 4.2 MEQ/L (3.5-5.3)

--------------------------------------------------------------------------------
RUN:  AUG 9                    CLINICAL LABORATORY                    PAGE 1
      3:07 PM

DOE, JANE  0652159  89  F

0819:0233S  RESULTED RECV:  8/9    8:47 AM  COLL:  8/9     6:40 AM

   ORDERED:  URINALYSIS

COLOR = YELLOW                          CHARACTER = CLEAR
SPEC. GRAVITY = 1.010 (1.003-1.030)    PH = 5* PH (5.5-6.5)
PROTEIN = 0                            GLUCOSE = 0
KETONES = 0                            BILIRUBIN = 0
OCCULT BLOOD = 0                       UROBILINOGEN = 0
RBC, URINE - NEG                       WBC, URINE = NEG

--------------------------------------------------------------------------------
```

```
RUN:  AUG 1                    CLINICAL LABORATORY                      PAGE 1
      8:35 PM

DOE, JANE    0652159  89  F

0820:0330S   HBO ORDER # 1 RESULTED RECV:  8/1    3:36 PM  COLL: 8/1    2:46 PM
    COMMENT:  DOSE @ 9 AM 8/01, DRAWN @ 2:46 PM
    ORDERED:  DIGOXIN LEVEL

DIGOXIN = 2.6** NG/ML (0.5-2.0)

-------------------------------------------------------------------------------

RUN:  AUG 1                    CLINICAL LABORATORY                      PAGE 1
      8:35 PM

DOE, JANE   065219  89  F

0802:0172S   RESULTED RECV:  8/1    3:40 PM  COLL:  8/1     2:45 PM
    ORDERED:  ELECTROLYTES

[ELECTROLYTES D]
    SODIUM = 137 MEQ/L (135-148)            POTASSIUM = 2.9* MEQ/L (3.5-5.3)
    CHLORIDE = 93* MEQ/L (95-105)

-------------------------------------------------------------------------------

RUN:  AUG 3                    CLINICAL LABORATORY                      PAGE 1
      5:00 PM

DOE, JANE   065219  89  F

0801:0321S   RESULTED RECV:  8/3    3:51 PM  COLL:  8/3     3:10 PM
    COMMENT:  DOSE @ 9:00 AM
    ORDERED:  DIGOXIN LEVEL

DIGOXIN = 1.9 NG/ML  (0.5-2.0)

-------------------------------------------------------------------------------
```

```
RUN:   AUG 1                    CLINICAL LABORATORY                      PAGE 1
       8:37 AM

DOE, JANE   065219   89   F

0814:071198  HBO ORDER  COMPLETE RECV: 7/30      8:00 AM COLL: 7/30     7:35 AM
   SOURCE:   URINE
   ORDERED:  CULTURE AND SENSITIVITY

URINE - 1D 21H - PRELIM
      ...HEAVY GROWTH OF STAPHYLOCOCCUS AUREUS
      ...PROTEUS MIRABILIS
      ...PSEUDOMONAS AERUGINOSA AST TO FOLLOW
      ...NO ANAEROBES GREW

SENSITIVITY - MIC (MIC SYSTEMIC)
   ORGANISM:  PROTEUS MIRABILIS
```

ANTIBIOTIC	MIC LEVEL	DOSE
AMIKACIN	<1-S	IM,IV Q8-12H;15MG/KG/DA
AMPICILLIN	0.5-S	PO 0.25 GM Q6H
CEFAMANDOLE NAFATE	<1-S	IM,IV 0.5-1.0 GM Q6-8H
CEPHALOTHIN	<1-S	PO, 0.25 Q6H;IV 1GM Q4H
CHLORAMPHENICOL	2-S	PO 0.25-0.5 GM Q6H
GENTAMYCIN	<0.5-S	IM,IV Q6-8H;3-5MG/KG/DA
MOXALACTAM	<1-S	IM 0.25-1 GM Q8-12H
PIPERACILLIN	<8-S	IV 3-4 GM Q4-6H
SULFAMETHOXAZOLE/TRIME	<0.5-S	PO 1-2 TABS Q12H
TETRACYCLINE	>4-R	
TOBRAMYCIN	<0.5-S	IM,IV Q8H;3-5MG/KG/DA

```
SENSITIVITY - MIC (MIC STAPHYLOCOCCUS)
   ORGANISM:  STAPHYLOCOCCUS AUREUS
```

ANTIBIOTIC	MIC LEVEL	DOSE
AMPICILLIN	0.5-R	BETA LACTAMASE POSITIVE
CEPHALOTHIN	<1-S	PO 0.25 Q6H;IV 1GM Q4H
CHLORAMPHENICOL	4-S	PO 0.25-0.50M Q6H
ERYTHROMYCIN	<0.25-S	PO 0.25-0.5MG Q6H
GENTAMYCIN	<1-S	IM,IV Q6-8H;3-5MG/KG/DA
NAFCILLIN	<0.12-S	PO 0.5GM;IV 1-3GM Q4H
NITROFURANTOIN	<16-S	PO 0.05-.1GM Q6H,LUTI
PENICILLIN	0.25-R	BETA-LACTAMASE POSITIVE
SULFAMETHOXAZOLE/TRIME	<0.25-S	PO 1-2 TABS Q12H
TETRACYCLINE	<0.25-S	PO 0.25-0.5GM Q6H
VANCOMYCIN	<1-S	IV 0.5GM Q4-6H

```
RUN:   AUG 1                    CLINICAL LABORATORY                        PAGE 2
       8:37 AM

DOE, JANE   065219   89   F

URINE - 2D - **FINAL**
     ...HEAVY GROWTH OF STAPHYLOCOCCUS AUREUS
     ...PROTEUS MIRABILIS
     ...PSEUDOMONAS AERUGINOSA
     ...NO ANAEROBES GREW


     SENSITIVITY - MIC (MIC P.AERUGINOSA)
     ORGANISM:  PSEUDOMONAS AERUGINOSA
```

ANTIBIOTIC	MIC LEVEL	DOSE
AMIKACIN	4-S	IM,IV Q8-12H;15MG/KG/DA
CARBENICILLIN	64-S	PO,IV 1-4GM Q4-6H
CEFOPERAZONE	4-S	IV,IM 1-4GM Q12H
CEFOTAXIME	16-VR	
CEFOXITIN	>16-R	
GENTAMYCIN	4-S	IM,IV Q6-8H;3-5MG/KG/DA
MOXALACTAM	8-S	IM 0.25-1 GM, Q8-12H
PIPERACILLIN	<8-S	IV 3-4 GM Q4-6H
TETRACYCLINE	>4-VR	
TOBRAMYCIN	<0.5-S	IM,IV Q8H;3-5MG/KG/DA

```
RUN:   JUL 30                 CLINICAL LABORATORY                        PAGE 1
       1:57 PM

DOE, JANE    0652159  89  F

0819:0151S  HBO ORDER # 1 RESULTED  RECV:7/30     7:56 AM COLL:7/30     6:40 AM

   ORDERED:  THYROID PROFILE

T3 UPTAKE - 35.5 % (30-40)                  T4-RIA = 6.0 MCG% (4.5-11.5)
FTI = 6.1 (5-11)

-------------------------------------------------------------------------------

RUN:   JUL 30                 CLINICAL LABORATORY                        PAGE 1
       9:13 AM

DOE, JANE  065219  89  F

0813:0159S  RESULTED RECV:  7/30     8:35 AM  COLL:  7/30     7:35 AM
   ORDERED:  URINALYSIS

COLOR = YELLOW                        CHARACTER = HAZY
SPEC. GRAVITY = 1.005 (1.003-1.030)  PH = 8.5* PH (5.5-6.5)
PROTEIN = TRACE                      GLUCOSE = 0
KETONES = 0                          BILIRUBIN = 0
OCCULT BLOOD = 1+*                   UROBILINOGEN = 0
BACTERIA = 3+*                       RBC, URINE = 1-2
WBC, URINE = 25-50
NITRITE = POS*
```

```
RUN:  JUL 30                    CLINICAL LABORATORY                        PAGE 1

DOE, JANE      0652159      89  F

0817:01458     HBO  ORDER #/1  RECV:  7/30     8:07 AM  COLL:  7/30     6:40 AM

         ORDERED:  CHEMISTRY PROF., CBC, URINALYSIS
         CHEMISTRY PROF.
 =>        SMA T. PROTEIN           6.1     G/DL         (6-8.0)
 =>        SMA ALBUMIN              3.2     G/DL         (2.7-4.8)
 =>        SMA CALCIUM              8.5     MG/DL        (8.5-10.5)
 =>        SMA INORG PHOS           4.4     MG/DL        (2.5-4.5)
 =>        SMA CHOLESTEROL          148*    MG/DL        (160-330)
 =>        SMA CREATININE           1.1     MG/DL        (0.7-1.4)
 =>        SMA BILIRUBIN            0.4     MG/DL        (0.1-1.2)
 =>        SMA ALK PHOS             56      U/L          (30-100)
 =>        SMA CPK                  104     U/L          (50-250)
 =>        SMA LDH                  155     U/L          (100-225)
 =>        SMA SGPT                 3       U/L          (0-40)
 =>        SMA SGOT                 11      U/L          (7-40)
 =>        SMA SODIUM               141     MEQ/L        (135-148)
 =>        SMA POTASSIUM            4.3     MEQ/L        (3.5-5.3)
 =>        SMA GLUCOSE              85      MG/DL        (70-115)
 =>        SMA BUN                  27*     MG/DL        (10-26)
 =>        SMA URIC ACID            5.4     MG/DL        (2.2-7.7)
 =>        SMA TRIG.                60      MG/DL        (30-190)
 =>        SMA A/G                  1.1*                 (1.5-1.9)
 =>        SMA BUN/CREA             25*                  (15-24)
 =>        WBC                      10.8    X10^3        (4.8-10.8)
 =>        RBC                      3.96*   X10^6        (4.2-5.4)
 =>        HGB                      11.4*   G/DL         (12.0-16.0)
 =>        HCT                      34.7*   %            (37-47)
 =>        MCV                      89.9    UM^3         (81-99)
 =>        MCH                      30.3    UUG          (27.0-31.0)
 =>        MCHC                     33.7    G/DL         (33.0-37.0)
 =>        RDW                      16.0*                (11.5-14.5)
 =>        MPV                      10.6*   UM^3         (7.4-10.4)
 =>        TOTAL CELL CNT           100
 =>        POLYS                    57      %
 =>        BAND                     2       %
 =>        LYMPHOCYTE               34      %
 =>        EOSINOPHIL               3       %
 =>        REACTIVE LYMPH           4       %
 =>        ANISOCYTOSIS          SL-MOD
 =>        COMMENT 1          PLATELETS APPEAR ADEQUATE
```

DEPARTMENT OF RADIOLOGY

```
DATE  7/29                    07/29          22100A
NAME  DOE, JANE                              AGE  089Y
FILE NO.  112112                             PT TYPE:  I
```

ADDRESS	PROCEDURE

```
1012 BROWN STREET                  TECHNICIAN:  RAL  LML
LAFAYETTE       IN      47904
DR. J. OMAR                        TRANSCRIPTION DATE:  7/29
DIABETES MELLITUS, CARDIOMEGALY    WTRANSCRIBED BY:          JIA

DR. CASEY
```

DIAGNOSIS

7/29

AP SUPINE CHEST. COMPARISON IS MADE TO PREVIOUS STUDY FROM 7/22.
AGAIN, A LEFT PLEURAL EFFUSION IS IDENTIFIED. IT HAS DECREASED SLIGHTLY
FROM THE PATIENT'S PREVIOUS STUDY. THE LUNGS ARE OTHERWISE CLEAR.

X. Y. Zimmerman, MD
RADIOLOGIST ELECTRONIC SIGNATURE

■ Medication Administration Record (MAR)

This section of the patient's medical chart or medication record contains a comprehensive list of all current medication the patient is receiving either on a routine or on prn schedule. In some facilities, the duration of time for this record may range from a few days up to 1 month. Routine and prn oral medications may be separated on the MAR to aid the person's documentation of medication administered. When medication is administered to a patient, the person administering the medication must sign his or her initials and the administration time on the MAR to indicate that a dose of the medication was administered at a specific time. When a patient refuses to take a medication, the same documentation as above is required plus the initials must be circled and a note written in the progress notes that the patient refused to take the medication. When a medication is discontinued (d/c) or the drug strength, dose or dosage interval, dosage form, or route of administration is changed, the d/c medication listed on the MAR must be highlighted (usually a red, pink, or yellow felt marker), dated and initialed by the medication person. When the schedule of a medication is changed, the medication should be discontinued on the MAR and the new order should be rewritten on the MAR.

With some medication that may be particularly harmful or have frequent dosage changes, there may be special drug administration sheets (e.g., insulin, warfarin, parenteral therapy). These special drug administration sheets are used when a patient's condition or therapy may be unstable, and the medication dose is changed or titrated to obtain the proper clinical response in the patient or in the laboratory test. Some examples of drugs and special records include: warfarin dose adjusted to patient's daily prothrombin time; insulin dose adjusted based upon fasting blood glucose or 4 PM blood glucose levels; and intravenous therapy. The administration of external medication may be either recorded on the MAR or on a separate record along with the treatments (e.g., topical creams or ointments, bladder irrigations, enemas).

Information presented in the medication administration record usually includes:

1. Medication, strength, dose, dosage interval, route of administration, original start date, and length of therapy;
2. Record of routine and prn medication administration times (e.g., routine medication is usually administered at 9 AM, 1 PM, 5 PM and 9 PM);
3. Record of medication refused by the patient;
4. Daily record of the specific individual administering the medication (e.g., person's initials after the administration date and time);
5. Patient allergies/drug sensitivities;
6. Instances when medication is to be crushed and/or given with applesauce;
7. Dates on which medication was started and/or discontinued;

8. Initials/names of all persons administering medication during the shift (e.g., days, evenings, nights);

9. Limitations or contraindications to administrating medication as ordered (e.g., hold the dose of digoxin if patient has apical pulse less than 60, hold antihypertensive if systolic blood pressure is less than 100 mm Hg, hold the dose of morphine if respirations are less than 12);

10. Patient's diagnosis(es).

Before going on to the next section of Jane Doe's medical chart, read through the following pages of her Medication Administration Record example and locate the previously mentioned patient information.

FIGURES 1.27-1.33   MEDICATION ADMINISTRATION RECORD

NURSE'S MEDICATION NOTES

DATE	TIME	INITIALS	MEDICATION	REASON/REMARKS
8/1	5:00p	DS	Tylenol 10gr.	c/o headache/tylenol
	9:00p	EE	Restoril 15mg	"can't sleep"
	10:00p	EE	—	pt sleeping
8/3	9:00a	LS	Tylenol 10gr.	c/o pain in (R) arm
	10:00a	LS	—	pain better
8/4	10:30a	NL	Tylenol 10gr.	c/o pain in (R) arm
	11:00a	NL	—	pain better
	11:55a	BR	Rigan 2cc IM	c/o nausea/vomiting
	12:10p	BR	—	N+V relieved

NURSE'S SIGNATURE	INITIALS
Jerry Williams, RN	JW
Carol Nicholas, RN	CN
Norma White, RN	NW
Donna Small, LPN	DS

NURSE'S SIGNATURE	INITIALS
April Phelps, RN	JW
Carrie Riggs, RN	CR
Nellie Long, LPN	NL
Lisa Strong, RN	LS

NURSE'S SIGNATURE	INITIALS
Laura Hart, RN	LH
Susan Hanson, LPN	SH
Brenda Ranger, RN	BR

PRN MEDICATIONS	HR.	1	2	3	4	5	6	7	8	9	10	11	12	13	14	15	16	17	18	19	20	21	22	23	24	25	26	27	28	29	30	3
7/29 Tylenol 325 mg Tab ii: take q 3 hr prn pain	P R N					NL																											
		DB	LS																														
7/31 Tigan 2cc IM q 4 hr prn nausea	P R N						CK																										
7/29 B+O Suppositories prn bladder spasm x 14 days (D/c 8/11/85)	P R N											X X	X X																				
												X X	X X																				
7/31 Restoril 15 mg hs prn sleep (may repeat x1)	P R N	NEE																															
No alcohol																																	

PRN MEDICATIONS	HR.	1	2	3	4	5	6	7	8	9	10	11	12	13	14	15	16	17	18	19	20	21	22	23	24	25	26	27	28	29	30	3

DOCTOR Omar, J.

PATIENT'S NAME Doe, Jane

Aug.
148A

• DIET
• ALLERGIES NKA
• DIAGNOSIS
• FACILITY

ROUTINE MEDICATIONS	HR.	1	2	3	4	5	6	7	8	9	10	11	12	13	14	15	16	17	18	19	20	21	22	23	24	25	26	27	28	29	30
7/29 Lanotin 0.125mg tab ↑ p.o. q.o.d. (Hold if AP < 60)	P	BR X	CR X		BR X		X																									
	AP	92 X		88 X		80 X																										
7/29 Septra -DS tab ↑ tab BID × 14d	9	BR BR	CR	LP	BR	BR							X																		
DISC DATE	9	DS	06	PC	EL	FS	C8						X																		
7/29 Lasix 40mg p.o. d	9	BR	BR	CR	LP	BR	BR						X																		
DISC DATE													X																		
8/3 Slow-K tab ↑ tab BID	9	X	X	CR	LP	BR	BR																								
DISC DATE	5	X	X	EL	EL	FS	C8																								
ORDER DATE																																
DISC DATE																																
ORDER DATE																																
DISC DATE																																
ORDER DATE																																
DISC DATE																																
ORDER DATE																																
DISC DATE																																
ROUTINE MEDICATIONS	HR.	1	2	3	4	5	6	7	8	9	10	11	12	13	14	15	16	17	18	19	20	21	22	23	24	25	26	27	28	29	30

DOCTOR Omar, J.

PATIENT'S NAME Doe, Jane

Aug.

146 A

• DIET
• ALLERGIES   NKA
• DIAGNOSIS
• FACILITY

PARENTERAL FLUID SHEET

Name: Doe, Jane
Room No.
Patient No.
Physician: Omar, J.
Date: 8/6

Date	No.	Solution / Amount Additive	Site	Device	Time	Signature	Rate	I.V. CARE — DATE & TIME Tubing Chngd	Dressing Chngd	Site Insp	Signature
8/6	#1 Bag	D_5W – 100 cc/hr × 2000 cc	L arm	Angio cath.	Start	M. Miller	24 gtt/m	8/6	—	MM	M. Miller
					Finish 2:30/am	X. Bordman	"			XB	X. Bordman
8/7	#2 Bag	D_5W – 100 cc/hr	L hand	#22 Angio	Start 2:30 am	X. Bordman	24 gtt/m			XB	X. Bordman
					Finish						
8/7		6:30 am Order recd to D/C IV			Start						
					Finish						
					Start						
					Finish						
					Start						
					Finish						
					Start						
					Finish						
					Start						
					Finish						
					Start						
					Finish						
					Start						
					Finish						
					Start						
					Finish						
					Start						
					Finish						

NURSE'S MEDICATION NOTES

DATE	TIME	INITIALS	MEDICATION	REASON/REMARKS	DATE	TIME	INITIALS	MEDICATION	REASON/REMARKS
7/29	10¹⁵	OP	B+O supp. nee?	for bladder spasms					
	10³⁰	OP		spasms relieved					
7/29	10¹⁵	CR	Tylenol gr. X	c/o (R) arm pain					
	11¹⁰	CR		arm pain relieved					
7/30	1²⁵	CR	Tylenol gr. X	c/o (R) arm pain					
	2³⁰	CR		arm pain relieved					
7/31	6³⁰	NL	Ativan 2cc IM	c/o nausea					
	7⁰⁰	NL		nausea relieved					
7/31	9⁰⁰	NL	Restoril 15mg	pt. couldn't sleep					
	10⁰⁰	NL		pt. sleeping					

PRN MEDICATIONS	HR.	1	2	3	4	5	6	7	8	9	10	11	12	13	14	15	16	17	18	19	20	21	22	23	24	25	26	27	28	29	30	31
7/29 B+O Suppositorium prn bladder spasm x 14 days (DC 8/11)	P / R / N																												X	X / DV		
7/29 Tylenol 325 mg tab ii po q 3 hr prn pain	P / R / N																												X	X / RCR		
7/31 Tigan 2 cc q 4 hr prn nausea IM																														X / X / X	X / NL	
7/31 Restoril 15 mg cap i hs prn sleep (may repeat x1)	P / R / N																												X	X / X	X / NL	

PRN MEDICATIONS	HR.	1	2	3	4	5	6	7	8	9	10	11	12	13	14	15	16	17	18	19	20	21	22	23	24	25	26	27	28	29	30	31

DOCTOR Omar, J.

PATIENT'S NAME Doe, Jane

July 1468A

- DIET
- ALLERGIES N/KA
- DIAGNOSIS
- FACILITY

ROUTINE MEDICATIONS	HR.	1	2	3	4	5	6	7	8	9	10	11	12	13	14	15	16	17	18	19	20	21	22	23	24	25	26	27	28	29	30	31
7/29 Lanoxin 0.125 mg po ÷ tab qd (✓ apical pulse)	9																												X	X	CR PB	
	AP																												X	X		
7/29 Septra-DS tab po ÷ tab BID ×14d D/c p 9 am dose on 8/12	9																												X	X	72/70	
										⑨																			X	X	CR PB	
																													X	X		
																													X	CP	DS/CE	
7/29 Lasix 40 mg tab po ÷ tab qd	9																												X	X	CR PB	

ROUTINE MEDICATIONS	HR.	1	2	3	4	5	6	7	8	9	10	11	12	13	14	15	16	17	18	19	20	21	22	23	24	25	26	27	28	29	30	31

DOCTOR Oman, J.J.   July 19

'IENT'S NAME Doe, Jane   148A

• DIET
• ALLERGIES   NKA
• DIAGNOSIS
• FACILITY

■ Graphic Section or Patient Data Sheets

The graphic section of a patient's medical chart typically contains patient data recorded either by a nurse or nurse's aid. These subjective and objective data help to document the frequency and extent of various body functions and help to illustrate trends or patterns that may represent therapeutic or adverse effects of medication. These data may be recorded on a variety of schedules, depending upon the patient's medical status (e.g., every 8-hr shift, daily, weekly, monthly). Information in the graphic section usually includes:

1. Vital signs (e.g., temperature, apical pulse, respirations, blood pressures);
2. Current weight;
3. Eating habits;
4. Continence (bowel and bladder);
5. Sleeping habits;
6. Oral intake of fluids;
7. Urinary output;
8. Body movement, joints exercise, etc.;
9. Hygiene.

Before going on to the next section of Jane Doe's medical chart, read through the following pages of her Graphics Section or Patient Data Sheets example and locate the previously mentioned patient information.

FIGURES 1.34-1.38   GRAPHIC SECTION/PATIENT DATA RECORD

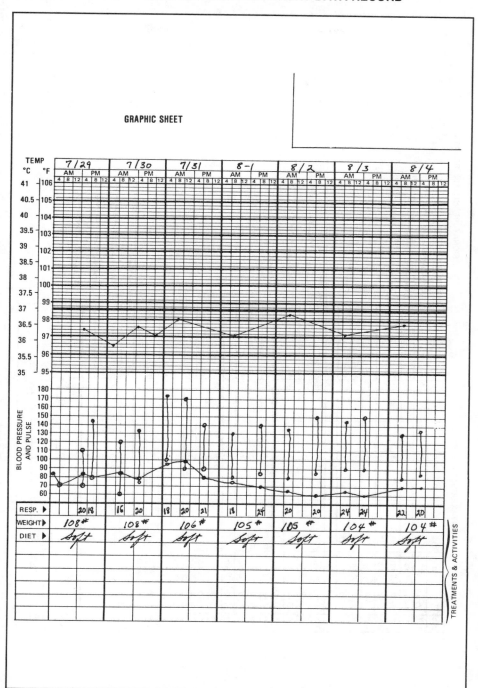

GRAPHIC SHEET

INTAKE/OUTPUT RECORD

DS	I	O	DS	I	O	DS	I	O	DS	I	O
1 N	100		9 N			17 N			25 N		
D	150	100	D			D			D		
E	200	200	E			E			E		
T	450	300	T			T			T		
2 N	60	100	10 N			18 N			26 N		
D	200	200	D			D			D		
E	30		E			E			E		
T	290	300	T			T			T		
3 N	—	150	11 N			19 N			27 N		
D	300	200	D			D			D		
E	200	200	E			E			E		
T	500	650	T			T			T		
4 N	100	100	12 N			20 N			28 N		
D	400	350	D			D			D		
E	200	400	E			E			E		
T	700	850	T			T			T		
5 N	300	150	13 N			21 N			29 N		
D	450	500	D			D			D		
E	300	275	E			E			E		
T	1050	925	T			T			T		
6 N	100	150	14 N			22 N			30 N		
D	400	400	D			D			D		
E	300	200	E			E			E		
T	800	750	T			T			T		
7 N			15 N			23 N			31 N		
D			D			D			D		
E			E			E			E		
T			T			T			T		
8 N			16 N			24 N					
D			D			D					
E			E			E					
T			T			T					

N = Night
D = Day/Date
E = Evening
T = Total
S = Shift

SIGNATURE/INITIALS RECORD

NIGHT SHIFT
Rhonda Silver (RS) NA
Karen Marks (KM) NA
Solly Bachus (SB) NA

DAY SHIFT
Debra Marks (DM) NA
Jackie Dower (JD) NA
Diane McCory (DM) NA

EVENING SHIFT
Darlene Western (DW) NA
Tony Warren (TW) NA
Mary Owens (MO) NA

TREATMENT RECORD

ORDER DATE	TREATMENTS	HR.	1	2	3	4	5	6	7	8	9	10	11	12	13	14	15	16	17	18	19	20	21	22	23	24	25	26	27	28	29	30	31
8/1	Change cath. q 6 weeks and prn	P R N																															
8/1	V.S. Daily		98 98 98 98																														
8/1	Daily Weight		101 102 101 105 104																														
8/5	Enap lotion BID to sacral area and (L) heel	7-3 3-11 11-7																															
8/5	Urge oral fluids	7-3 3-11 11-7																															
ORDER DATE																																	

NURSE'S SIGNATURE	INITIALS	NURSE'S SIGNATURE	INITIALS	NURSE'S SIGNATURE	INITIALS	NURSE'S SIGNATURE	INITIALS

Dr. Oman
Doe, Jane
Aug.
Room 148
Allergies: NKA

TREATMENT RECORD

ORDER DATE	TREATMENTS	HR.	28	29	30	31
7/29	Sling for (R) arm				CB MM MM	
7/29	Up in chair c asst. TID to tolerance (pasty while up)	9 5		CR MM MM L CR CB EE EE CR CB		
7/29	Vital signs	T P R BP		97⁴ 99⁴ 98 78 84 80 20 28 20 149 132 146	78 78 140	
7/29	Monthly weight			108		
7/29	Vaseline Std. Care Lotion to dry skin prn	P R N				
ORDER DATE						

NURSE'S SIGNATURE	INITIALS	NURSE'S SIGNATURE	INITIALS	NURSE'S SIGNATURE	INITIALS
Mary Miller	MM				
Sandy Godwin	SG				
Ellen Ensley	EE				
Carol Ringer	CR				
Connie Black	CB				

Dr. Omar 7/29

Doe, Jane Room 148

ALL ENTRIES MUST BE INITIALED AND INITIALS IDENTIFIED BY FULL NAME IN SIGNATURE AREA

	HR	1	2	3	4	5	6	7	8	9	10	11	12	...	32
Sleep: Document: G = Good F - Fair P = Poor		F	G	G	G	G	G								
Bath/Shower: Type: Days:		BS	S	S	BS	S	S								
Shampoo:															
Nails: ✓ if podiatrist															
A.M. Care: Includes Oral Care, Hair Care, Peri Care		C	C	C	C	C	C								
P.M. Care: Includes Oral Care, Peri Care		C	C	C	C	C	C								
Food Intake: Record % Eaten, Record Assistance Given — B	B	30	30	20	20	20	10								
L	L	10	10	7d	30	15	10								
D	D	40	30	50	70	90									
Bladder: Document — N	N	N	N	N	N	N	N								
D	D	N	N	N	N	N	N								
E	E	N	N	N	N										
Bowel: Document — N	N	O	O	O	O	O	O								
D	D	✓	O	✓	✓	✓	O								
E	E	O	O	✓	O	O	✓								
Staff Initials — N	N														
D	D														
E	E														

A.M. Care / P.M. Care legend:
S = Self c Supervision
M = Minimal Assistance
P = Partial Assistance
C = Complete Assistance

Food Intake legend:
S = Feeds Self c Superv.
M = Moderate Superv.
P = Partial Assistance
C = Complete Assistance
T = Tube Feed

Bladder — Document:
C = Continent
I = Incontinent
N = Indwelling
S = Suprapubic

Bowel — Document:
✓ = B.M.
O = No B.M.
I = Involuntary

N = Night
D = Day
E = Evening

Month/Year: Aug
Last Month Date: 8-1
This Month Date: 9-1
Date:

Weight: 108 / 107
B/P 140/80

Patient Name: Doe, Jane

Physician: Omen

Rm. # 148
Pt. # 4227

■ Interdisciplinary Care Plan/Patient Care Plan

Some health care facilities, especially long-term care facilities and hospitals with specialized departments or units such as a hemodialysis unit or a hospice unit, may have a special committee to formulate patient care plans. The committee usually has a representative from each health care discipline directly involved with the patient's care, (e.g., physician, nurse, pharmacist, physical therapist, occupational therapist, dietician, and representatives from social services, patient activities). Its purposes are to meet regularly to identify any diagnosed and un-diagnosed problems (e.g., medical, social, psychological, physical, dietary) of the patient and to identify measures to resolve or alleviate each problem. After the patient's care has been reviewed, subsequent committee meetings may discuss the degree of resolution of each patient's problems and identify any new problems. Sometimes patient information discussed by various individuals is not recorded in the patient's medical chart. It is very important for all health care professionals to participate on this committee, so that they may provide input on the patient care plan and be informed of how other health care professionals interact with the patient. For example, a therapist may mention that a patient has been very lethargic in the mornings and ask if this lethargy could be related to the patient's drug therapy. This type of information should alert the pharmacist and nurse to look for drugs or drug interactions that may cause lethargy or sedation as an adverse drug side effect. If no medication can be associated with causing the lethargy, the committee should investigate other possibilities, such as an undi-agnosed medical problem (e.g., anemia or hypokalemia).

Although these patient care plans may or may not be included as a written part of the patient medical chart, it is imperative for the pharmacist to utilize the information contained in them.

■ Summary

Monitoring drug therapy is an ongoing process involving continuous review, assessment, and evaluation of the patient's continually changing medical status as reflected in the patient's medical chart. The pharmacist must have a thorough understanding of the medical chart and its contents so that valuable time will not be lost searching for specific patient information. Pharmacists should keep in mind that it is not enough to be a problem identifier. One must also be a problem solver.

■ Chapter 1 Review Questions

Directions: Indicate the correct response for each of the following by sup-plying the information requested or by choosing *True* or *False*.

1.   List five types of patient information that can be found in the Ad-
     mission Record section of a patient's medical chart.

     a. _____

     b. _____

c. _____

d. _____

e. _____

2. List five types of patient information that can be found in the History and Physical Examination section of a patient's medical chart.

a. _____

b. _____

c. _____

d. _____

e. _____

3. List five types of patient information that can be found in the Physician's Orders section of a patient's medical chart.

a. _____

b. _____

c. _____

d. _____

e. _____

4. List five types of patient information that can be found in the Physician's Progress Notes section of a patient's medical chart.

a. _____

b. _____

c. _____

d. _____

e. _____

5. List five types of patient information that can be found in the Universal Progress Notes or Nurse's Notes section of a patient's medical chart.

a. _____

b. _____

c. _____

d. _____

e. _____

6. List five types of patient information that can be found in the Medication Administration Records section of a patient's medical chart.

    a. _____

    b. _____

    c. _____

    d. _____

    e. _____

7. List four types of patient information that can be found in the Laboratory Tests section of a patient's medical chart.

    a. _____

    b. _____

    c. _____

    d. _____

8. List five types of patient information that can be found in the Graphic Section of Patient Data Sheets sections of a patient's medical chart.

    a. _____

    b. _____

    c. _____

    d. _____

    e. _____

9. The Interdisciplinary Care Plan only deals with a patient's diagnosed medical problems.

    True / False

10. The physician's therapeutic goals for the patient may provide directions for appropriate monitoring of drug therapy.

    True / False

Check your responses on page 299.

Chapter 2
Process of Drug Therapy
Monitoring and Assessment

Monitoring drug therapy in either a small or large health care facility is an ongoing process involving a great number of patient-, disease-, and drug-monitoring parameters. When it is not possible for a clinical pharmacist to monitor all patients, it may be necessary to monitor only those patients who are at a significantly higher risk of developing drug-induced problems. Types of such patients to be selected for monitoring include: (*a*) pediatric patients; (*b*) elderly patients with multiple chronic disease states; (*c*) cancer patients; (*d*) patients with heart disease, renal failure, liver failure, or chronic lung disease; (*e*) patients who are taking potent medications with low therapeutic and toxic serum drug levels; and (*f*) patients taking medications with a high risk of toxicity, such as aminoglycosides, antiarrhythmics, anticonvulsants, antineoplastics, theophylline, and lithium. In general, patients who appear to be the most seriously ill as well as those that receive the most medication should have their drug therapy monitored by a clinical pharmacist. Some of these patients will need to be monitored weekly or monthly; others will require monitoring several times daily (1, 2).

After the types of patients to be monitored are identified, the pharmacist can begin collecting data on those patients and information on each patient's drug therapy and begin organizing it in a meaningful manner. To accomplish this task, the pharmacist must determine and understand fully all factors that led up to the patient's present medical status and influenced the patient's admission to the facility. The pharmacist should also know what previous medical problems the patient has had and the therapeutic measures that were used to treat them. Therefore, the patient's medical chart or past medical history must be thoroughly examined. It is also important to interview the patient, whenever possible, as well as to read all patient care information and notes in the chart by nurses, therapists, or aides or by the patient's physician.

All essential information involving the patients to be monitored, such as past and present medical histories and past and present medication utilization, should be documented on a patient medical profile and drug therapy profile or be written up as a patient case profile. This profile may be used to document the completeness of the clinical pharmacist's review of the patient's drug therapy and to communicate any pertinent information to other health care professionals. Although a great deal of patient data will have been evaluated, the case write-up itself should be a condensation of the patient's medical chart. When completed, the patient's medical profile should provide the pharmacist with a comprehensive overview of the patient's past and present medical conditions and all therapeutic measures being taken to help improve the patient's medical status. The patient case write-up should include:

1. Baseline patient data (e.g., age and/or birth date, sex, height, weight, blood pressure, temperature, apical heart rate, and respiration rate);
2. Chief complaint, history of present illness, previous medical history, family history, and social history;
3. Drug allergies and/or hypersensitivities;
4. Diagnosis(es);
5. Current listing of all routine and prn medication;
6. Diet;
7. Date and results of relevant clinical laboratory tests;
8. Facility course summary;
9. Patient problem list;
10. Evaluation of the patient and his or her disease state(s) and drug therapy using the SOAP format.

The essential patient data should be organized into a readily retrievable form which can be easily accomplished by utilizing the above format.

The pharmacist should also collect and evaluate general monitoring parameters on all patients. Many times, progression or regression of a patient's medical condition will be reflected in these parameters. Abnormal general monitoring parameters may be the first signs or symptoms of adverse drug effects, the onset of an acute illness, or exacerbation of a chronic disease. These general patient monitoring parameters include:

1. Chief complaint (e.g., pain, diarrhea, upset stomach, nausea, or vomiting);
2. Mental status (e.g., cheerful, happy, sad, depressed, agitated);
3. Physical activity (e.g., tired, lethargic, sleepy);
4. Sleeping habits (e.g., sleeps well, is restless, has insomnia, awakes early in the morning);
5. Eating habits (e.g., eats well, not hungry, is a picky eater);
6. Skin appearance (e.g., pallor, pink, warm, dry, moist, turgor);
7. Continence of bowel and bladder;
8. Urine appearance (e.g., color, cloudy, mucus strands, crystals, bloody);
9. Height;
10. Weight;

11. Age and/or birthdate;
12. Vital signs (e.g., temperature, rectal, etc.; apical/radial heart rate; respiration rate);
13. Blood pressure (e.g., sitting and/or standing);
14. Hydration status (e.g., fluid intake and output);
15. Edema (e.g., 1+, 2+, 3+, or 4+ edema, pitting edema, sacral, pedal, facial);
16. Diet (e.g., no added salt, 2 g sodium, salt substitute, 1500 kcal, American Diabetes Association (ADA));
17. Drug allergies or hypersensitivities;
18. Clinical laboratory tests (e.g., complete blood count, electrolytes, chemistry profile, urinalysis, culture and sensitivity, x-rays);
19. Signs and symptoms of disease state(s);
20. Drug-monitoring parameters.

By collecting and evaluating these types of patient data, the clinical pharmacist can better determine how well the patient is responding to medical treatment.

The following systematic approach to performing a drug therapy assessment has been designed to help the clinical pharmacist monitor and evaluate drug therapy more effectively and efficiently. This step-by-step approach to the drug therapy monitoring process focuses on a series of statements about the patient's past and present medical problems and about current medication. These steps are designed to lead the pharmacist through the patient's medical chart and to allow him or her to review and evaluate all aspects that are relevant to the patient's medical status and drug therapy.

To help illustrate the various steps involved in compiling a patient's medical and drug therapy profile and in performing an initial drug therapy assessment, the case of Jane Doe, described in Chapter 1, will be reviewed in a systematic fashion. The thought processes involved in each step of Jane Doe's drug regimen and drug therapy will be presented below, along with a sample patient case write-up of the requested information. Before this task can be performed efficiently and effectively, some experience or practice by the pharmacist would be helpful. In time, the pharmacist will be able to determine which patient information is essential and which is important but not vital for the patient's overall drug therapy evaluation. While all patient information needs to be collected and reviewed by the pharmacist, only essential patient information needs to be included in the case write-up.

■ Step 1
Identifying the Reason(s) for the Patient's Admission to the Facility

To determine why the patient was admitted to the facility, the clinical pharmacist should review the patient's current medical problem(s) and/or disease state(s) as determined by the physician at the time of admission. The pharmacist should keep in mind that this information may not be totally accurate. Possible inaccuracies may occur due to one or more of the following factors:

1.　Incomplete listing of pertinent medical problems;
2.　Existing medical problem for which there is no documented diagnosis;
3.　Undiagnosed medical problem for which the patient may or may not be taking medication.

Each of these situations need to be reviewed and evaluated.

In performing an initial drug therapy review, the pharmacist must consider all medical problems as factors contributing to the patient's admission to a facility. Usually, a patient will have one acute medical problem (e.g., drug toxicity, pneumonia, stroke, heart attack, broken bone) that is cited in the clinical record as the primary reason for admission. However, if this acute medical condition is considered to be the patient's only problem, other potentially major medical problems, such as diabetes or hypertension, may be neglected by the pharmacist and other professional staff caring for the patient.

Why Was The Patient (Jane Doe) Admitted To the Facility?

Patient information needed to enable the pharmacist to determine the reason for Jane Doe's admission to the facility may be found in the Admission Record and the Past Medical History sections of the patient's medical chart. This information will also help the pharmacist begin to compile a patient's medical profile and drug therapy profile and to understand the patient's overall medical status. To accomplish this task and begin writing up the patient's case, the pharmacist should refer to these sections of Jane Doe's medical chart in Chapter 1.

CHIEF COMPLAINT (CC)

The patient's CC is usually written as a brief statement of the patient's primary complaint(s) and an indication of the duration of the complaint(s). Quite often, the patient's CC is a manifestation of a medical problem and contributes to the patient's admission to the facility.

HISTORY OF PRESENT ILLNESS (HPI)

The patient's HPI is usually written as a brief description of all signs and symptoms of the medical illness/problem in chronological order.

A.　Data needed
　　1.　Onset of CC—date and manner (i.e., sudden, gradual, insidious);
　　2.　Characteristics—quality, severity, location, temporal relationships (i.e., continuous, intermittent), aggravating and relieving factors, and associated symptoms;
　　3.　Course (i.e., continuous, progressive, intermittent);
　　4.　Results of drug therapy initiated.

B.　Questions to consider
　　1.　Are the signs and symptoms the patient is exhibiting characteristic of a self-limiting medical problem or an acute exacerbation of a chronic disease?

2. Has the patient had this problem before and if so, how was it resolved?

PAST MEDICAL HISTORY (PMH)

The PMH is usually a brief description of all known medical problems from the past and appear in a reverse chronological order.

A. Data needed

1. General health and level of activity;
2. Growth, development and childhood diseases;
3. Immunizations;
4. Previous illnesses, injuries, and surgical procedures;
5. Drug allergies and drug sensitivities;
6. New and previous medications taken on a routine schedule.

B. Questions to consider

1. Do these previous medical problems affect current drug therapy?
2. Does any past problem indicate a contraindication for a drug or drug class?

After reviewing these sections of Jane Doe's chart and after thinking about the types of information needed, the pharmacist may begin writing up a patient case by completing the following requested information.

PATIENT WRITE-UP OF JANE DOE

CC: _____

_____

HPI: _____

_____

_____

_____

_____

_____

_____

_____

_____

_____

_____

PMH: _____

_____

_____

_____

_____

ALLERGIES: _____

After completing all requested information, see page 87 and compare this portion of your patient case write-up of Jane Doe with the example case write-up provided. If you experience difficulty completing this exercise, please refer to the examples and try to pattern your write-up after the example. It is not necessary that your patient case write-up be exactly like the example provided. Overall content should be similar; however, statements will vary from one person to another. As mentioned before, developing the skills involved in collecting patient data and putting them into this type of patient medical and drug profile format requires time and experience.

■ Step 2
Reviewing the Patient's Social and Medical Histories

A patient's family and social history may help the pharmacist understand why a patient is in his or her present condition. These histories may provide information regarding both past psychological or sociological problems and genetic illness patterns (e.g., diabetes, hypertension, alcoholism). A patient's past medical history will help the pharmacist determine what medical problems the patient has contracted and the extent to which the patient has recovered from these problems.

In some instances, the patient admitted to the facility may have been recently discharged from another hospital or long-term care facility (LTCF). In this type of situation, a discharge summary (typewritten as dictated by a physician or handwritten) of the patient's medical and social histories may be in the patient's chart and should provide much of this needed information. In those instances where the patient's past medical history information is still current, this recent discharge summary may serve as the patient's admitting history and physical (H & P) exam. Often, complete copies of previous laboratory tests may be included by the physician along with a record of the patient's progress while in the previous facility. Many times, impressions (not necessarily diagnoses) will be listed by the physician when he or she is not completely sure of the patient's total medical status. Often these impressions refer only to acute medical problems that contributed to the patient's admission to the facility or were detected after a series of laboratory tests and a physical exam. These impressions may ultimately turn out to be medical problems and should not be overlooked or considered unimportant by the pharmacist.

If the patient was not discharged from a hospital or LTCF but was admitted from his or her residence, the physician will generally see the patient in the hospital's emergency room or shortly after admission to the facility and perform a history and physical examination. It should be noted that patient information collected in the H & P may be incomplete. The admitting H & P performed by the physician may lack complete medical history and social history as most information will be gathered from the patient who may not be a good historian. To obtain a more complete picture, it may be helpful to integrate pertinent information from the social worker's evaluation, the nursing assessment, and the pharmacist's drug history interview with the physician's history and physical.

Reviewing Jane Doe's Family, Social, and Medical Histories

Patient information needed to enable the pharmacist to review Jane Doe's family, social, and medical histories may be found in the Admission Record, Family History, Social History, Past Medical History, and History and Physical Examination sections of the patient's medical chart. The clinical pharmacist should refer to these sections of Jane Doe's medical chart in Chapter 1. The following directions will help give the pharmacist an idea of the types of patient information usually contained in these areas of the patient case write-up.

FAMILY HISTORY (FH)

A.   The patient's FH usually includes

    1.   Summary of age and state of health or cause of death for immediate family members;

    2.   Family members with similar diseases or similar clinical signs and symptoms;

    3.   Presence of infections or chronic diseases in family members.

B.   Questions to consider

    1.   Are any diseases of family members genetically transmitted?

    2.   Are any diseases of family members a direct result of the environment in which the patient (family) resided?

SOCIAL HISTORY (SH)

A.   The SH usually includes

    1.   Personality patterns or behavior;

    2.   Marital and sexual history;

    3.   Social and economic status, education, occupation, standard of living, and environment;

    4.   Social habits and recent changes in habits in sleep, diet, exercise, drugs, coffee or caffeinated beverages, tobacco, and alcohol.

B.   Questions to consider

    1.   How many packs of cigarettes does the patient smoke each day?

    2.   How much alcohol does the patient drink each day/week?

    3.   How much caffeinated beverage does the patient drink each day?

    4.   Will any of the above contribute to the patient's problems?

    5.   Will any of the above items significantly change drug metabolism and/or excretion of drugs?

6. Which drugs that the patient takes may be affected by the use of alcohol, caffeine, tobacco?

PHYSICAL EXAMINATION (PE) AND REVIEW OF SYSTEMS (ROS):

Depending on the type of patient, the nature of the illness, and the completeness of the physical exam, some of the following information on various body systems or organs may not be included in the PE.

General Appearance: apparent health, developmental status, apparent physiologic age, habitus, nutrition, gross deformities, mental state and behavior, facies, posture;

Vital Signs: temperature, pulse or apical heart rate, respiration rate, blood pressure, weight, height;

Skin: pallor, texture, moisture, turgor, eruptions, abnormalities of hair and nails, pigmentation, cyanosis, clubbing, edema, petechiae;

Head: symmetry, deformities of cranium, face and scalp tenderness, bruits;

Eyes: visual acuity, visual fields, extraocular movements, conjunctiva, sclera, cornea, pupils, including size, shape, equality, and reaction; ophthalmoscopic examination, including lens, media, disks, retinal vessels, and macula; tonometry, pallor, jaundice, proptosis, ptosis;

Ears: hearing acuity, auricles, canals, earwax, tympanic membranes, mastoid tenderness, discharge;

Nose: nasal mucosa and passages, septum, turbinates, transillumination of sinuses (tenderness over sinuses);

Breasts: symmetry, nodules (include size), consistency, tenderness, mobility, dimpling, nipple discharge, and lymph nodes;

Thorax and Lungs: configuration, symmetry, expansion, type of respiration, excursion of diaphragm, resonance, breath sounds (e.g., retraction, labored breathing, prolonged expiration, cough, sputum, adventitious sounds including rales, wheezes, rhonchi, and rubs);

Cardiovascular System: precordial activity, apical pulse, size, rate, rhythm, heart sounds (e.g., thrills, murmurs, friction rubs, bruits, central venous distention, abnormal venous pulsations), abdominal aorta, peripheral arterial pulses, including carotid, radial, femoral, posterior tibial, and dorsalis pedis pulsations;

Abdomen: contour, bowel sounds, abdominal wall tone, palapable organs, including spleen, kidney, bladder, uterus, liver (scars, dilated veins, tenderness, rigidity, masses, distention, ascites, pulsations, bruits);

Back and Extremities: symmetry, range of motion, joints, peripheral arterial pulses, color, temperature, curvatures of spine, costovertebral angle tenderness, joint deformities, muscle tenderness, edema, ulcers, varicosities;

Neurological Exam: cranial nerves, gait, coordination, sensory and motor systems, muscle stretch reflexes (paresthesias, weakness, muscle atrophy, fasciculations, spasticity), abnormal reflexes (paresthesias, weakness, muscle atrophy, fasciculations, spasticity, abnormal reflexes, tremors);

Genitalia:

Female: external genitalia, vagina, cervix, cytology smear, fundus, adnexa, rectovaginal examination, vaginal discharge, tenderness;

Male: penis, scrotal contents, urethral discharge, hernias;

Rectum: sphincter tone, prostate, test for occult blood, hemorrhoids, fissures, masses;

Personality Status: affect, intellectual functions, thought content and processes, motor behavior, patterns of adjustment, ability to handle life crises, and behavior during the interview.

After reviewing these sections of Jane Doe's medical chart and after thinking about the many different types of patient data, begin completing the requested information in the space provided below:

PATIENT CASE WRITE-UP OF JANE DOE—CONTINUED

FH: No past family history _____
_____
_____

SH: The patient was a homemaker who lived in this area ___
_____
_____
_____
_____
_____

ADMITTING
PE and ROS: The patient is an alert and oriented elderly female _____
_____
_____
_____
_____

VS: BP 110/70, _____
_____

HEENT: Pupils are pinpoint and _____
_____
_____

_____
_____
_____
_____

LUNGS: Grunting respirations _____
_____
_____
_____

BREASTS: _____
_____

HEART: Heart rate regular _____
_____
_____

ABDOMEN: Abdomen appeared to be WNL _____
_____
_____

EXTREMITIES: Patient has a bruised, abraded area _____
_____
_____
_____
_____
_____
_____
_____

IMPRESSIONS/
DIAGNOSIS(ES): Fractured dislocation of _____
_____
_____
_____
_____
_____
_____

After completing all requested information, refer to page 87 and compare this portion of your patient case write-up of Jane Doe with the example provided. If you experience difficulty, please refer to the example and pattern your write-up after the example.

▪ Step 3
Assessing Diagnostic Tests Results

Serum and/or urine clinical laboratory test values may be used by the pharmacist as: (*a*) direct indicators of a patient's medical condition; (*b*) a guide for the clinician to rapid and thorough understanding of a patient's medical condition; and (*c*) as a diagnostic tool in determining the status of vital body systems of metabolism and excretion. In some instances, laboratory tests are essential for the pharmacist to monitor properly and assess how well a patient's disease is being controlled or to prevent drug toxicity when there are no physical signs and symptoms present. Abnormal laboratory values are usually an indication of present or impending complications that may require immediate medical attention. The pharmacist must be concerned with the meaning and significance of abnormal laboratory values and must always attempt to correlate laboratory value with clinical signs and symptoms exhibited by the patient. Too often, clinicians may end up treating an abnormal laboratory value rather than treating the patient.

To obtain meaningful test results and avoid charging the patient for laboratory tests that may need to be repeated, these tests must be conducted at the proper times. The pharmacist can be helpful in working with nurses and physicians in determining the most appropriate times for serum drug levels. For example, due to a patient's altered physiological condition (e.g., decreased renal function) and a drug's pharmacokinetic profile, the half-life ($t_{1/2}$) of the drug may increase when renal function decreases. Extending the half-life of a drug means it will take a longer period of time than normal to achieve steady state level in the blood. If a serum drug level were to be run when the drug is not in steady state, the serum drug level value would be in error and the true value that the drug would achieve on the present dose would be greater than the measured value. With such classes of drugs as aminoglycosides, this type of error could cause the patient to lose hearing or cause kidney damage. This type of professional cooperation would help assure that blood and/or urine specimens are collected and run at proper times during the day based upon the specific drug and laboratory test being conducted. Table 2.1 contains a listing of selected drugs whose serum drug levels are often measured to help determine their therapeutic effectiveness and to help avoid toxicity problems. This table may be used by the pharmacist to help determine the most appropriate times to draw serum drug samples.

In monitoring the results of these laboratory tests, the pharmacist should always check to be sure that the physician has either seen the laboratory test results or has been given the test results over the telephone. If the physician has not responded to a patient's abnormal laboratory test value, it may be because the test results were never seen by the physician or that the results were not communicated to him or her. The clinical pharmacist should follow up on these situations to bring about a positive response.

Assessing Diagnostic Test Results

Information needed to assess Jane Doe's clinical laboratory tests may be found in the Laboratory Section of her medical chart. Please refer to this section in

TABLE 2.1 SERUM DRUG LEVELS—WHEN TO DRAW SAMPLE[3-30]

Drug	Half Life (t$_{1/2}$) (normal renal function)	Time Required to Achieve Steady State (normal renal function)	Time to Draw Sample	Adult Therapeutic Level	Potential Toxic Level
Amikacin (AMIKIN)	2 hr	8.0 hr	Trough—prior to dose Peak—0.5 hr postdose (IV) 1–1.5 hr postdose (IM)	Trough <10 µg/ml Peak 20–30 µg/ml	>10 µg/ml >30 µg/ml
Aminoglycosides (Gentamicin and Tobramycin)	0.5–3 hr (<30 yr) 1.5–15 hr (<30 yr)	2.5–15 hr (<30 yr) 7.5–15 hr (>30 yr)	Trough—prior to dose Peak—15–30 min postdose (IV) 1–1.5 hr postdose (IM)	<2.0 µg/ml 4–10 µg/ml	Trough >2.0 µg/ml Peak >10 µg/ml
Carbamazepine (TEGRETOL)	9–15 hr	36–75 hr	6–12 hr postdose (oral)	4–8 µg/ml	>8 µg/ml
Digoxin (LANOXIN)	1.6 days	1–2 weeks	5–8 hr postdose (oral)	0.8–2.0 ng/ml	>2.0 ng/ml
Lidocaine (XYLOCAINE)	1.5 hr	6–8 hr	During continuous infusion	2–4 µg/ml	>5 µg/ml
Lithium (LITHOBID)	18–36 hr	3–7 days	8–12 hr postdose	0.6–1.4 mEq/L	>1.5 mEq/L
Primidone (MYSOLINE)	10–12 hr	50–60 hr	4 hr postdose	5–12 µg/ml	>12 µg/ml
PHENOBARBITAL	50–120 hr	10–25 days	4 hr postdose	15–40 µg/ml	>40 µg/ml

Drug	Half-life	Sampling	Therapeutic range	Toxic level
Phenytoin (for DILANTIN brand only)	20–40 hr	Trough—prior to dose Peak—oral—3–9 hrs IV—2–4 hrs	10–20 µg/ml	>20 µg/ml
Procainamide (PROCAN-SR, PRONESTYL)	3–4 hr	Trough—prior to dose Peak—0.75–2.5 hr (oral)	4–10 µg/ml	>10 µg/ml
Quinidine (Various brands)	6–7 hr	Trough—prior to dose Peak—sulfate: 1 hr postdose gluconate: 5 hr postdose	2.3–5 µg/ml	>5 µg/ml
Theophylline (Various brands)	4.4 hr (smoker) 8.7 (4–16) hr (nonsmoker)	Peak—2 hr (sol/solid dosage) —4–6 hr (slow release dosage) —12 hr after start IV infusion; then every 24 hours	10–20 µg/ml	>20 µg/ml
Valproic acid (DEPAKENE)	11–15 hr	4 hr postdose (oral)	60–100 µg/ml	>100 µg/ml
Warfarin (COUMADIN)	42 hr	PT drawn preferably in the morning. *Stat* PTs can be drawn at any time although not as accurate	Patient value 1½–2 times control time	Patient value >2.5 times control time

Chapter 1 and begin completing the patient information requested below. When laboratory tests values are normal, time and space may be reduced by listing only the abnormal laboratory test values and indicating that all others were within normal limits (WNL). However, when a laboratory test value has changed from an abnormal value to a normal value, it may be helpful to record both values to show a trend or improvement in the situation.

LABORATORY/TEST RESULTS

A.   Data needed

   1.   What are the results of current clinical laboratory tests?
   2.   What is the physician's evaluation of any x-ray information?
   3.   Are there any previous laboratory tests to use as a basis of comparison?

B.   Questions to consider

   1.   Were the blood and/or urine specimens obtained at the proper time(s)?
   2.   How do test results impact on the patient's status or on current drug therapy?
   3.   Are there any significant drug-laboratory interactions?
   4.   When will these tests be repeated or are other tests needed?

PATIENT CASE WRITE-UP OF JANE DOE—CONTINUED

Clinical Diagnostic
Laboratory Tests: August 9, Urinalysis was WNL except for pH of 5.0

August 6, Serum K^+ 4.2 mEq/liter (3.5—5.0)

_____

_____

_____

_____

_____

_____

_____

_____

_____

_____

_____

_____

_____

_____

_____

After completing all requested information, refer to page 88 and compare this portion of your patient case write-up of Jane Doe with the example provided. If you experience difficulty, please refer to the example and pattern your write-up after the example.

Information about which diagnostic laboratory tests were run and their results may be found in the Laboratory Report or Tests section of the patient's medical chart. For further information on the laboratory tests and the significance of their results, refer to Chapter 4.

■ Step 4
Compiling the Patient's Current List of Medications/Treatments and Diet

The complete drug regimen of the patient may be divided into two groups: 1) those medications being administered on a routine basis and 2) those given only on a prn basis. Some assessment needs to be made of the patient's use of prn medications and their concurrent use with routine medication. It is essential that the pharmacist determine which medications were actually taken by the patient before admission to the facility and compare that list with the patient's present list of medications. To accomplish this task, the pharmacist should examine the patient's medication administration record.

Sometimes a medication dosage form may need to be crushed to help patients swallow it more easily. The pharmacist should monitor this practice, because crushing some drug dosage forms can interfere with the drug's effectiveness, cause toxicity, or cause adverse effects. For further information on drug products that should not be crushed, refer to Chapter 7.

The pharmacist should also be aware that institutionalized patients may keep medication at their bedside, and some of this medication may be mislabeled or may not be exactly what the physician has ordered. These medications may not present a hazard to the patient when taken alone, but when taken in combination with other medication, a potentially serious situation could result. Therefore, allowing patients to keep unknown or unordered medication at bedside should be discouraged except for authorized emergency medication (e.g., nitroglycerin sublingual tablets).

Once a complete list of medication has been compiled, all medication orders should be checked to assure that each of the following is indicated: *a*) complete name of drug; *b*) dosage form; *c*) drug strength; *d*) dose; *e*) dosage interval; and *f*) duration of treatment. It should be noted that the duration of therapy for some medication may be governed by facility stop-order policies (e.g., a 10-day stop-order policy for antibiotics). Therefore, facility stop-order polices should also be considered by the pharmacist.

Compiling the Patient's Current List of Medications Treatment

Information needed for the pharmacist to compile Jane Doe's current Medication/Treatments may be found on the medication Administration Record and Physician's Orders sections of her medical chart. Please refer to these sections in Chapter 1 and begin to complete the patient information requested below:

MEDICATION HISTORY

A.   Data needed

1. For the current list of medical problems what drug therapy has proven effective?
2. Has the patient ever experienced an allergic reaction or an adverse reaction to any drug? (Describe characteristics, duration and drug)
3. Has some organ system been permanently altered by drug therapy, aging or other cause?

B. Questions to consider
1. What impact do the above data have on the selection of drugs and dosages?
2. Was the adverse drug reaction (either positive or negative) adequately documented?

PRESENT MEDICATIONS
A. Data needed
1. What medications does the patient currently receive?
2. How is the patient receiving the drug (dosage form), and what is the dose and time interval?
3. How long has the patient been receiving the medication?
4. What over-the-counter drugs does the patient receive?

B. Questions to consider
1. Could one or more of these drugs be causing the medical problem?
2. What organ functions may be affected by these medications?
3. Are drug dosages, intervals of administration, and dosage forms correctly delivering the drug to this patient?
4. What is the potential for clinically significant drug interactions in this patient's drug therapy?

DRUG ALLERGIES
A. Data needed
1. What allergies does the patient have (drug, food, pollen)?
2. What were the characteristics of any allergic reaction?

B. Questions to consider
1. How do these data influence future drug therapy?
2. What drugs might need to be avoided in this patient?

COMPLIANCE
A. Data needed
1. Is the patient taking his or her medications as prescribed?
2. What are the social and living conditions surrounding this patient that may affect drug-taking behavior?

B. Questions to consider
    1. Could therapeutic failures be a result of poor compliance?
    2. Could adverse drug reactions be a result of poor compliance?
    3. How reliable is the information concerning compliance?
    4. What can be done to improve compliance in this patient?

DIET

C. Data needed and questions to consider
    1. Does the patient require a special diet as a result of a specific disease or condition? Example: American Diabetes Association diet for patients with diabetes mellitus.
    2. Should the patient have certain dietary restrictions as a result of a specific disease or condition? Example: 2–g sodium diet for congestive heart failure.
    3. Is the patient allergic or sensitive to certain foods or have an intolerance for specific types of foods? Example: Intolerance to lactose in dairy products due to a deficiency of lactase enzyme.

PATIENT CARE WRITE-UP OF JANE DOE—CONTINUED

Current Medication/Treatments List

Routine Medication: LANOXIN 0.125 mg orally 1 tablet every day

PRN Medication:

Treatments (topical or external preparations):

Diet: _____

After completing all requested information refer to page 88 and compare this portion of your patient case write-up of Jane Doe with the example provided. If you experience difficulty, please refer to the example and pattern your write-up after the example.

▪ Step 5
Using Drug- and/or Disease-Monitoring Parameters

Specific drug- and/or disease-monitoring parameters should be used by the pharmacist to help determine therapeutic effectiveness and the occurrence of drug-related problems.

In general, a drug- and/or disease-monitoring parameter could be any of the following:

1.   Clinical improvements in the patient's medical condition(s);
2.   Clinical signs and/or symptoms of the onset of an acute medical problem;
3.   Clinical signs and/or symptoms of a failure to reverse a disease process;
4.   Clinical signs and/or symptoms of a lack of response to appropriate drug therapy;
5.   Adverse and/or toxic side effects of the drug regimen;
6.   Clinical laboratory values or diagnostic tests that indicate serum and/or urine drug levels, blood chemistry, and body and/or organ functions.

For example, general drug-monitoring parameters for antibiotics may include: white blood count; elevated temperature; blood, tissue or urine culture and sensitivity report; patient response, new rashes, dosage and schedule, and oral, intramuscular, or intravenous bioavailability. It is important that the pharmacist evaluate a patient's drug therapy for both adverse effects and therapeutic effects. That is to say, the pharmacist should be concerned with monitoring the patient's response or lack of response to his or her drug therapy as well as being concerned with drug interactions and allergies.

When the pharmacist performs a drug regimen review, drug-monitoring parameters for each routine or prn medication being used should be evaluated. After compiling a list of all the medication a patient takes, the pharmacist should identify the appropriate drug-monitoring parameters for each medication. Unless these parameters can be immediately recalled from memory, they should be written out to aid the evaluation process. If a drug that is unfamiliar to the pharmacist is being taken by the patient, the drug should be thoroughly researched in a current drug information reference. A listing of drugs by therapeutic classes and their drug-monitoring parameters is included in Chapter 3. Although not all drugs are specifically listed, once the drug's class or category is determined, general drug-monitoring parameters may be derived from those in that particular drug class. When these parameters have been identified for each medication, the pharmacist should determine which parameters are relevant to the patient's medical condition.

After the pharmacist has identified all appropriate drug-monitoring parameters for the patient's medication, he or she should then determine which disease-monitoring parameters should be followed. Using this combined approach should enable the pharmacist to determine if the disease process is being reversed, maintained at the present level, or continuing to progress. With most patients, these two sets of parameters will be an accurate representation of their overall medical status. For example, disease-monitoring parameters for congestive heart failure may include: general monitoring parameters for the patient and disease-related parameters such as heart and lung sounds; exertional fatigue; signs and symptoms (shortness of breath, chest congestion, edema); laboratory tests (serum digoxin level, serum electrolytes, serum creatinine); and drug and nondrug therapy. A listing of selected common diseases and their specific monitoring parameters is included in Chapter 3 so that the pharmacist may better evaluate drug and nondrug therapy's intervention with a disease process. As with drug-monitoring parameters, disease-monitoring parameters should be written out by the pharmacist until he or she is able to recall them accurately from memory. As a minimum, the pharmacist should be able to provide at least four drug- and/or disease-monitoring parameters and at least one laboratory test for each drug or disease state.

The information needed to identify and evaluate drug- and disease-monitoring parameters may be obtained from the Physician's Orders, Physician's Progress Notes, Universal Progress Notes, Medication Administration Record, Laboratory Tests and Graphic Sections of the patient's medical chart, as well as the Drug- and Disease-Monitoring Parameters for Therapeutic and Adverse Effects section in Chapter 3.

■ Step 6
Preparing a Patient Problem List

The next step in performing a drug therapy assessment is to monitor the facility course summary and prepare a patient problem list. It is essential for the pharmacist to know exactly what diseases or medical disorders the physician has diagnosed when he or she routinely visits the patient so that all necessary drugs or disease parameters may be monitored. As not all medical problems may be diagnosed, and some admitting diagnoses from the patient's past medical history may no longer be valid, the clinical pharmacist must compile his or her own patient problem list from all patient data available. By monitoring the patient's progress on a daily basis, the pharmacist might find medical or drug-related problems documented in the Nurse's Notes or Progress Notes and/or the Physician's Progress Notes sections of the medical chart. At times, drug-related problems may be exhibited by the patient as nausea, vomiting, confusion, or lethargy, and sometimes another drug may be prescribed to treat these drug-induced adverse effects. If a new drug- or disease-related problem is detected by the pharmacist, he or she must confirm and determine its significance. If warranted, it should be added to the patient's problem list. Other patient information that could prove useful includes the patient's history of compliance with medication regimens.

Preparing a Patient Problem List

Information needed for the pharmacist to prepare Jane Doe's Patient Problem List may be found in the History of the Present Illness, Past Medical History, and the History and Physical Examination, Physician's Progress Notes, and Nurse's Notes or Progress Notes sections of Jane Doe's medical chart. Please refer to all new sections of the chart selections in Chapter 1. The following statements should be considered by the pharmacist to help formulate a patient problem list and facility course summary.

A. Data to collect
1. Vital signs;
2. Drugs added or deleted;
3. Administration of prn medication;
4. Eating and sleeping patterns;
5. Alertness, confused, lethargic;
6. Signs and/or symptoms of diseases;
7. Therapeutic effectiveness of drug therapy;
8. Adverse effects of drugs.

B. Questions to consider
1. What are the medical problems listed by the physician?
2. What are the chief complaints of the patient?
3. What are the physician's initial impressions?
4. Are there any undiagnosed problems?
5. Is there a problem in determining a specific indication for drug therapy?
6. Could drugs be causing the above noted problems?
7. What effect might these problems have on drug therapy?
8. What significant things are happening to the patient on a day-to-day basis?

After reviewing these sections of Jane Doe's medical chart, begin completing the requested information in the space provided below.

PATIENT CASE WRITE-UP OF JANE DOE—CONTINUED

Facility Course
Summary (FCS):

Day 7–29   Patient was admitted to the facility with some pain in right shoulder and chest congestion. She is alert and oriented to TPPE. She has a poor appetite and ate only 10% for supper. BP 110–114/80–90, T 97.4, P 86–96, R 18–20.

Day 7–30 _____
_____
_____
_____
_____
_____
_____
_____
_____
_____
_____
_____
_____
_____
_____
_____
_____
_____
_____
_____
_____
_____
_____

Patient Problem
List (PPL):   1. Fractured dislocation of right humeral head
2. Pain in right shoulder
3. Congestive heart failure with atherosclerotic heart
disease
_____
_____
_____
_____
_____
_____
_____
_____
_____
_____

After completing all requested information, refer to page 89 and compare this portion of your patient case write-up of Jane Doe with the example provided. If you experience difficulty, please refer to the example and pattern your write-up after the example.

■ Step 7
Matching Diagnosis(es) with Medication(s)

Ideally, each drug or set of drugs being administered to the patient should correspond to at least one diagnosis. In performing a drug therapy assessment, the pharmacist will begin with the patient's problem list (see Step 6) and attempt to match medications to specific medical problems or disease states. A review and assessment of the patient's physiological systems may be very helpful in establishing these relationships.

The pharmacist should question the use of all medication that cannot be directly connected to one or more of the patient's medical problems. As mentioned earlier, some potential medical problems may be undiagnosed. It is therefore essential that the pharmacist identify these medical problems early so that the patient receives only the medication needed to assure proper medical care. All medication being consumed that cannot be matched to a medical problem should probably be considered unnecessary. The pharmacist should discuss the use of these drugs with the patient's physician to determine their need or to have them discontinued. If untreated medical problems have been identified through the drug therapy assessment process, they should be brought to the attention of the patient's attending physician.

After the pharmacist has determined that use of the drug is appropriate for the medical condition, then other monitoring activities should proceed. These activities include making sure that the drug's dose is correct for the patient's sex, weight, and age, and may include such other factors as metabolic status (e.g., liver function) and excretion status (e.g., renal function). The process of determining appropriate doses of medication for patients involves the application of basic pharmacokinetic principles. When a patient does not respond appropriately to drug therapy, it may be necessary for the pharmacist to recommend adjustments in a patient's drug therapy or calculate new drug doses and/or dosage intervals to help achieve therapeutic objectives and prevent drug toxicities. Drugs for which the application of pharmacokinetic principles are essential in achieving safe and therapeutic drug doses and/or dosage intervals include: digoxin, aminoglycoside antibiotics, theophylline, quinidine, procainamide, phenytoin, barbiturates, and lithium. Along with achievement of safe and effective drug doses, it is also important for the pharmacist to assess a patient's clinical response to drug therapy.

In addition to determining the types of medication that should be taken by the patient, the pharmacist should review and evaluate the following for each new medication: dose, patient drug allergies, drug sensitivities, drug administration time(s), dosage interval, route of administration, dosage form, and therapeutic, physical, or chemical incompatibilities and interactions.

The process of analyzing the relationship between diagnosis and treatment will help the pharmacist to discover inappropriate, inadequate, or excessive use of drugs or drug-dosing problems and help him or her formulate a therapeutic plan based upon current patient data.

Information needed for this process may be gathered from the patient interview, the History and Physical Examination, the Physician's Orders, the medication administration record, and the Progress Notes sections of the patient's medical chart.

■ Step 8
Evaluating the Drug Therapy and Documenting Findings

After a sufficient data base has been collected on the patient's past medical history and present medical status, the final steps of the drug regimen review process of evaluating the drug regimen and documenting findings can be completed. To a great extent, this process has already begun in the previously mentioned steps of the drug therapy assessment process.

The concept of associating drug use with a corresponding diagnosis or disease state was first implemented by Lawrence Weed, M.D., and is known as the Problem-Oriented Medical Record (POMR) or SOAP (Subjective, Objective, Assessment, and Plans or recommendations) format. This system involves a four-step approach to problem solving that attempts to identify (subjective data), quantify (objective data), assess (synthesis and analysis of the data), and solve (formulate therapeutic plans or recommend corrective measures) the medical problem. Although the SOAP format was originally designed to aid physicians in documenting and solving medical problems, it can be easily adapted and used by the pharmacist in assessing overall achievement of therapeutic objectives of a patient's drug regimen and in evaluating and solving problems related to the drug therapy.

By using the SOAP format in performing drug therapy assessments, the pharmacist can evaluate patient data and document significant findings in the same process. To accomplish this, patient data for each patient problem must be grouped into either subjective or objective categories for analysis by the pharmacist.

Subjective—S

Subjective patient data for each identified patient problem may help the pharmacist to identify current and potential medical problems. These data, which cannot be counted or measured very well, may include such patient information as:

1. Chief complaint (e.g., complaints of pain, backache, shortness of breath);
2. Mental status (e.g., happy, cheerful, anxious, depressed);
3. Medical status (e.g., no significant change, clinical signs of improvement or regression of a medical condition);
4. Eating habits;
5. Nausea, vomiting, diarrhea;
6. Shortness of breath or dyspnea;
7. Sleeping habits;

8.   Skin color and appearance (e.g., pale, pink, dry, turgor, rash);
9.   Urine color and appearance (e.g., clear, cloudy or turbid, foul odor, bloody);
10.   Bowel and bladder control;
11.   Activity level (e.g., active, lethargic, tired, sleepy);
12.   Orientation (e.g., disoriented, confused);
13.   Coughing;
14.   Upset stomach;
15.   Relief of symptoms following prn or routine medication administration.

These types of subjective information are usually recorded in the patient's medical chart in the Universal or Nursing Progress Notes or Physician Progress Notes sections, graphics, and patient data sheets. Because nurses and/or nurse's aides are with the patient on a 24–hr/day basis, they will be recording much of this information as a result of their daily observations of the patient. The pharmacist may use these subjective findings to help monitor therapeutic or beneficial effects and adverse effects of drug therapy. The pharmacist may also use them to identify early signs or symptoms of the onset of an acute medical problem.

Objective—O

Objective patient data for each identified patient problem are helpful to the pharmacist in quantifying the extent to which the patient is being affected by the disease and/or medication. These data can be counted or measured and may include such patient information as:

1.   Temperature—oral or rectal;
2.   Apical, carotid, or radial pulse;
3.   Respiration rate;
4.   Blood pressure;
5.   Height;
6.   Weight;
7.   Fluid intake and urine output, diet (e.g., 1500 kcal, American Diabetes Association, 2 g sodium, no added salt);
8.   Clinical laboratory tests (e.g., blood chemistry profile, complete blood count, prothrombin time, partial thromboplastin time, urinalysis laboratory reports, x-rays, electrocardiograms);
9.   Urine diagnostic tests (e.g., glucose, ketone, pH, hematest);
10.   Bacteria culture and antibiotic sensitivity reports;
11.   Time of day and/or dates when data were documented.

These types of patient information may be recorded either by the patient's physician, nurses and/or nurse's aides and may be reported by the clinical laboratory. Human error (in obtaining the specimen) as well as laboratory error (in analyzing the specimen) may cause these laboratory values to be inaccurate. Therefore, it is usually helpful to have a range of values, for example, blood pressure ranged from 140/60 mm Hg to 168/94 mm Hg, apical pulses ranged from 54–70 bpm, and fasting blood glucose ranged from 100–150 mg/dl. In some instances, a patient's response to drug therapy can be monitored and evaluated by objective data only (e.g., temperature, pulse, respiration rate, blood pressure, renal clearance). As objective data can be accurately measured, it is more desirable to use these data in monitoring a patient's response to drug therapy.

Objective data are usually recorded in the patient's medical chart and may be located in the History and Physical, Progress Notes, Graphics Section, or Patient Data Sheets and Laboratory Data Sections.

Assessment—A

After all pertinent patient data for each identified patient problem have been collected, classified, and categorized as either subjective or objective, the pharmacist is ready to begin analyzing and synthesizing the data to assess how well the patient is responding to therapy. Whenever possible, a patient's subjective complaint or problem should be quantified with objective data to help determine the extent or severity of the problem. Objective data will also help to determine how quickly or how aggressively corrective therapeutic measures should be initiated. By having both subjective and objective data to support the pharmacist's assessment of the existence of a problem, a much stronger argument can be presented to convince other health care professionals that measures should be initiated to correct or treat the problem.

The pharmacist should always be aware that in some patients, especially the elderly, there may be objective data (e.g., abnormal laborabory value) that tend to indicate the presence of a problem but no apparent subjective data (e.g., patient complaints) to support the assessment and vice versa. In these situations, good professional judgment and clinical experience must be combined to permit the pharmacist to make the best decision or assessment. These instances will require the pharmacist to do some creative thinking to determine more definite drug- or disease-monitoring parameters to help explain confusing data. When appropriate, the pharmacist may need to recommend that some laboratory work be done to help clarify an unclear or problematic situation. Such cases may also require the pharmacist to monitor the problem more frequently or for longer periods of time before the best decision can be made.

It should be noted that some acute medical or problematic situations are self-limiting and will not require medication. Sometimes a conservative approach is more advisable rather than an aggressive short- or long-term treatment. At times, the pharmacist must decide if resolution of the situation he or she has defined as problematic will really make a difference in the patient's overall condition. In some cases, the cure may be worse for the patient than the medical problem. The pharmacist should monitor these situations closely so that he or she can determine when drug therapy is rational, determine the appropriate length of therapy, and see that the medication is discontinued after the problem situation is stabilized or the patient is asymptomatic. If the medication is not discontinued when the patient is asymptomatic, continued use of the medication may cause other acute problems. After the patient becomes asymptomatic, the physician should be consulted to reevaluate the situation. Through this process, active pharmacist participation in performing drug therapy assessments can prevent patients from taking unnecessary medications.

As mentioned earlier, the pharmacist may need to request certain laboratory tests to evaluate and determine the significance of the test results as they relate to the patient's medical status and therapy. Patients who take medication over a long period of time will usually need to have some routine lab tests performed. These medications and lab tests include:

1.   Oral anticoagulants (prothrombin time, preferably every 1–2 weeks until patient is stabilized, then at least every month);
2.   Oral hypoglycemic agents or insulin (urine glucose/acetone daily and fasting blood sugar at least monthly when patient is stabilized);
3.   Digitalis products with a potassium-depleting diuretic (serum electrolytes at least every 3 months);
4.   Hematinics, such as iron, B_{12}, and folic acid (complete blood count within 30 days of initiating therapy, then every 3–6 months) (30).

For a better understanding of which drugs may require laboratory tests for proper monitoring, see Chapter 5.

Many times laboratory test values may appear to be within the normal range of values as established by the laboratory. In such instances, two or more sets of tests could be necessary to help identify a trend or a change occurring over an appropriate time period. Laboratory test results must always be evaluated with regard to the patient's sex, age, and clinical signs and symptoms. For example, a normal (WNL) serum creatinine level for a younger adult may accurately represent normal renal function, but the same value for an elderly patient may represent renal insufficiency. As mentioned before, sometimes laboratory tests are treated rather than patients. Therefore, the pharmacist should determine what is "normal" for the particular patient or type of patients being monitored rather than what is "normal" for the entire patient population. Sometimes patients will present with toxic signs or symptoms when serum drug levels are WNL or within the therapeutic range. Other patients may do quite well and not exhibit adverse effects when test values are elevated above the normal limits.

When changes or trends are identified, they may be indications of an acute medical problem, and clinical signs and symptoms of the problem (subjective data) may follow very soon. Many times, immediate medical attention may be needed to prevent a critical situation. Pharmacists can play a vital role in alerting nursing and medical staff to these situations before the patient suffers the discomfort or pain that may be associated with the problem. Often, the pharmacist may be the first professional person to detect the presence of a patient's acute medical problem. Sometimes, professional staff members may interpret abnormal patient behavior as merely another sign of getting older and may not perceive the abnormal patient response as a treatable medical problem or as an adverse response to a medication.

The pharmacist's assessment of the patient should follow extensive evaluation of all available patient data. Each patient problem identified on the patient problem list should be assessed on an individual basis. Positive (e.g., hypertension appears to be well controlled) or negative statements (e.g., hypertension is not well controlled and blood pressure varies greatly) should be listed that reflect the pharmacist's opinion concerning the patient's present medical status, including progress being made in treating previously identified medical problems (refer to patient problem list), untreated acute or chronic problems, adverse drug reactions, medication being administered to the patient that appears to be unnecessary or unwarranted, as well as appropriate nondrug therapy.

Plans (P) or Recommendations

After problems have been identified, quantified, and assessed by the pharmacist to be clinically significant, the next procedure is to list some plans or formulate some realistic recommendations for each problem to:

1. Correct or treat medical or drug-related problems (e.g., provide an alternative therapy or drug and/or discontinue drugs, modify drug dose or dosage interval, change the route of drug administration, advise the patient not to take drugs together, advise taking drugs with or without food as appropriate);
2. Request clinical laboratory tests;
3. Change diet contents and/or use parenteral or enteral nutrition;
4. Request vital signs be taken more frequently;
5. Request more nursing measures;
6. Educate the patient on disease states and on the need to take medication and to take it properly;
7. Continue to monitor unclear or problematic situations;
8. When appropriate, to continue present drug and nondrug therapies.

It should be noted that plans and recommendations formulated by the pharmacist may not be realistic or may not be implemented if they are not in harmony with the physician's therapeutic goals for the patient.

Evaluating the Drug Therapy and Documenting Findings

One approach the pharmacist can use in writing up the evaluation portion of a patient case is to note each patient problem that was identified in the patient problem list and evaluate it individually (e.g., Problem 1, congestive heart failure, Problem 2, hypertension) as if it were the only problem the patient had. All subjective (S) patient data that are specifically related to this problem are grouped together. All objective (O) patient data that are related will follow. Next, the patient problem is assessed. Finally, any recommendations or plans (P) for the problem are listed. These four steps (SOAP) complete the initial evaluation of the problem. Followup monitoring of the problem should follow the same processes. For the purpose of this text, this approach will be called "Evaluation of All Problems on an Individual Basis."

Another approach that can be used in writing up the evaluation portion of the patient case is to combine all patient information. For example, all subjective patient data for all identified patient problems could be arranged under the appropriate heading. Objective patient data would be grouped in a similar manner.

Each problem could be assessed and listed in the same numerical order as it appears in the patient problem list. The plan(s) or recommendation(s) pertaining to each problem could be listed in a similar fashion. For the purpose of this text, this approach will be called "Collective Evaluation of All Patient Problems."

To illustrate these two methods of patient evaluation further, the sample patient case, Jane Doe, has been evaluated using the collective and individual evaluation approaches. As there is generally more than one correct way to write up a patient case evaluation, the pharmacist may review each approach and determine its merits. Each evaluation approach may have its perceived advantages as well as disadvantages. In time, the pharmacist may prefer one approach over the other or modify one approach to meet the drug therapy monitoring needs of patients in his or her practice environment.

Information needed to evaluate Jane Doe's case may be collected from the Physician's Progress Notes, Nurse's Notes or Progress Notes, Laboratory Tests, Graphics or Patient Data Sheets and History and Physical sections of her chart. With this information in mind, begin using the SOAP format and writeup your evaluation of Jane Doe using the collective and/or individual evaluation approaches.

PATIENT CASE WRITE-UP OF JANE DOE—CONTINUED

Subjective (S)
Evaluation of
Patient: _____

_____

_____

_____

_____

_____

_____

Objective (O)
Evaluation of
Patient: _____

_____

_____

_____

_____

_____

_____

_____

_____

Assessment (A) of
Patient: _____

_____

_____

_____

_____

_____

_____

_____

_____

_____

Plans (P) For The
Patient: _____

_____

_____

_____

_____

_____

_____

_____

_____

_____

After completing all requested information, refer to pages 89 or 92 and compare this portion of your patient write-up of Jane Doe with the examples provided. If you experience difficulty, please refer to the examples and pattern your write-up after the example.

■ Step 9
Communicating Review Findings and Following-Up

When the pharmacist has performed his or her assessment of the patient's problems and the patient's drug therapy and has documented pertinent findings in the patient's medical chart, these plans or recommendations should be communicated to the appropriate health care professional to ensure immediate follow-up. If these findings involve recommendations for better drug administration, the pharmacist should communicate these recommendations directly to the medication administration nurse and/or director of nursing. With other recommendations involving physicians, it may be necessary, and perhaps best, for the pharmacist to see the physician personally when he or she is in the facility or to telephone him or her to obtain some positive action or response to specific recommendations. In such cases, it would be wise for the pharmacist to have formulated several possible alternatives in advance and be ready to present what he or she feels is the best solution to the problem. It should be noted that some physicians may be more receptive to unsolicited requests from nurses than from pharmacists. In this situation, the health care person who has the best rapport with the physician and who can accurately communicate appropriate information to the physician should follow-up on the pharmacist's recommendation(s). As the nurse may not have gone through the thought process involved in arriving at the recommendation(s), it is very important that the nurse knows why the recommendation(s) is needed for the patient so that the nurse will be supportive. The pharmacist should always keep in mind that his or her primary goal is to provide optimum drug therapy. Providing quality patient care must supercede both the pride of having done everything one's self as well as the idea of receiving credit for the patient's improved medical status as a result of his or her recommendation(s). It is by working together with other health care professionals that pharmacists become more effective members of the health care team.

■ Summary

Monitoring drug therapy is an ongoing process that involves reviewing and monitoring a patient's medication as well as assessing and evaluating all patient information. The initial review of a patient's drug regimen and the assessment of his or her medical condition will require a fair amount of time on the part of the pharmacist. However, once a sufficient patient data base has been established, subsequent monitoring should require much less time. Subsequent monitoring of the patient's drug therapy should focus on follow-up, monitoring of the results of previous recommendations, the changes in drug therapy, the changes in the patient's medical condition (subjective and objective), and monitoring for significant changes or trends in the patient's behavior or medical status. Follow-up monitoring of the drug therapy should build upon the pharmacist's initial assessment. The SOAP notes could also be used to follow any subsequent medical problem the patient encounters.

As the pharmacist becomes more familiar with the medical chart contents, more comfortable working with various health care professionals, and more confident of his or her ability to review and assess a patient's drug therapy, the pharmacist will find himself or herself actively involved as a health care team member. The pharmacist will also receive professional reward for his or her contributions in helping provide quality health care.

The pharmacist should read through the following condensed patient cases and evaluate the patients, their medical problems, and their drug therapies using the SOAP approach. For self-evaluation purposes, sample evaluations (using the individual and collective evaluation methods) of each patient are included to assist the pharmacist in developing his or her approach to the review process. Some cases have portions of the evaluation that are incomplete; the pharmacist should attempt to complete any incomplete or missing information. Obviously, successful intervention can take several difficult routes. This format represents only one method in which essential patient data may be identified, quantified, assessed, and presented in a meaningful manner. With some practice and clinical experience, the pharmacist will soon learn how to approach drug therapy assessment in any patient and be able to perform routine drug therapy monitoring.

■ Chapter 2 Review Questions

Directions: Indicate the correct response in each of the following by choosing *True* or *False* or by supplying the information requested.

1. When clinical laboratory tests are run, collection time for serum drug levels must be individualized for each drug.

    True / False

2. In which two sections of the medical chart will the pharmacist find patient information that will help determine why the patient was admitted to the health care facility?

    a. _____

    b. _____

3. List two ways in which a patient's past family and social history may be very helpful to the pharmacist in evaluating drug therapy.

    a. _____

    b. _____

4. List three types of patient information included in a patient's past medical history, present history, and physical examination that may be helpful to the pharmacist.

    a. _____

    b. _____

    c. _____

5. When evaluating drug therapy, why is it important for the pharmacist to compile his or her own patient problem list?

    _____

    _____

6. List three ways in which serum and/or urine laboratory values may be utilized by the pharmacist.

    a. _____

    b. _____

    c. _____

7. Ideally, each drug or set of drugs being administered to the patient should correspond to at least one of the patient's diagnoses.

    True / False

8.   All medications being taken by the patient that cannot be matched to medical problems should be considered as probably unnecessary.

       True / False

9.   List four types of drug- and/or disease-monitoring parameters.

       a. _____

       b. _____

       c. _____

       d. _____

10.   Subjective patient data cannot be measured very well, but may help the pharmacist in identifying real and potential medical problems.

       True / False

11.   Objective patient data can be counted or measured and may help the pharmacist quantify the extent to which the patient is being affected by the disease and/or medication.

       True / False

12.   Patients may present signs and/or symptoms of drug toxicity when serum drug levels are within the normal range.

       True / False

13.   The pharmacist's assessment of a patient's drug therapy could contain both positive and negative conclusions that represent the pharmacist's evaluation of the patient's drug therapy, and overall medical status.

       True / False

14.   List four types of plans or recommendations that may be presented by the pharmacist.

       a. _____

       b. _____

       c. _____

       d. _____

15.   Drug therapy recommendations from the pharmacist should be communicated to the appropriate health care professional only by the pharmacist.

       True / False

Check your answers on page 302. Be sure that you understand the information presented in this portion as well as the answers to each of these questions.

■ References

1. Young WW, Bell JE, Bouchard VE, Duffy MG, Clinical pharmacy services: prognostic criteria for selective patient monitoring, Part 1. *Am J Hosp Phar* 1974; 31:562–568.

2. Young WW, Bell JE, Bouchard VE, Duffy MG, Clinical pharmacy services: prognostic criteria for selective patient monitoring, Part 2. *Am J of Hosp Pharm* 1974; 31:667–676.

3. Bigger JT, Hoffman BF, Antiarrhythmic drugs. In: Goodman LS, Gilman A, eds. *The Pharmacological Basis of Therapeutics,* 7th ed, Macmillan, New York, 1985, pp 748–783.

4. Gibaldi M, Levy G. Pharmacokinetics in clinical practice. *JAMA* 1976; 235:1987–1992.

5. Powell JR, Vozeh S, Hopewell P, Costello J, Steiner LB, Riegelman S. Theophylline disposition in acutely ill hospitalized patients. *Am Rev Respir Dis* 1978; 118:229–238.

6. Hendeles L, Weinberger M, Johnson G. Monitoring serum theophylline levels. *Clin Pharmacokinet* 1978; 3:294–312.

7. Laursen LC, Johannesson N, Sondergaard I, Weeke B. Maximally effective plasma concentrations of enprofylline and theophylline during constant infusion. *Br J Clin Pharmacol* 1984; 18:591–595.

8. Jacobs MH, Senior RM, Kessler G. Clinical experience with theophylline. *JAMA* 1976; 235:1983–1986.

9. Smith TW. Digitalis in the management of heart failure. *Hosp Pract* 1984; 19:67–92.

10. Lee TH, Smith TW. Serum digoxin concentration and diagnosis of digitalis toxicity. *Clin Pharmacokinet* 1983; 8:279–285.

11. Doherty JE. How and when to use the digitalis serum levels. *JAMA* 1978; 239:2594–2596.

12. Lasagna L. How useful are serum digitalis measurements? *N Engl J Med* 1976; 294:898–899.

13. Atkinson AJ, Lertora JJL, Kushner W, Chao GC, Nevin MJ. Efficacy and safety of N-acetylprocainamide in long-term treatment of ventricular arrhythmias. *Clin Pharmacol Ther* 1983; 33:565–576.

14. Kates RE. Plasma level monitoring of antiarrhythmic drugs. *Am J Cardiol* 1983; 52:8–13C.

15. Edelbroek PM, de Wolff FA. The quinidine-fluorometry dilemma. *Clin Chem* 1981; 27:1778–1784.

16. Drayer DE, Lorenzo B, Reidenberg MM. Liquid chromatography and fluorescence spectroscopy compared with a homogeneous enzyme immunoassay technique for determining quinidine in serum. *Clin Chem* 1981; 27:308–310.

17. Roden DM, Woosley RL. Class I antiarrhythmic agents: quinidine, procainamide and N-acetylprocainamide, disopyramide. *Pharmacol Ther* 1984; 23:179–191.

18. Anderson JL, Harrison DC, Meffin PJ, Winkle RA. Antiarrhythmic drugs: clinical pharmacology therapeutic uses. *Drugs* 1978; 15:271–309.

19. Burgess ED, Friel PN, Blair AD, Raisys VA. Serum phenytoin concentrations in uremia. *Ann Intern Med* 1981; 94:59–60.

20. Troupin AS. The measurement of anticonvulsant agent levels. *Ann Intern Med* 1984; 100:854–858.

21. Richens A. Clinical pharmacokinetics of phenytoin. *Clin Pharmacokinet* 1979; 4:153–169.

22. Letteri JM, Mellk H, Louis S, Kutt H, Durane P, Glazko A. Diphenylhydantoin metabolism in uremia. *N Engl J Med* 1971; 285:648–652.

23. Noone P, Parsons TMC, Pattison JR, Slack RCB, Garfield-Davies D, Hughes K. Experience in monitoring gentamicin therapy during treatment of serum gram-negative sepsis. *Br Med J* 1974; 1:477–481.

24. Barza M, Lavermann M. Why monitor serum levels of gentamicin? *Clin Pharmacokinet* 1978; 3:202–215.

25. Yee GC, Evans WE. Reappraisal of guidelines for pharmacokinetic monitoring of aminoglycosides. *Pharmacotherapy* 1981; 1:55–75.

26. Amdisen A. Serum level monitoring and clinical pharmacokinetics of lithium. *Clin Pharmacokinet* 1977; 2:73–92.

27. Taylor WJ, Finn AL. *Individualizing Drug Therapy*. Gross, Townsend, Frank, Inc, New York, 1981, pp 11–15, 23–28, 38–41, 42–46, 62–71.

28. Knoben JE, Anderson PO. *Handbook of Clinical Drug Data*. Drug Intelligence Publications, Inc, Hamilton, IL, 1983, pp 251–256, 412–414, 475–476, 477–478, 478–479, 602–605.

29. Evan WC, Jusko JJ, Shentag WJ. *Applied Pharmacokinetic*. Applied Therapeutics, Inc, San Francisco, 1985, pp 95, 174, 275, 319.

30. Department of Health and Human Services, Health Care Financing Administration, *State Operations Manual-Provider Certification,* Sections 3160 and 3161, January, 1982, pp 3-113–3-114.

■ Case Study 1: Write-Up of Jane Doe

CC: Pain in right shoulder for the past few hours and has grunting respirations of 52 per minute.

HPI: The patient is an 89 YOWF, who was admitted to the emergency room at 9:00 PM as a result of falling off a step at home earlier in the evening. She denied any LOC prior to or after the fall. A chest x-ray revealed a fracture dislocation of the right humerus, pleural effusion, a consolidated area in the anterior segment of the left lower lobe, and cardiomegaly. An ECG revealed a LBBB and some PVCs.

PMH: The patient has a positive history of diabetes mellitus, CHF, ASHD, cardiomegaly, osteoarthritic deformities of both knees, and she has episodic pain in the hip area. While living at home she took BUMEX 1 mg daily.

ALLERGIES: NKA

FH: No past medical history available on parents or causes of death.

SH: The patient was a homemaker who has lived in this area all of her life and has been a widow for the past 10 years. She has two daughters and one son, all are living and well. She graduated from high school and was living with her son. She has been active all of her life and enjoys watching sports.

PE & ROS
Upon Admission: The patient is an alert and oriented elderly female in some respiratory distress and C/O severe pain and tenderness in the area of her right shoulder. Ht., 5'3", Wt., 108 lb.

VS: BP 110/70, T 98.6 (o), AP 82, RR 20.

HEENT: Pupils are pinpoint and constrict to light. Decreased hearing acuity bilaterally. Tympanic membranes could not be visualized well due to cerumen buildup. The patient is edentulous.

LUNGS: Grunting respirations and markedly elevated respiratory rate. Decreased breath sounds in left pleural base as compared to the right.

BREASTS: No masses.

HEART: Heart rate regular on PE with no murmur detected. Cardiomegaly and LBBB with PVCs.

ABDOMEN: Abdomen appeared to be WNL with no organomegaly, tenderness, or fluid elicited.

EXTREMITIES: Patient has a bruised, abraded area over the lateral aspect of the left elbow and a small tear of paper thin skin on her right elbow. She has a circumferential ring just above her knees where she held her stockings. It was also noted that she had osteoarthritic deformities of both knees. Neither leg was foreshortened. Good ROM of both hip sockets.

IMPRESSIONS:
1. Fracture dislocation of the right humeral head
2. Cardiomegaly

3. LBBB with PVCs
4. Left pleural effusion
5. Diabetes mellitus

LABORATORY TESTS:
August 9, Urinalysis was WNL except pH of 5.0
August 6, Serum K$^+$, 4.2 mEq/L (3.5–5.3)
August 4, 2HPPBG, 229 mg/dl (50–120)
August 3, 4PMBG, 145 mg/dl
August 3, Serum digoxin level, 1.9 ng/dl (0.5–2.0)
August 1, Serum digoxin Level, 2.6 ng/dl (0.5–2.0)
August 1, Serum Na$^+$, 137 mEq/L (135–148), Serum K$^+$, 2.9 mEq/L, Serum Cl$^-$, 93 mEq/L (95–105),
August 1, Urine C & S revealed *Proteus mirabilis* and *Staphylococcus aureus* that are only sensitive to aminoglycosides, cephalosporins, and SMX/TMP, and *Pseudomonas aeruginosa* only sensitive to aminoglycosides and cephalosporins.
July 30, Thyroid T$_3$ uptake, T$_4$ and FTI were WNL
July 30, Urinalysis was WNL except:
Protein, trace
Occult blood, 1+
Bacteria, 3+
WBCs, 25–50
Nitrite, positive
Character, hazy
pH, 8.5
July 30, Blood chemistry profile was WNL except:
Cholesterol, 148 mg/dl (160–330)
BUN, 27 mg/dl (10–26)
BUN/Creat ratio, 25 (15–24)
July 30, CBC was WNL except:
C, 3.96 × 10^6 mm^3 (4.2–5.4)
HGB, 11.4 g/dl (12–16)
HCT, 34.7% (37–47)
July 30, FBS, 166 mg/dl
July 29, Chest x-ray compared to one on file 2 years ago. Film shows left pleural effusion again, but it has decreased slightly in size from before. Lungs are otherwise clear.

ADMITTING
MEDICATIONS: *Routine Medications:*
LANOXIN 0.125 mg p.o. 1 tablet qd
SEPTRA-DS p.o. 1 tablet bid
LASIX 40 mg p.o. 1 tablet qd
SLOW-K 8 mEq p.o. 1 tablet bid
PRN Medications:
B & O Supp. 1 Supp. rect. prn bladder spasm × 14 d
TYLENOL 325 mg p.o. 2 tablets q 3 hr prn pain
TIGAN 200 mg IM q 4 hrs. prn nausea
RESTORIL 15 mg p.o. 1 capsule h.s. prn sleep (may repeat × 1)

HALEYS-MO p.o. 30 ml prn constipation (if no result use
FLEET enema)
DIET: 1 g sodium

Facility Course Summary

July 29, Patient was admitted to the facility with some pain in right shoulder and chest congestion. She is alert and oriented to TPPE. She has a poor appetite and ate only 10% for supper. BP, 110–114/80–90; T, 97.4; AP, 82–84; R, 18–20; Wt. 108 lb.

July 30, Patient is A & O without any c/o pain during the night but did not sleep well. TYLENOL 10 gr, p.o. given for arm pain during afternoon. Eating better now (about 10–50%). Foley catheter is patent. Hgb, 11.4; FBS, 166; BP, 110–174/70–100; T, 97; AP, 86–96; R, 18–20.

July 31, No c/o pain this morning. Foley catheter draining amber-colored urine. Patient seemed confused this morning and awoke early stating that she can't sleep. Patient c/o nausea about mid-morning with small amount of emesis of undigested food. TIGAN IM given to help relieve nausea. Seemed more confused after supper. RESTORIL given for sleep. BP, 140–176/90–100; AP, 80–96; R, 18–21.

August 1, No more N and V during night. Physician concerned about patient's electrolyte imbalance and serum digoxin level. Patient seemed very confused and disoriented. Patient yelling and trying to climb over side rails of bed. Patient still not eating well. BP, 130–140/80–84; T, 97; P, 70–76; R, 20.

August 2, Patient alert and confused and very agitated and yelling loudly. Serum K^+ 2.9 mEq/L, digoxin level 2.6 ng/ml; BP, 136– 150/80–86; T, 97; AP, 60–66; R, 20.

August 3, Takes fluids well but c/o mouth feeling dry. Patient still not eating well. BP, 144–150/90; T, 97; AP, 66–64; R, 24.

August 4, Serum digoxin level is 1.9 ng/ml today.

August 6, Patient still has nausea and eating only 10%, skin turgor poor, IV of D_5W started to rehydrate patient. No swelling or infiltration at IV site at 11 PM. At 11:20 PM, patient pulled out IV line.

August 7, IV restarted at 12:15 AM. No signs of redness at IV site. Patient had trouble sleeping even after taking RESTORIL. Patient seems agitated and is yelling. IV was infusing well, but pt. pulled IV line out at 2:45 AM. IV line reinserted and infusing well. VALIUM ordered to help calm patient down. Serum K^+ 4.2 mEq/L.

August 8, Patient pulled out Foley catheter this afternoon. Catheter reanchored without difficulty.

August 9, Patient A & O and ate 75% of supper this evening; c/o pain in right arm.

Pharmacist's Evaluation of Jane Doe's Case

Patient Problem List

1. Fractured dislocation of right humeral head;

2. Pain in right shoulder;
3. Congestive heart failure with athrosclerotic heart disease;
4. Left bundle branch block and premature ventricular contractions;
5. Osteoarthritis of both knees;
6. Diabetes mellitus;
7. Urinary tract infection;
8. Poor appetite;
9. Digoxin toxicity;
10. Confused, disoriented, agitated, and yelling;
11. Low blood counts;
12. Left pleural effusion;
13. Hypokalemia and hypochloremia;
14. Decreased renal function;
15. Dehydration;
16. Difficulty sleeping;
17. Blood pressure elevated at times.

Collective Evaluation of All Patient Problems

Subjective Evaluation of Patient
1. Upon admission, patient was alert and oriented, but lately has become more agitated, confused, and disoriented, yelling at times;
2. Patient c/o pain in right shoulder;
3. Patient c/o nausea and vomiting;
4. Patient not eating well (ranges 10–75%);
5. Patient has poor skin turgor and c/o mouth feeling dry;
6. Patient has had some problems sleeping;
7. Urine appearance reported as hazy.

Objective Evaluation of Patient
1. VS are T, 97; AP, 60–90; R, 18–24; BP, 110–176/70–100; Wt 108 lbs;
2. Serum K^+ on August 6 was WNL at 4.2 mEq/L;
3. Urinalysis on August 9 was WNL;
4. 2HPPBG level on August 4 was elevated at 229 mg/dl and a 4PMBG level on August 3 was elevated at 145 mg/dl;
5. SrCr 1.1 mg/dl, estimated CrCl <30 ml/min, and BUN of 27 mg/dl;
6. Thyroid function tests were WNL;
7. C & S run on August 1 revealed three organisms: *Proteus mirabilis*, *Staphyloccus aureus*, and *Pseudomonas aeruginosa*, sensitive to aminoglycosides and some cephalosporins;
8. Serum digoxin level was 1.9 ng/ml on August 3 and 2.6 ng/ml on August 1.

Assessment of Patient
1. Pain associated with fracture dislocation of right humeral head appears to be controlled with TYLENOL. No plans to correct fracture due to patient's age and medical condition.

2. Continue to use TYLENOL on a prn basis to control shoulder pain.
3. CHF and ASHD should improve when patient's serum digoxin level decreases to WNL.
4. LBBB and PVCs appear not to be problematic at this time.
5. Patient does not appear to be bothered much from osteoarthritis.
6. DM not well controlled (blood glucose elevated) on diet alone.
7. UTI being treated with SEPTRA-DS appears to be resolving. However, the drug is not effective against *Pseudomonas aeruginosa.*
8. Poor appetite should improve when serum digoxin level is WNL.
9. Digoxin toxicity should be resolved on the new dose of digoxin, 0.125 mg every other day.
10. Confusion, disorientation, and agitation could possibly be related to digoxin toxicity.
11. Low RBCs and Hgb not being treated at the present time, could be exacerbating her CHF.
12. Left pleural effusion appears to be improved somewhat from previous reports.
13. Hypokalemia and hypochloremia improving with KCl supplement.
14. Renal function is low. Estimated creatinine clearance from serum creatinine is <30 ml/min.
15. Dehydration appears to be resolving with the IV D_5W and encouraging patient to increase intake of fluids.
16. Patient's difficulty sleeping may resolve when pain from shoulder decreases and when her overall mental status improves. Continue to use RESTORIL on a prn basis.
17. Continue to monitor BP on a weekly basis. If elevated BP continues, drug therapy may be needed.

Plans for the Patient
1. Monitor patient for problems associated with dislocation of right humeral head.
2. Monitor patient for pain of right shoulder.
3. Monitor patient for S and Sx of CHF and ASHD.
4. Continue to monitor LBBB and PVCs with periodic ECG.
5. Continue to monitor osteoarthritis knee problems.
6. Request patient be put on an ADA diet and continue to monitor FBSs. If FBS elevated, consider adding insulin or an oral hypoglycemic agent to control DM.
7. Since patient has a Foley catheter, monitor for S & Sx of UTI. Repeat UA, C & S after ATB therapy.
8. Monitor patient for weight loss/gain.
9. Repeat serum digoxin level (about 2–3 weeks) when new steady state achieved and run serum electrolytes and serum creatinine levels. Monitor for S and Sx of digoxin toxicity.
10. Monitor excessive sedation and lethargy that could result from use

of VALIUM prn to control confusion, disorientation, agitation, and yelling.

11. Encourage oral intake of food and fluids. Repeat CBC next month. A multiple vitamin/mineral supplement may be needed.

12. Continue to monitor left pleural effusion with periodic chest x-ray.

13. Monitor serum electrolytes, serum creatinine, potassium intake, and drugs that conserve or deplete potassium.

14. Monitor for signs and symptoms of renal insufficiency. Monitor drugs that are renally excreted.

15. Monitor fluid intake and output, S and Sx of dehydration (e.g., skin turgor, dry skin).

16. Monitor use of hypnotic to help prevent dependence.

17. Monitor BP on a weekly basis. If elevated BP continues, drug therapy may be needed.

End of Evaluation

Evaluation of All Problems on an Individual Basis

Problem 1—Fractured dislocation of right humeral head

S – No current related problems;

O – No current information;

A – Right arm fracture appears not to be bothering patient at present time;

P – Monitor pain or other problems with right arm.

Problem 2—Pain in right shoulder

S – Patient c/o pain in right shoulder upon admission (July 29);

O – TYLENOL 10 gr given for arm pain on July 30, pain relieved;

A – Pain in shoulder appears to be decreasing and can be cotrolled with the use of TYLENOL;

P – Continue to use TYLENOL prn to control shoulder pain.

Problem 3—CHF with ASHD

S – Patient c/o chest congestion upon admission (July 29);

O – Admission PE on patient revealed cardiomegaly; serum digoxin level, 1.9;

A – CHF and ASHD should improve when serum digoxin level WNL;

P – Continue to monitor serum digoxin level, renal function and S and Sx of CHF and ASHD.

Problem 4—LBBB and some PVCs

S – No current related problems;

O – ECG run on admission revealed LBBB and PVCs;

A – LBBB and PVCs appear not to be problematic at this time;

P – Continue to monitor periodic ECG for PVCs.

Problem 5—Osteoarthritis of both knees

S – No current related complaints;

O – No data available;

A – Osteoarthritis appears to be controlled;

P – Continue to monitor patient for knee problems.

Problem 6—Diabetes mellitus

S – No current related complaints;

O – FBS 166 on July 30, 4PMBG 145 on August 3 and 2HPPBG was 229 on August 4;

A – Blood glucose elevated;

P – Put patient on an ADA diabetic diet; if DM not well controlled, drug therapy may be needed;

 – Run FBS on a weekly basis to determine DM control.

Problem 7—Urinary tract infection

S – Urine appearance hazy.

O – Urinalysis on July 30 showed: bacteria 1 +, WBCs 25–50, nitrite positive, trace protein and blood, and pH of 8.5. C & S on August 1 identified three bacteria $>10^5$ col/ml: *Proteus mirabilis, Staphylococcus aureus* sensitive to aminoglycosides, cephalosporins and SMX/TMP; *Pseudomonas aeruginosa* only sensitive to aminoglycosides and some cephalosporins. Oral temperatures range from 97—98.6 (F).

A – Tx with SMX/TMP not effective against *Pseudomonas aeruginosa* and another drug may be needed. However, by treating the other two organisms, the infection by this bacteria may resolve on its own.

 – Due to decreased renal function, therapeutic concentrations of SMX/TMP may not be achieved in the urine.

P – Monitor patient for S & Sx of UTI. Following therapy, repeat urinalysis and C & S.

Problem 8—Poor appetite

S – Patient not eating well (ranges 10—75%);

O – Weight 108 lb upon admission;

A – Poor appetite may be related to digoxin toxicity and should resolve when serum digoxin level is WNL, and N and V resolve;

P – Monitor patient for weight loss more closely; encourage oral intake of food and fluids; a multiple vitamin/mineral supplement may be needed.

Problem 9—Digoxin toxicity

S – Patient c/o nausea and vomiting that began on July 31. Not eating well and appears to be more confused and agitated.

O – Serum digoxin level of 2.6 on August 1 and 1.9 on August 3, AP range, 64–96.

– Patient received TIGAN 200 mg (2 ml) IM on July 31 to help control nausea.

A – Digoxin toxicity appears to be resolving. Confusion and agitation may also improve as the digoxin toxicity resolves.

P – Monitor renal function (SrCr, BUN), serum digoxin level, AP, orthopnea; ECG and S and Sx of digoxin toxicity.

Problem 10—Confused, disoriented, and agitated

S – Patient confused, disoriented, agitated, and yelling on August 1 and August 2;

O – VALIUM given to calm patient down;

A – These problems may be related to digoxin toxicity (CNS effects) and may resolve on their own when serum digoxin level is WNL;

P – Monitor excessive sedation and lethargy from use of VALIUM prn.

Problem 11—Low blood counts

S – Patient not eating well (ranges 10–75%);

O – RBCs 3.96; Hgb 11.4; and Hct 34.7 on July 30; wt is 108 lb;

A – Low blood counts may be related to poor nutrition or anemia;

P – Encourage oral intake of food and fluids, repeat CBC next month; A multiple vitamin/mineral supplement may be needed; Check stools for occult blood.

Problem 12—Left pleural effusion

S – No related complaints;

O – Chest x-ray on July 29 indicates that the area has decreased in size from 2 years ago;

A – Left pleural effusion appears to be improving;

P – Continue to monitor with chest x-rays.

Problem 13—Hypokalemia and hypochloremia

S – No related complaints;

O – Serum K^+ 2.9 mEq/L on August 1 and 4.2 on August 6; Serum Cl⁻ was 93 on August 1;

A – Serum potassium now WNL, serum chloride probably also WNL;

P – Monitor serum electrolytes, serum creatinine, potassium intake, and drugs that conserve or deplete potassium.

Problem 14—Decreased renal function

S – No related complaints;

O – SrCr 1.1 mg/dl, estimated CrCl <30 ml/min, BUN of 27;

A – Renal function probably improving with oral and IV fluids;

P – Continue to encourage fluids;
– Repeat serum creatinine and BUN;
– Monitor renally excreted drugs (present and future).

Problem 15—Dehydration

    S – Patient c/o nausea and vomiting on July 31, mouth feeling dry on day August 3, and skin turgor poor on day August 3;

    O – AP, 90, BP, 140–176/90–100;

    A – Dehydration appears to be improving;

    P – Monitor fluid intake and output, S & Sx of dehydration (e.g., skin turgor, dry skin), and BP.

Problem 16—Difficulty sleeping

    S – Patient having difficulty sleeping (July 31);

    O – Patient got RESTORIL for sleep on July 31;

    A – Difficulty sleeping may resolve after patient calms down and gets used to institutionalization;

    P – Continue using RESTORIL on a prn basis and monitor for excessive sedation.

Problem 17—Elevated blood pressure

    S – No related complaints;

    O – BP ranges 110–176 / 70–100;

    A – BP WNL at times and elevated at other times;

    P – Continue to monitor BP on a weekly basis; if elevated BP continues, drug therapy may be needed.

End of Evaluation

▪ Case Study 2

Chief Complaint (CC):	Confusion, dizziness, some pain in hands, moderate N-V-D and lethargy for the past 4–6 weeks.
History of Present Illness (HPI):	The patient is a 67 YOWF, who presents with N-V-D, lethargy, and difficulty with ADLs due to dizziness and some pain in hands. She states that her present problems began about 4–6 weeks ago when some new medications were prescribed for her stomach and lung problems.
Past Medical History (PMH):	She has a long Hx of COPD, mild HTN, ASHD, CHF, and was hospitalized 6 weeks ago for GI bleeding. She was diagnosed as having a duodenal ulcer and RA in her hands and shoulders. There is no Hx of diabetes, TB, or cancer. Allergies: PCN and sulfa. Medications PTA include Aspirin, ISORDIL, MAALOX, BRONKOTABS, and SERAPES. She also took EX-LAX tablets prn for relief of constipation.
Family History (FH):	Father died at the age of 67 from a heart attack. She has a younger brother with cancer of the liver. Her mother is living and has mild HTN and a CVA with right hemiparesis.
Social History (SH):	The patient is a social drinker and has smoked two packs of cigarettes per day for the past 20 years. She worked as a sales clerk in a local department store. She is trying to quit smoking.
Physical Examination (PE) and Review of Systems (ROS) Upon Admission:	Anxious female who looks older than her age. Moderate difficulty in mobility and in some respiratory distress. Ht., 5′ 3″; Wt., 45 kg.

VS:	T(o), 100.2 (F); AP 106; R, 28; BP, 186 / 98 mm Hg.
HEENT:	PERLA, EOMs are full, ears reveal normal TMs.
NECK:	Supple.
CHEST:	Shallow breathing through the mouth, slightly rounded, protruding chest.
CARDIAC:	Heart regular, tachycardia without gallop or murmur.
ABDOMEN:	Soft and tender.
GU and RECTAL:	Negative.
SKIN:	Pale skin color, no rashes
EXTREMITIES:	Slight pedal edema, limited ROM, and legs are weak.
NEUROLOGICAL:	WNL.

Admitting Laboratory Tests:

Blood Chemistry profile (Chem-19) was WNL except:

TP, 4.7 g/dl (6.0–8.0 g/dl)	Na, 134 mEq/L (135–148 mEq/L)
Alb, 2.5 g/dl (2.7–4.8 g/dl)	K, 3.2 mEq/L (3.5–5.3 mEq/L)

SrCr, 1.9 mg/dl (0.7–1.5 mg/dl)   Cl, 94 mEq/L (98–108 mEq/L)
BUN, 36 mg/dl (10–20 mg/dl)

CBC was WNL except:
WBC, 18.1×10^3 (4.8–10.8 $\times 10^3$ MCV, $80mm^3$ (80–94 mm^3)
RBC, 3.8×10^6 (4.7–6.1 $\times 10^6$)   Segs, 68% (40–60%)
Hgb, 11.8 g/dl (14–18 g/dl)   Bands, 14% (0–5%)

Urinalysis report was WNL except:
Appearance, cloudy   Nitrite, positive
Protein, 1^+ Bacteria, 3^+
RBC, trace   Urine pH, 8.5
WBC, > 50

Urine C & S report, pending.

Current Medications: Prednisone, 5 mg p.o. 1 tablet tid;
GAVISCON, p.o. chew 1 tablet qid prn;
METAMUCIL, 1 teaspoonful in water/juice p.o. bid;
Theophylline (THEO-DUR), 200 mg p.o. 1 tablet bid;
Prazosin (MINIPRESS), 2 mg 1 capsule p.o. bid;
Ibuprofen (MOTRIN), 400 mg 1 tablet p.o. tid;
Digoxin (LANOXIN), 0.25 mg 1 tablet p.o. daily;
MAALOX, 30 ml p.o. with each dose of MOTRIN and prn upset stomach;
Cimetidine (TAGAMET), 300 mg 1 tablet p.o. bid;
Acetaminophen (TYLENOL), gr X p.o. or rectal Q 4 hr prn pain or elevated temperature >100.

Diet: 1500 kcal.
Impressions:
1. COPD;
2. RA;
3. Hx of duodenal ulcer;
4. ASHD with CHF;
5. HTN;
6. Probable UTI.

Facility Course Summary (FCS):

Day 1, Patient admitted to the facility with some SOB and c/o being nauseated, especially after eating. Urine was cloudy and had a foul odor. Cephalexin (KEFLEX), 250 mg p.o. qid and O_2 per NC at 2–4 L/min prn were prescribed. Acetaminophen 10 gr rectal suppository given for elevated temperature.

Day 2, Patient is not eating well and c/o nausea, vomiting, and pain and burning upon urination. Diarrhea × 3. SrCr ordered by physician. VS: BP, 182/96; T (O), 101.8 (F); AP 98; R, 30.

Urine culture and sensitivity report:
Organism: *Proteus mirabilis*
Greater than 100,000 col/ml.

Antibiotic sensitivity (MIC in mcg/ml):
Sulfamethoxazole/Trimethoprin   (MIC < 2/32)
Gentamicin   (MIC < 2)

Tobramycin　　　　(MIC < 0.5)
Nitrofurantoin　　　(MIC < 32)
Carbenicillin　　　　(MIC > 64)

Organism is resistant to all other antibiotics/antibacterial agents.

Physician D/C cephalexin (KEFLEX) order and ordered tobramycin (NEBCIN) at 80 mg IM every 8 hours. Tobramycin consult requested by the physician.

Day 3,　Nausea and diarrhea unchanged. Patient alert and somewhat agitated. C/O a bad headache. VS: BP, 170/94; AP, 96; R, 28; T(o), 100. D/C prazosin (MINIPRESS) order and start enalapril (VASOTEC) 2.5 mg daily. Physician waiting for tobramycin consult from the clinical pharmacist. SrCr laboratory report came back and was 2.1 mg/dl.

End of Patient Case Write-up

Proceed to Patient Case Evaluation Exercise

Patient Case Study Evaluation Exercise Number Two

The following represents an evaluation of the patient's drug therapy using the problem oriented medical record or SOAP format. The evaluation example illustrates the "Collective Evaluation Of All Patient Problems."

First, the reader should thoroughly review this sample patient case write-up. Then, provide appropriate information in each of the blank spaces below for the example of the Pharmacist's Evaluation of the Patient Case. The pharmacist may refer back to the patient case write-up whenever needed to review patient data or to use these data in evaluating the patient case. The exact order of information provided in the blanks in the reader's evaluation need not conform precisely to the suggested answers. However, the reader's answers should be similar. If the pharmacist experiences difficlulty with either example, *briefly* refer to the answer sheet that follows each example evaluation for a little help or go back and review the SOAP format evaluation processes discussed in Chapter 2.

Pharmacist's Evaluation of the Patient Case

Collective Evaluation of All Patient Problems
A.　**Patient problem list**
　　1.　Nausea, vomiting, and diarrhea;
　　2.　Bad headache;
　　3.　Chronic obstructive pulmonary disease and possible theophylline toxicity;
　　4.　Shortness of breath;
　　5.　Agitation;

6. Urinary tract infection;
7. _____
8. _____
9. _____
10. _____
11. _____
12. _____
13. _____
14. _____
15. _____
16. _____
17. _____

B. Subjective Evaluation of Patient
1. Patient c/o N, V, and D, lethargy, bad HA and SOB;
2. Patient is alert and becoming more agitated;
3. Patient has slight pedal edema;
4. _____
5. _____
6. _____
7. _____

C. Objective Evaluation of Patient
1. VS are: T range, 100–101.8 (F);
                 AP range, 76–106 bpm;
                 R range, 24–28 per minute;
                 BP range, 170–186 / 94–98 mm Hg.
2. CBC shows MCV 80; RBCs, 3.8; Hgb, 11.8; Hct, 36.8;
3. WBC of 18.1 and bands of 14%;
4. _____
5. _____
6. _____
7. _____
8. _____
9. _____

D. Assessment of Patient
1. N, V, D, and agitation may be due to:
   a. Theophylline toxicity;
   b. Digoxin toxicity;
   c. Ibuprofen use;
   d. Diarrhea may be due to MAALOX use;
2. Bad headache possibly related to elevated BP or to ibuprofen use;
3. COPD appears to be under control although patient has elevated AP and RR; Possible theophylline toxicity due to high dose of theophylline and being used concurrently with cimetidine;

4. SOB appears to have resolved (only reported on day 1);
5. Agitation of patient appears to be minor;
6. Patient has UTI, and allergic to PCN and sulfa; MICs for other ATBs are too high to be effective for UTI in this patient; therefore, DOC is an aminoglycoside; the present dose of tobramycin is high and may be toxic for the patient;
7. _____
8. _____
9. _____
10. _____
11. _____
12. _____
13. _____
14. _____
15. _____
16. _____
17. _____

E. Plans For The Patient
1. Monitor N, V, D, skin turgor, and other S and Sx of dehydration; Encourage fluid intake;
2. Use TYLENOL to help relieve bad headache;
3. Obtain serum theophylline level (adjust dose accordingly) and monitor for S and Sx of SOB; Try to wean patient off oxygen; Have patient quit smoking; D/C cimetidine and replace with rinetidine, famotadine or nizatidine to avoid inhibition of hepatic microsomal enzyme metabolism.
4. Monitor patient for SOB;
5. Monitor patient agitation;
6. _____
7. _____
8. _____

9. _____
   _____
10. _____
    _____
11. _____
    _____
12. _____
    _____
13. _____
    _____
14. _____
    _____
15. _____
    _____
16. _____
    _____
17. _____
    _____

End of Evaluation

To check your responses, compare your evaluation with the example.

Possible Answers for Patient Case Study Number Two

Collective Evaluation of All Patient Problems

A.   **Patient Problem List**
1.   N, V, D;
2.   Bad headache;
3.   Chronic obstructive pulmonary disease with possible theo-phylline toxicity;
4.   Shortness of breath;
5.   Agitation;
6.   Urinary tract infection;
7.   Elevated temperature;
8.   Hypertension;
9.   Pedal edema;
10.   Low blood counts;
11.   ASHD and CHF with possible digoxin toxicity;
12.   Duodenal ulcer;
13.   Impaired renal function;
14.   Rheumatoid arthritis;
15.   Poor nutrition;
16.   Possible tobramycin nephrotoxicity and ototoxicity;

17. Hypokalemia, hyponatremia, and hypochloremia.

B. Subjective Evaluation of Patient
1. Patient c/o N, V, D, lethargy, bad HA, and SOB;
2. Patient is alert and becoming agitated;
3. Patient has slight pedal edema;
4. Patient c/o pain and burning upon urination;
5. Urine reported as cloudy and has foul odor;
6. Patient not eating well;
7. Patient c/o pain in hand.

C. Objective Evaluation of Patient
1. VS ranges: T, 100–101.8 (F); AP, 76–106; RR, 24–28; and BP, 170–186/94–98 mm Hg;
2. CBC shows MCV, 80; RBCs, 3.8×10^6; Hgb, 11.8 g/dl; Hct, 36.8 %;
3. WBCs, 18.1×10^3; and bands 14%;
4. TP, 4.7 g/dl and albumin 2.5 g/dl;
5. Serum creatinine of 2.1 mg/dl (est. CrCl 19 ml/min) on day 3; BUN was 36 mg/dl upon admission;
6. Urinalysis shows urine cloudy; 1+ protein; WBC >50; 3+ bacteria; pH of 8.5; and nitrite, positive;
7. C & S report indicates *Proteus mirabilis* sensitive to gentamicin; tobramycin, and SMX/TMP;
8. Serum electrolytes were Na^+, 134 mEq/L; K^+, 3.2 mEq/L; Cl^-, 94 mEq/L;
9. Three episodes of diarrhea were noted on day 2.

D. Assessment of Patient
1. N, V, D, and agitation may be due to:
   a. Theophylline toxicity;
   b. Digoxin toxicity;
   c. Ibuprofen and/or prednisone use;
   d. Diarrhea may be a result of the MAALOX or theophylline therapy;
2. Bad headache possibly related to elevated BP;
3. COPD appears to be under control although patient has elevated AP and RR; Possible theophylline toxicity due to high dose of theophylline and being used concurrently with cimetidine;
4. SOB appears to have resolved (only reported on day 1);
5. Patient agitation appears to be minor in nature;
6. Patient has UTI and allergic to PCN and sulfa. MICs for other ATBs are too high to be effective for UTI in this patient; therefore, the DOC in this patient is an aminoglycoside; the present dose is possibly toxic for the patient;
7. Elevated temperature appears to be resolving;

8. HTN is uncontrolled;
9. Pedal edema will probably resolve when cardiac status improves;
10. Low blood counts may be due to malnourishment, bleeding ulcer, or rheumatoid arthritis;
11. ASHD with CHF possibly aggravated by decreasing renal function and possible digoxin toxicity;
12. Duodenal ulcer may be aggravated by present drug therapy, e.g., prednisone, theophylline, and ibuprofen;
13. Impaired renal function has gotten worse; possibly due to nephrotoxicity from high dose of NEBCIN;
14. RA appears to be controlled;
15. Poor nutrition should improve when N, V, and diarrhea are resolved, and the loss of appetite may be a result of digoxin toxicity; Current drug therapy may be irritating the GIT leading to N, V, and D;
16. Nephrotoxicity and ototoxicity are likely with present dose of NEBCIN.
17. Hypokalemia, hyponatremia, and hypochloremia should resolve when vomiting and diarrhea improve. A KCl supplement may be needed even though VASOTEC will help conserve potassium.

E. **Plans For The Patient**
1. Monitor frequency of N, V, and D; encourage fluid intake; monitor skin turgor, and other S and Sx of dehydration;
2. Use TYLENOL to help relieve bad headache;
3. Obtain serum theophylline level (adjust dose accordingly) and monitor S and Sx of COPD such as SOB; Try to wean patient off of oxygen; Have patient quit smoking; D/C cimetidine and replace with rinetidine, famotadine, or nizatidine
4. Monitor patient for SOB;
5. Monitor patient agitation;
6. Obtain serum peak and trough levels of tobramycin and serum creatinine level (adjust dose and dosage interval accordingly); Monitor patient for ototoxicity and nephrotoxicity; Monitor for S and Sx of UTI and repeat urinalysis following therapy; Encourage fluid intake;
7. Control elevated temperature with TYLENOL; Continue to monitor oral temperature;
8. Obtain daily BP to monitor effectiveness of VASOTEC and request a NAS diet; Consider changing MAALOX to RIOPAN to help decrease sodium intake;
9. Monitor patient for pedal edema; Have patient elevate legs when sitting and reclining to improve venous return to heart;
10. Encourage nutritional intake; a dietary supplement may be

required; Repeat CBC to monitor low blood counts and to determine if an iron supplement is needed (low MCV); Monitor stools for occult blood loss; Give ibuprofen with meals to help decrease GI upset;

11. Monitor for S and Sx of ASHD and CHF; Obtain postdistribution serum digoxin level (5–8 hours postdose) and serum creatinine levels; Adjust digoxin dose and dosage interval accordingly;

12. Monitor for S and Sx of duodenal ulcer; Hematest stools for occult blood loss; Endoscopy may be performed to view presence of ulcer; If open ulcer present, sucralfate may be of value; Give ibuprofen with meals to help decrease GI upset and irritation; Consider use of misoprostol (CYTOTEC);

13. Monitor renal function by measuring serum creatinine, and BUN and estimate creatinine clearance; monitor all drugs that are renally excreted;

14. Monitor for RA S and Sx; sulindac may be a better choice of NSAID when renal function is low;

15. Encourage dietary intake and monitor body weight; A dietary supplement may be needed;

16. Run serum tobramycin trough and peak levels (adjust dosage accordingly); monitor serum creatinine and BUN;

17. Repeat serum electrolytes; if potassium and chloride are still low, consider adding a KCl supplement; Monitor potassium closely in patients with poor renal function.

End of Evaluation Answers

Pharmacist' Evaluation of Patient Case Number Two

The following represents an evaluation of the patient's drug therapy using the problem-oriented medical record or SOAP format. The evaluation example illustrates the "Evaluation Of All Patient Problems on an Individual Basis."

First, the reader should thoroughly review this sample patient case write-up. Then, provide appropriate information in each of the blank spaces below for the example of the Pharmacist's Evaluation of the Patient Case. The pharmacist may refer back to the patient case write-up whenever needed to review patient data or to use these data in evaluating the patient case. The exact order of information provided in the blanks in the reader's evaluation need not conform precisely to the suggested answers. However, the reader's answers should be similar. If the pharmacist experiences difficulty with either example, *briefly* refer to the answer sheet that follows each example evaluation for a little help or go back and review the SOAP format evaluation processes discussed in Chapter 2.

Evaluation of All Problems on an Individual Basis
Patient Problem List
1. Nausea, vomiting, and diarrhea;

2. Bad headache;
3. Chronic obstructive pulmonary disease and possible theophylline toxicity;
4. Shortness of breath;
5. Agitation;
6. Urinary tract infection;
7. _____
8. _____
9. _____
10. _____
11. _____
12. _____
13. _____
14. _____
15. _____
16. _____
17. _____

Patient Problem 1—Nausea, Vomiting, and Diarrhea

S – Patient c/o N,V, and D, reportedly as a result of some new medications;
O – Problems have been present for approximately 4–6 weeks;
A – N, V, and D may be a result of:
  1. Theophylline toxicity;
  2. Digoxin toxicity;
  3. Ibuprofen and/or prednisone use;
  4. Diarrhea may be due to MAALOX therapy;
P – _____
    _____

Patient Problem 2—Headache

S – Patient c/o a bad headache on day 3;
O – No related patient information except for BP of 170/94 mm Hg;
A – Bad HA possibly related to elevated BP;
P – _____

Patient Problem 3—Chronic Obstructive Pulmonary Disease

S – Patient c/o SOB on day 1 and uses O_2 prn;
O – Respiration rate ranges from 24–28 bpm and heart rate ranges from 76–106 bpm;
A – _____
    _____
    _____
P – _____
    _____

_____
_____

Patient Problem 4—Shortness of Breath

    S – Patient c/o SOB on day 1;
    O – No related patient information present;
    A – SOB appears to have resolved (only reported on day 1);
    P – _____

Patient Problem 5—Agitation

    S – Patient reported as agitated on day 3;
    O – No related patient information present;
    A – _____
    P – _____

Patient Problem 6—Urinary Tract Infection

    S – _____
       _____

    O – _____
       _____
       _____
       _____

    A – UTI is being treated effectively with NEBCIN. However, the
        present dose is possibly toxic for the patient;
    P – Obtain serum peak and trough levels of tobramycin and serum
        creatinine level (adjust dose and dosage interval accordingly);
        Repeat urinalysis and C and S (if needed) following therapy for
        UTI; Monitor patient for nephrotoxicity, ototoxicity, and S and
        Sx of UTI; Encourage fluid intake.

Patient Problem 7—Elevated Temperature

    S – _____
    O – Oral temperature ranges from 100–100.8 (F);
    A – Elevated temperature appears to be resolving;
    P – _____
       _____

Patient Problem 8—Hypertension

    S – _____
    O – _____
    A – _____
    P – _____
       _____

Patient Problem 9—Pedal Edema

    S – _____
    O – _____

A – Pedal edema will probably resolve when cardiac status improves;

P – Monitor patient for pedal edema; When possible, have patient elevate legs and feet to improve venous return to heart.

Patient Problem 10—Low Blood Counts

S – Patient is not eating well and has lethargy;

O – CBC upon admission shows RBC, 3.8×10^6; Hgb, 11.8 g/dl; Hct, 36.8 %; MCV, 80 mm^3;

A – _____

P – _____
  _____
  _____
  _____
  _____

Patient Problem 11—ASHD and CHF With Possible Digoxin Toxicity

S – _____

O – _____
  _____

A – ASHD and CHF possibly aggravated by decreasing renal function and possible digoxin toxicity;

P – Monitor for S and Sx of ASHD and CHF; Obtain postdistribution serum digoxin level (5–8 hours postdose); Obtain serum creatinine level; Adjust digoxin dose and dosage interval accordingly.

Patient Problem 12—Duodenal Ulcer

S – _____

O – _____

A – _____
  _____

P – Monitor for S and Sx of duodenal ulcer; Hematest stools for occult blood loss; Endoscopy may be performed to view presence of ulcer; If open ulcer present, sucralfate may be of value; Give ibuprofen with meals to help decrease GI upset and irritation; Consider misoprostol (CYTOTEC) therapy.

Patient Problem 13—Impaired Renal Function

S – No related patient information present;

O – SrCr, 2.1 mg/dl on day 3 (est. CrCl < 20 ml/min); SrCr upon admission was 1.9 mg/dl and BUN of 36 mg/dl;

A – _____
  _____

P – _____
  _____

Patient Problem 14—Rheumatoid Arthritis

S – _____

O – _____

A – _____

P – _____

_____

Patient Problem 15—Poor Nutrition

S – _____

O – _____

_____

A – Poor nutrition (loss of appetite) may be a result of digoxin toxicity; Appetite should improve when serum digoxin level is WNL; Current drug therapy may be irritating the GIT, leading to N,V, and D;

P – _____

_____

Patient Problem 16—Possible Tobramycin Nephrotoxicity and Ototoxicity

S – _____

O – _____

_____

A – Ototoxicity and nephrotoxicity is likely on present dose;

P – Obtain serum tobramycin peak and trough levels, serum creatinine, and BUN; Adjust dose and dosage interval of tobramycin accordingly;

Patient Problem 17—Hypokalemia, Hyponatremia, and Hypochloremia

S – Patient c/o lethargy;

O – _____

A – _____

_____

_____

_____

_____

P – _____

_____

_____

_____

End of Evaluation Exercise

To check your responses, compare your evaluation with the example.

Possible Answers For Patient Case Study Exercise Number Two

Evaluation of All Problems on an Individual Basis
Patient Problem List

1. N, V, D;

2.   Bad headache;
3.   Chronic obstructive pulmonary disease with possible theophylline toxicity;
4.   Shortness of breath;
5.   Agitation;
6.   Urinary tract infection;
7.   Elevated temperature;
8.   Hypertension;
9.   Pedal edema;
10. Low blood counts;
11. ASHD and CHF with possible digoxin toxicity;
12. Duodenal ulcer;
13. Impaired renal function;
14. Rheumatoid arthritis;
15. Poor nutrition;
16. Possible tobramycin nephrotoxicity and ototoxicity;
17. Hypokalemia, hyponatremia, and hypochloremia.

Patient Problem 1—Nausea, Vomiting, and Diarrhea

S – Patient c/o N, V, and D, reportedly as a result of some new medications;

O – Problems have been present for approximately 4–6 weeks;

A – N, V, and D may be a result of:
   Theophylline toxicity;
   Digoxin toxicity;
   Ibuprofen and/or prednisone use;
   Diarrhea may be due to MAALOX therapy;

P – Monitor frequency of N,V and D, skin turgor, and other S and Sx of dehydration; encourage fluid intake.

Patient Problem 2—Bad Headache

S – Patient c/o a bad headache on day 3;

O – No related patient information except for BP of 170/94 mm Hg;

A – Bad HA possibly related to elevated BP;

P – Use TYLENOL to control HA.

Patient Problem 3—Chronic Obstructive Pulmonary Disease with Possible Theophylline Toxicity

S – Patient c/o SOB on day 1 and uses O_2 prn;

O – Respiration rate ranges from 24–28 bpm and apical heart rate ranges from 76–106 bpm;

A – COPD appears to be under control although patient has elevated RR and AP; Possible theophylline toxicity could be due to high dose of theophylline and concurrent use of high dose of cimetidine;

P – Obtain a serum theophylline level and adjust dose accordingly; D/C cimetidine and replace with appropriate dose of rinetidine, famotadine, or nizatidine to avoid inhibition of hepatic microsomal enzyme metabolism; Monitor for S and Sx of COPD; Try to wean patient off of oxygen; Have patient quit smoking.

Patient Problem 4—Shortness of Breath

S – Patient c/o SOB on day 1;
O – No related patient information present;
A – SOB appears to have resolved (only reported on day 1);
P – Monitor patient for SOB.

Patient Problem 5—Agitation

S – Patient reported as agitated on day 3;
O – No related patient information present;
A – Agitation appears to be minor in nature;
P – Monitor patient agitation.

Patient Problem 6—Urinary Tract Infection

S – Patient c/o pain and burning upon urination; Urine reported as being cloudy and has foul odor;
O – Urinalysis shows: urine cloudy, 1+ protein; WBC, > 50; bacteria, 3+; nitrite, positive; and urine pH of 8.5; C and S report indicates *Proteus mirabilis* sensitive to gentamicin, tobramycin and SMX/TMP; CBC shows: WBCs, 18.1 x 10^3; and bands, 14%;
A – UTI is being treated effectively with NEBCIN; however, the present dose is possibly toxic for the patient;
P – Obtain serum peak and trough levels of tobramycin and serum creatinine level (adjust dose and dosage interval accordingly); Repeat urinalysis and C and S (if needed) following UTI therapy; Monitor patient for nephrotoxicity, ototoxicity, and S and Sx of UTI; Encourage fluid intake.

Patient Problem 7—Elevated Temperature

S – No related patient information present;
O – Oral temperature ranges from 100–100.8 (F);
A – Elevated temperature appears to be resolving;
P – Use TYLENOL to help control elevated temperature; Continue to monitor oral temperature.

Patient Problem 8—Hypertension

S – Patient c/o bad HA on day 3;
O – BP ranges from 170–186/94–98 mm Hg;
A – Hypertension is uncontrolled;
P – Obtain BP daily to monitor effectiveness of VASOTEC; Request NAS diet; Consider changing MAALOX to RIOPAN to help decrease sodium intake.

Patient Problem 9—Pedal Edema

S – Patient had slight pedal edema upon admission but not reported lately;

O – No related patient information present;

A – Pedal edema will probably resolve when cardiac status improves;

P – Monitor patient for pedal edema.When possible have patient elevate legs and feet to improve venous return to heart.

Patient Problem 10—Low Blood Counts

S – Patient is not eating well and has lethargy;

O – CBC upon admission shows: RBC, 3.8 × 10 ^{6}; Hgb, 11.8 g/dl; Hct, 36.8%; MCV, 80 mm^3;

A – Low blood counts may be due to malnourishment, a bleeding ulcer, or RA;

P – Improve dietary intake; a liquid dietary supplement may be needed; Monitor stools for occult blood loss; Repeat CBC to monitor low blood counts and to determine if iron therapy needed (low MCV); Give ibuprofen with meals to help decrease GI upset.

Patient'Problem 11—ASHD and CHF with Possible Digoxin Toxicity

S – Patient has N, V, D, lethargy, agitation, and SOB;

O – AP, 106; RR, 28; SrCr, 2.1 mg/dl (est. CrCl < 20 ml/min); Digoxin dose of 0.25 mg Q D;

A – ASHD and CHF possibly aggravated by decreasing renal function and possible digoxin toxicity;

P – Monitor for S and Sx of ASHD and CHF; Obtain postdistribution serum digoxin level (5–8 hours postdose); Obtain serum creatinine level; Adjust digoxin dose and dosage interval accordingly.

Patient Problem 12—Duodenal Ulcer

S – Patient c/o N, V, and lethargy;

O – CBC upon admission shows: RBCs 3.8 × 10^6; and Hct, 36.8%;

A – Duodenal ulcer may be aggravated by present drug therapy, e.g., prednisone, theophylline, and ibuprofen;

P – Monitor for S and Sx of duodenal ulcer; Hematest stools for occult blood loss; Endoscopy may be performed to view presence of ulcer; If open ulcer present, sucralfate may be of value; Give ibuprofen with meals to help decrease GI upset and irritation; Consider misoprostol (CYTOTEC) therapy.

Patient Problem 13—Impaired Renal Function

S – No related patient information present;

O – SrCr 2.1 mg/dl on day 3 (est. CrCl < 20 ml/min); SrCr upon admission was 1.9 mg/dl and BUN of 36 mg/dl;

A – Impaired renal function has gotten worse; possibly due to nephrotoxicity from high dose of NEBCIN;

P – Continue to monitor serum creatinine and BUN; Monitor the doses of drugs that are primarily renally excreted.

Patient Problem 14—Rheumatoid Arthritis

S – Patient c/o pain in hands upon admission;

O – No related patient information present;

A – RA appears to be controlled;

P – Monitor for S and Sx of RA; Sulindac may be a better choice of NSAID when renal function is low.

Patient Problem 15—Poor Nutrition

S – Patient not eating well and has lethargy;

O – TP, 4.7 g/dl; and albumin, 2.5 g/dl; RBC, 3.8×10^6; Hgb, 11.8 g/dl; and Hct, 36.8%;

A – Poor nutrition (loss of appetite) may be a result of digoxin toxicity; Appetite should improve when serum digoxin level is WNL; Current drug therapy may be irritating the GIT leading to N, V, and D;

P – Encourage dietary intake; a dietary supplement may be needed; Monitor body weight.

Patient Problem 16—Possible Tobramycin Nephrotoxicity and Ototoxicity

S – No related patient information present;

O – SrCr has increased from 1.9 mg/dl upon admission to 2.1 mg/dl on day 3; tobramycin 80 mg, IM Q 8 hours for a 45-kg patient;

A – Ototoxicity and nephrotoxicity is likely on present dose;

P – Obtain serum tobramycin peak and trough levels, serum creatinine, and BUN; Adjust dose and dosage interval of tobramycin accordingly.

Patient Problem 17—Hypokalemia, Hyponatremia, and Hypochloremia

S – Patient c/o lethargy;

O – Na^+, 134 mEq/L; K^+, 3.2 mEq/L; and Cl^-, 94 mEq/L;

A – Serum electrolytes low, possibly due to prolonged vomiting and diarrhea; Hypokalemia, hyponatremia, and hypochloremia should improve when N, V, and diarrhea are resolved; a KCl supplement may be needed; VASOTEC will help conserve potassium;

P – Repeat serum electrolytes; If serum potassium and chloride are still low, consider adding a low dose KCl supplement; monitor serum potassium closely in patients with poor renal function.

End of Exercise

■ Case Study 3

CC: Severe pain in chest and left lower leg for the past few days.

HPI: The patient is a 74 YOWF, who was admitted to the facility as a result of increasing knee joint and leg pain, edema of the left lower leg, anterior chest pain upon exertion, and SOB when reclining.

PMH: The patient was diagnosed with diabetes mellitus about 5–6 years ago and was controlled with diet and oral medication before this admission to the facility. Medications PTA include: TYLENOL, MAALOX, LANOXIN, HCTZ, DIABINESE, and PAVABID. She has a history of a large hiatal hernia and diverticulosis of the colon for which she was treated as an outpatient. She had a D & C 23 years ago and also has a history of arteriosclerotic heart disease with CHF and marked vascular hypertension. During the past year, she had recurring edema in both ankles and lately has pain and edema in the LLE which became intolerable.

Allergies: NKA

FH: Maternal aunt had diabetes. Mother had severe arteriosclerotic cerebral vascular disease.

SH: The patient was born and grew up in Lafayette, Indiana. She completed the eighth grade and worked as a dental assistant. She and her husband had no children and lived in the same house for 43 years. Her husband cared for her at home and anxiously plans for her return to home.

PE and ROS: An elderly, obese female with a great deal of pain in her left lower leg. Ht., 5'2"; Wt., 175.5 lb.

Upon Admission:

VS: T(o), 96.4(F); AP, 78; R, 20; BP, 120/60;

HEENT: Vision/hearing good. Patient wears eyeglasses. Nose and throat are clear. Wax on eardrums.

RESP: CHF history, lungs clear, SOB noted and no rales.

CIRC: Nailbeds blanche easily. Patient has had thrombophlebitis in left lower leg, which is now edematous.

GIT: No problems. Patient has had a hiatal hernia which does not seem to bother her. She had a peptic ulcer 3 years ago.

Skin: Has dry patches (like rash) on lower left extremity.

URIN: Continent with no voiding problems.

NEUR: Reflexes good. Patient is alert and oriented to TPPE.

MUSC: ROM to all extremities with no discomfort.

ADL: Patient feeds herself. Needs assistance with wheelchair for bathroom use. Can bathe herself except for back, legs, and feet. Uses wheelchair to avoid weightbearing on left leg.

Impressions:
1. Phlebitis LLE;
2. Diabetes mellitus;
3. CHF 2° to ASHD;

Laboratory Tests:

March 30

Chest and Left Hip Exam and X-rays

Conclusions:
1. No acute abnormality of left hip or pelvis.
2. Chest shows large hiatal hernia with no cardiopulmonary abnormality.

Doppler Ultrasound Exam

Conclusion:

No spontaneous flow in left femoral vein; therefore, definite evidence of left femoral thrombosis.

ESR (Westergren) 68 (0–20 mm/hr.)

DATES	FBS (70–110 mg/dl)	PT (control 11 sec)	PTT
March 28,	230 mg/dl	11.2 sec	18.6, 28.6 sec
March 30,	-----	14.2 sec	39.4 sec
March 31,	-----	16.0 sec	44.8 sec
April 1,	119 mg/dl	18.8 sec	
April 2,	104 mg/dl	30.2 sec	
April 3,	92 mg/dl	34.3 sec	
April 4,	-----	27.6 sec	
April 5,	81 mg/dl	22.9 sec	
April 6,	82 mg/dl	20.4 sec	
April 7,	99 mg/dl	21.5 sec	
April 8,	-----	23.9 sec	
April 9,	79 mg/dl	25.8 sec	
April 10,	-----	25.4 sec	
April 11,	151 mg/dl	26.5 sec	
April 12,	93 mg/dl	28.9 sec	
April 13,	94 mg/dl	38.6 sec	

April 11

Blood Chemistry Profile-19

All tests were WNL except the following:

T. Protein	5.4 g/dl	(6–8 g/dl)
Albumin	3.4 g/dl	(2.7–4.8 g/dl)
Calcium	8.7 mg/dl	(8.5–10.5 mg/dl)
In. Phos.	5.1 mg/dl	(2.5–4.5 mg/dl)
Creatinine	2.6 mg/dl	(0.7–1.4 mg/dl)
LDH	245 U/L	(100–225 U/L)
Na^+	134 mEq/L	(135–148 mEq/L)
K^+	3.5 mEq/l	(3.5–5.3 mEq/L)
Glucose	151 mg/dl	(70–110 mg/dl)
BUN	46 mg/dl	(10–26 mg/dl)
Uric acid	9.1 mg/dl	(2.2–7.7 mg/dl)
CrCl (est.)	13 ml/min	(100–120 ml/min)

Hematology

The CBC was WNL except for RBCs low normal and a slight increase in the WBCs (13.1×10^3)

Urinalysis Culture and Sensitivity

The urine pH was 8.5, appearance was pale and cloudy. There were moderate bacteria (2+), WBCs >50 were present and nitrite positive, but everything else was WNL. Hematest was positive. C and S pending.

Admitting Medications:

Chlorpropamide (DIABINESE) 100 mg	2 tablets q AM
Piroxicam (FELDENE) 20 mg	1 capsule q AM

Hydrochlothiazide (HYDRODIURIL) 50 mg	1 tablet q d
Papaverine (PAVABID) 150 mg	1 capsule q 8°
MOM Susp.	30ml q hs prn
Temazepam (RESTORIL) 15 mg	1 capsule q hs prn
Propoxyphene Napsylate-APAP (DARVOCET-N) 100 mg	1 tablet q 4° prn pain

Heparin 5000 units IV as loading dose, then give 1500 units/hour routinely as maintenance dose.

Diet: 1200 kcal ADA & 2 g Na$^+$

Treatments (TX):
1. Keri Lotion, apply to left leg qid;
2. Wt. weekly;
3. Physical therapy twice weekly;
4. FBS daily;
5. BR with BRP only;
6. No walking or sitting in chair;
7. ROM exercises bid to all extremities;
8. Continue upper extremity strengthening with self exercise 4–5 times/week.

Facility Course Summary (FCS):

March 28, Upon admission to the facility, the patient had 4+ edema in her left lower extremity. She was alert and oriented to TPPE. She ate 75–100% of her meals. She complained frequently of severe pain in her left leg. FBS, 230 mg/dl; and PT, was 11.2/11 sec, PTT 18.6 and 28.6 sec. Pain usually controlled with DARVOCET-N 100 mg.

March 29, Medication changes: D/C HYDRODIURIL and begin LASIX 40 mg 1 tablet bid; K-TABS 1 tablet tid; D/C DIABINESE; start ORINASE 500 mg, 1 tablet tid; and start COUMADIN, 10 mg qd x 2 days, 7.5 mg qd x 2 days then 5 mg daily. Run daily PT, PTT and FBS. I/O 1200/2600 ml. PT 14.2, sec; PTT 32.8 sec.

March 30, Patient still complains of pain in left leg and knee. She also complained that they were trying to "starve her to death" and the food has "no taste" at all. C/O SOB with R 28. PT was 14.2/11 sec; and PTT 39.4 sec.

March 31, PT was 15.0 sec, PTT, 44.8 sec. Pain in leg some better. Decrease heparin dose to 1000 units/hour, for 2 days, then 800 units/hour for 3 days, then d/c.

April 1, FBS decreased to 119 mg/dl; and PT increased to 18.8/11 sec. Nurses state that the patient is usually pleasant, cheerful, and gets along well with everyone. VS were BP, 140/80; T, 97; AP, 80; R, 24. Edema seems improved, currently about 1–2+.

April 2, FBS was down to 104 mg/dl and PT increased to 30.2/11 sec. COUMADIN dose decreased to 4 mg daily. Swelling in LLE much improved.

April 3, FBS was down to 92 mg/dl and PT was 34.3/11 sec. COUMADIN dose decreased to 3 mg daily. BP, 146/84.

April 4, PT was 27.6/11 sec. and patient seemed to be having less pain. COUMADIN dose decreased to 2.0 mg daily. Patient complained of some hunger and upset stomach.

April 6, FBS was 82 mg/dl and the PT was 20.4/11 sec. Patient still complained of upset stomach, thought to be heartburn. MYLANTA, 30 ml 1/2 hr after breakfast, lunch, and dinner was prescribed. Occasional complaints of leg pain were noted.

April 9, Patient states that her stomach feels better now, but she is still hungry. FBS was 79 mg/dl; PT had increased to 25.8/11 sec. Hypoglycemic reaction x 1 noted. Orange juice and honey given. Patient feels much better. Dose of ORINASE was decreased to 500 mg bid.

April 12, Patient complained of pain and burning upon urination. Urine has pinkish tinge. UA, C & S were ordered. Patient was started on BACTRIM, 1 tab bid x 10 days for the UTI. T(o), 97°F; Wt., 171 lb; PT was 26.5/11 sec. C and S results pending. Lab tests ordered.

April 13, FBS was 94; and the PT has increased to 38.6/11 sec. Physician ordered nurses to hold the COUMADIN. VS were BP, 130/80, T, 98.4; AP, 68; R, 22. Hematest on urine was positive. C & S results show that *Proteus mirabilis* and *Pseudomonas aeruginosa* are present with >100,000 col/ml. No antibiotic sensitivity results available yet.

Pharmacist's Evaluation of Patient Case 3

The following represents an evaluation of the patient's drug therapy using the problem-oriented medical record or SOAP format. The evaluation example illustrates the "Collective Evaluation Of All Patient Problems."

First, the reader should thoroughly review this sample patient case write-up. Then, provide appropriate information in each of the blank spaces below for the example of the Pharmacist's Evaluation of the Patient Case. The pharmacist may refer back to the patient case write-up whenever needed to review patient data or to use these data in evaluating the patient case. The exact order of information provided in the blanks in the reader's evaluation need not conform precisely to the suggested answers. However, the reader's answers should be similar. If the pharmacist experiences difficulty with either example, *briefly* refer to the answer sheet that follows each example evaluation for a little help or go back and review the SOAP format evaluation processes discussed in Chapter 2.

Collective Evaluation of All Patient Problems

A. Patient Problem List
1. 4+ edema of LLE;
2. Knee joint and leg pain;
3. SOB when reclining;
4. Chest pain upon exertion;
5. Diabetes mellitus, type II;

6. Obesity;
7. Dry skin of LLE;
8. Phlebitis LLE;
9. _____
10. _____
11. _____
12. _____
13. _____
14. _____
15. _____
16. _____
17. _____
18. _____
19. _____
20. _____

B.   Subjective Evaluation of Patient
1. Patient is cheerful, alert, and oriented to TPPE;
2. Patient occasionally c/o left leg and knee joint pain;
3. Although she dislikes the food, she eats 75–100% of meals;
4. _____
5. _____
6. _____
7. _____
8. _____
9. _____
10. _____

C.   Objective Evaluation of Patient
1. Urinalysis of April 11 shows bacteria 2+, pH 8.5, and nitrite positive. C & S report shows *Proteus mirabilis* and *Pseudomonas aeruginosa*, each with >100,000 col/ml;
2. CBC was WNL on April 11 except for low RBCs and elevated WBC 13.1;
3. Elevated PT of 38.6 seconds (range 11.2–38.6) on April 17 PTT ranges from 18.6–44.8 seconds;
4. BUN, of 46; SrCr, 2.6 with est. CrCl of 13 ml/min I.Phos. 5.1 on April 11;
5. Uric acid level was 9.1 mg/dl on April 11;
6. FBS of 94–151 mg/dl for April;
7. VS ranges: T, 97–99.6; AP, 68–80; R, 20–28;
8. _____
9. _____
10. _____
11. _____
12. _____

13. _____
14. _____

D.   Assessment of Patient

1. Patient's LLE has improved but remains edematous (1–2 +);
2. Pain in left leg and knee joint appears to be controlled with DARVOCET-N 100 mg;
3. SOB appears to have resolved; no complaints during past 2 weeks;
4. No c/o chest pain since admission;
5. Diabetes seems under control with FBS in normal range, but patient still overweight; only one hypoglycemic episode noted;
6. Patient has lost 4.5 lb in about 16 days, but still is overweight. Rate of weight reduction seems reasonable;
7. Dry skin on LLE appears to be resolved;
8. Phlebitis appears to be resolving;
9. CHF and ASHD appear to be stable.;
10. Patient has a UTI and being treated with BACTRIM. No ATB sensitivity yet;
11. Patient is not stabilized on COUMADIN; Elevated PT probably due to COUMADIN and BACTRIM drug interaction. Warfarin is being displaced from protein-binding sites;
12. _____
13. _____
14. _____
15. _____
16. _____
17. _____
18. _____
19. _____
20. _____

E.   Plans for the Patient

1. Continue to monitor patient for edema in lower extremities and whenever possible keep legs elevated;
2. Since pain in knee can be controlled by DARVOCET-N, suggest d/c FELDENE. No other S or Sx of arthritis present;
3. Continue to monitor patient for SOB;
4. Monitor patient for chest pain and heartburn as possible signs of hiatal hernia or cardiac involvement;
5. Monitor FBS with laboratory at least monthly; check blood glucose twice weekly using fingerstick blood sample and glucose meter;
6. Monitor weight reduction and eating habits. Keep present diet;
7. Continue to observe patient for dry skin and use Keri Lotion;

8. Continue monitoring for S & Sx of phlebitis and monitor warfarin therapy with weekly PTs;

9. Monitor patient for S & Sx of CHF and ASHD;

10. Monitor urine C & S report for appropriateness of antibiotic therapy; assuming BACTRIM is appropriate, the dose may need to be altered due to decreased renal function; repeat urinalysis following therapy.

11. Hold dose of COUMADIN for one day and begin COUMADIN 1 mg daily; Monitor daily prothrombin times; D/C BACTRIM due to very low renal function and drug interaction. Begin amoxicillin 500 mg p.o. every eight hours; Monitor C and S report when available for effectiveness of amoxicillin; Monitor use of drugs that are highly protein bound or inhibit hepatic microsomal enzymes that could elevate PT times; Continue monitoring PTs weekly until stable;

12. _____

13. _____

14. _____

15. _____

16. _____

17. _____

18. _____

19. _____

20. _____

To check your responses, compare your evaluation with the example.

Possible Answers for Patient Case Study 3

A. Patient Problem List

1. 4+ edema of LLE;
2. Knee joint and left leg pain;
3. SOB when reclining;
4. Chest pain upon exertion;
5. Diabetes mellitus, type II;
6. Obesity;
7. Dry skin of LLE;
8. Phlebitis LLE;
9. CHF 2° and ASHD;
10. UTI;
11. Elevated PTs;
12. Hiatal hernia;
13. HTN;
14. Renal impairment;
15. Hypokalemia;

16. Elevated uric acid;
17. Elevated LDH level;
18. Elevated inorganic phosphorus level;
19. Low blood counts;
20. Elevated erythrocyte sedimentation rate.

B. Subjective Evaluation of Patient
1. Patient is cheerful, alert and oriented to TPPE;
2. Patient occasionally c/o left leg and knee joint pain;
3. Although she dislikes the food, she eats 75–100% of meals; She states that she is starved and the food has no taste;
4. C/O SOB and swelling of feet when reclining and anterior chest pain upon exertion;
5. C/O upset stomach;
6. LLE edema 1–2+ on April 1;
7. Patient occasionally c/o being hungry and having upset stomach and heartburn;
8. Patient c/o pain and burning upon urination; urine has pinkish tinge;
9. Patient had a hypoglycemic reaction on April 9;
10. Dry skin on left lower extremity noted on admitting PE.

C. Objective Evaluation of Patient
1. Urinalysis of April 11 shows bacteria 2+, pH 8.5, and nitrite positive; C and S report shows *Proteus mirabilis* and *Pseudomonas aeruginosa*, each with 100,000 col/ml;
2. CBC was WNL on April 11 except for low RBCs elevated WBC 13.1;
3. PT elevated at 38.6 seconds (range 18.8–38.6) on April 17; PTT ranges from 18.6–44.8 seconds;
4. BUN, 46; SrCr, 2.6 with est. CrCl of 13 ml/min; I.Phos, 5.1 on April 11;
5. Uric acid level was 9.1 mg/dl on April 11;
6. FBS of 94–151 mg/dl for April;
7. VS ranges: T, 97–99.6; AP, 68–80; R, 20–28;
8. Ht, 5'2"; Wt, 171 lb;
9. Doppler exam shows decreased blood flow in left femoral vein of left leg;
10. Elevated ESR of 68 on March 30;
11. BP ranges from 130–146/80–84;
12. TP low at 5.4 g/dl;
13. LDH elevated at 245 U/L;
14. Serum K^+ low at 3.5 mEq/L on April 11.

D. Assessment of Patient
1. Patient's LLE edema has improved but remains edematous (1–2+);

2. Pain in left leg and knee joint appears to be controlled with DARVOCET-N 100 mg;
3. SOB appears to have resolved; no complaints in past 2 weeks;
4. No c/o chest pain since admission;
5. Diabetes seems under control with FBS in normal range, but patient still overweight; only one hypoglycemic episode noted;
6. Patient has lost 4.5 lb in about 16 days, but is still overweight; rate of weight reduction seems reasonable;
7. Dry skin on LLE appears to be resolving;
8. Phlebitis appears to be resolving;
9. CHF and ASHD appear to be stable;
10. Patient has a UTI and is being treated with BACTRIM; no ATB sensitivity yet;
11. Patient is not stabilized on COUMADIN; elevated PT probably due to COUMADIN and BACTRIM drug interaction; warfarin is being displaced from protein-binding sites;
12. Hiatal hernia appears to be under control;
13. Hypertension appears to be controlled;
14. Estimated CrCl of 13 ml/min, SrCr of 2.6 mg/dl, and I.Phos. 5.1 indicate the patient has severe renal impairment;
15. Hypokalemia is probably a result of LASIX therapy; Current serum K^+ level unknown;
16. Patient may be experiencing S and Sx of gout as uric acid level is elevated; level may be elevated due to poor renal function;
17. Serum LDH level is mildly elevated but patient is asymptomatic; elevated level may be related to bone atrophy during postmenopause;
18. Elevated inorganic phosphorus may be related to severe renal impairment; at this point, probably no therapy required;
19. Low blood counts may be related severe renal impairment or poor nutrition;
20. Elevated ESR possible due to inflammatory response from infection and phlebitis.

E. Plans for the Patient
1. Continue to monitor patient for edema in lower extremities and keep legs elevated whenever possible; restrict OOB time and elevate extremities when possible;
2. Continue to use DARVOCET-N to control pain in leg and knee; Since pain can be controlled with DARVOCET-N 100 mg and patient has no S & Sx of arthritis, suggest D/C FELDENE;
3. Continue to monitor patient for SOB;
4. Monitor patient for chest pain and heartburn as possible signs of hiatal hernia or cardiac involvement;

5. Monitor blood glucose with FBS test at least monthly; check blood glucose twice weekly using fingerstick blood sample and glucose meter;

6. Monitor weight reduction and eating habits; keep present diet;

7. As pain in knee can be controlled by DARVOCET-N, suggest d/c FELDENE; no other S or Sx of arthritis present;

8. Continue monitoring for S & Sx of phlebitis and monitor warfarin therapy with weekly PTs;

9. Monitor patient for S & Sx of CHF and ASHD;

10. Monitor urine C & S report for appropriateness of antibiotic therapy; drug and dosage may need to be altered due to decreased renal function; repeat urinalysis following ATB therapy;

11. Hold dose of COUMADIN for one day and begin COUMADIN 1mg daily; Monitor daily prothrombin times until stable;
    D/C BACTRIM due to very low renal function and drug interaction;
    begin Amoxicillin 500 mg p.o. every eight hours;
    Monitor C & S report when available for effectiveness of amoxicillin;
    Monitor use of drugs that are highly protein bound or inhibit hepatic microsomal enzymes that could elevate PT times;

12. Reduce use of MYLANTA to prn use only; Monitor patient for S & Sx of hiatal hernia and GI upset;

13. Monitor blood pressure on weekly basis;

14. Continue to monitor serum creatinine, creatinine clearance, BUN, I & O and all drugs that are renally excreted or cause renal toxicity;

15. Monitor serum potassium levels closely; due to poor renal function, patient may not be excreting much potassium; patient may need an oral potassium chloride supplement;

16. Monitor patient for S & Sx of gout; repeat serum uric acid level;

17. Monitor serum LDH level with next blood chemistry profile;

18. Monitor serum inorganic phosphorus level with next blood chemistry profile;

19. Monitor blood counts with a repeat CBC; at this point, therapy is not required;

20. Repeat ESR following UTI course of therapy;

21. Consider using PERI-COLACE (which has a stool softener to help prevent straining or constipation) instead of MOM for laxative effect; D/C MOM as it may decrease warfarin absorption, contains salt, and has magnesium that may accumulate in patients with decreased renal function;

22. May need APAP to help keep temperature WNL;

23.   Consider D/C PAVABID; need for this drug is unclear.

End of Evaluation Answers

Patient Case Study Evaluation

The following represents an evaluation of the patient's drug therapy using the problem-oriented medical record or SOAP format. The evaluation example illustrates the "Evaluation Of All Patient Problems on an Individual Basis."

First, the reader should thoroughly review this sample patient case write-up. Then, provide appropriate information in each of the blank spaces below for the example of the Pharmacist's Evaluation of the Patient Case. The pharmacist may refer back to the patient case write-up whenever needed to review patient data or to use these data in evaluating the patient case. The exact order of information provided in the blanks in the reader's evaluation need not conform precisely to the suggested answers. However, the reader's answers should be similar. If the pharmacist experiences difficulty with either example, *briefly* refer to the answer sheet that follows each example evaluation for a little help or go back and review the SOAP format evaluation processes discussed in Chapter 2.

Pharmacist's Evaluation of Patient Case
Patient Problem List

1.   4+ edema of LLE;
2.   Knee joint and leg pain;
3.   SOB when reclining;
4.   Chest pain upon exertion;
5.   Diabetes mellitus, type II;
6.   Obesity;
7.   Dry skin of LLE;
8.   Phlebitis LLE;
9.   _____
10.   _____
11.   _____
12.   _____
13.   _____
14.   _____
15.   _____
16.   _____
17.   _____
18.   _____
19.   _____
20.   _____

Evaluation of All Problems on an Individual Basis

Patient Problem 1–4+ Edema of Left Lower Extremity

S – Patient had 4+ edema of left lower extremity upon admission, but it had improved to 1–2+; edema not mentioned again during facility course summary;

O – _____
A – _____
P – _____

Patient Problem 2—Knee Joint and Leg Pain

S – Patient occasionally c/o knee joint and leg pain, especially upon admission;
Initially, pain was severe but gradually improved;
O – _____
A – _____
P – _____

Patient Problem 3—Shortness of Breath When Reclining

S – _____
O – _____
A – _____
P – _____

Patient Problem 4—Chest Pain Upon Exertion

S – _____
O – _____
A – No c/o chest pain since admission
P – _____

Patient Problem 5—Diabetes Mellitus, Type II

S – Patient reportedly had hypoglycemic reaction on April 9;
No other related problems noted;
O – _____
A – _____
P – _____

Patient Problem 6—Obesity

S – _____
O – _____
A – _____
P – _____

Patient Problem 7—Dry Skin of Left Lower Extremity

S – Dry skin on left lower extremity noted upon admitting PE;
Problem not noted in facility course summary;
O – No related patient information available;
A – _____
P – _____

Patient Problem 8—Phlebitis of Left Lower Extremity

S – Patient c/o severe pain and had 4 + edema in LLE upon admission; Pain and edema noted as decreasing during facility course summary;

O – _____

A – _____

P – _____

Patient Problem 9—Congestive Heart Failure, Secondary to ASHD

S – _____

O – _____

A – _____

P – _____

Patient Problem 10—Urinary Tract Infection

S – Patient c/o pain and burning upon urination;
Urine has pinkish tinge;

O – _____

_____

_____

A – _____

P – _____

_____

_____

_____

Patient Problem 11—Elevated Prothrombin Times

S – _____

O – Hematest on urine was positive for RBCs;
PT, ranges were 11.2–34.3 sec during March 28–April 3;
PT, ranges were 27.6–38.6 sec during April 4–April 13;

A – _____

_____

_____

P – _____

_____

_____

_____

_____

_____

Patient Problem 12—Hiatal Hernia

S – Patient c/o heartburn on April 6; No other reports of heartburn
and GI upset;

O – _____

A – _____

P – _____

Patient Problem 13—Hypertension

S – _____

O – _____

A – _____

P – _____

Patient Problem 14—Renal Impairment

S – _____

O – BUN, 46; SrCr, 2.6 with estimated CrCl of 13ml/min; I.Phos, 5.1;

A – Estimated CrCl 13 ml/min; SrCr, 2.6; BUN, 46; I.Phos, 5.1 indicate patient has severe renal impairment;

P – _____
_____

Patient Problem 15—Hypokalemia

S – _____

O – Serum potassium was 3.5 mEq/L on April 11;

A – _____

P – _____
_____
_____

Patient Problem 16—Elevated Uric Acid Level

S – _____

O – _____

A – _____

P – _____

Patient Problem 17—Elevated Lactic Dehydrogenase Level

S – No related patient information available;

O – Serum lactic dehydrogenase level 245 U/L on April 11;

A – _____
_____

P – _____
_____

Patient Problem 18—Elevated Inorganic Phosphorus Level

S – No related patient information available;

O – Serum inorganic phosphorus level 5.1 mg/dl;

A – Serum inorganic phosphorus is mildly elevated, but patient is asymptomatic; the elevated level is probably due to poor renal function; at this point, probably no therapy required;

P – _____

Patient Problem 19—Low Blood Counts

S – Patient eats 75–100% of meals upon admission, but later states that she is starved and the food has no taste;

O – _____

A – _____
_____

P – _____
_____

Patient Problem 20—Elevated Erythrocyte Sedimentation Rate

    S – No related patient information available;

    O – Erythrocyte sedimentation rate 68 mm/hr;

    A – _____

          _____

          _____

    P – _____

To check your responses, compare your evaluation with the example.

Possible Answers for Patient Case Study 3

Individual Evaluation of Each Patient Problem
Patient Problem List

1.   4 + edema of LLE;
2.   Knee joint and left leg pain;
3.   SOB when reclining;
4.   Chest pain upon exertion;
5.   Diabetes mellitus, type II;
6.   Obesity;
7.   Dry skin of LLE;
8.   Phlebitis LLE;
9.   CHF 2° and ASHD;
10.   UTI;
11.   Elevated PTs;
12.   Hiatal hernia;
13.   HTN;
14.   Renal impairment;
15.   Hypokalemia;
16.   Elevated uric acid;
17.   Elevated LDH level;
18.   Elevated inorganic phosphorus level;
19.   Low blood counts;
20.   Elevated erythrocyte sedimentation rate;

Patient Problem 1–4 + Edema of Left Lower Extremity

    S – Patient had 4 + edema of left lower extremity upon admission, but it had improved to about 1–2 +; edema not mentioned again during facility course summary;

    O – No related patient information available;

    A – Edema seems to be resolving; this is possibly due to Lasix TX;

    P – Continue to monitor patient for edema in lower extremities, and keep legs elevated whenever possible.

Patient Problem 2—Knee Joint and Leg Pain

S — Patient occasionally c/o knee joint and leg pain, especially upon admission; initially, pain was severe but gradually improved;

O — No related patient information available;

A — Knee joint and leg pain appear to be resolving, and are controlled with Darvocet-N 100 mg;

P — Continue to use Darvocet-N 100 mg to control pain in leg and knee; as pain can be controlled with Darvocet-N 100 mg, and patient has no S & Sx of arthritis, suggest d/c FELDENE.

Patient Problem 3—Shortness of Breath When Reclining

S — Upon admission, the patient c/o shortness of breath when reclining;

O — Respiration rate 28 on March 30, and 22 on April 13;

A — Shortness of breath appears to have resolved;

P — Continue to monitor patient for SOB.

Patient Problem 4—Anterior Chest Pain upon Exertion

S — When admitted, the patient was c/o anterior chest pain upon exertion;

O — No related patient information available;

A — No c/o chest pain since admission;

P — Monitor patient for chest pain and heartburn as possible signs of hiatal hernia or cardiac involvement.

Patient Problem 5—Diabetes Mellitus, Type II

S — Patient reportedly had hypoglycemic reaction on April 9; No other related problems noted;

O — FBS ranges from 79–151 mg/dl;

A — Diabetes appears to be under control with FBSs generally WNL; Patient is still overweight; only one hypoglycemic episode noted;

P — Run FBS at least monthly, and check blood glucose twice weekly using fingerstick blood sample and glucose meter.

Patient Problem 6—Obesity

S — No related patient information available;

O — Patient is 5'2", female, whose weight was 175.5 lb upon admission, and on April 12, her weight was 171 lb;

A — Patient has lost 4.5 lbs in about 16 days, but still is overweight; Rate of weight reduction seems reasonable;

P — Monitor weight reduction and eating habits; keep present diet.

Patient Problem 7—Dry Skin on Left Lower Extremity

S — Dry skin on left lower extremity noted upon admitting PE; Problem not noted in facility course summary;

O — No related patient information available;

A — Dry skin on left lower extremity appears to have resolved;

P — Continue to observe patient for dry skin, and use Keri Lotion.

Patient Problem 8—Phlebitis of Left Lower Extremity

S – Patient c/o severe pain and had 4+ edema in LLE upon admission;
Pain and edema noted as decreasing during facility course summary;

O – Doppler exam shows decreased blood flow in left femoral vein of left leg;

A – Phlebitis appears to be resolving;

P – Continue monitoring for S & Sx of phlebitis and monitor warfarin therapy with weekly PTs.

Patient Problem 9—Congestive Heart Failure, Secondary to ASHD

S – Upon admission patient c/o SOB when reclining, and chest pain upon exertion;

O – AP, ranges 68–80; RR, 20–28;

A – CHF and ASHD appear to be stable;

P – Continue to monitor patient for S & Sx of CHF and ASHD.

Patient Problem 10—Urinary Tract Infection

S – Patient c/o pain and burning upon urination;
Urine has pinkish tinge;

O – Urinalysis on April 11, revealed bacteria 2+; pH, 8.5; and nitrite test was positive;
C & S report, shows *Proteus mirabilis* and *Pseudomonas aeruginosa*, each with 100,000 col/ml;
Temperature ranges, 97–99.6 degrees (F);
WBCs, 13.1;

A – Patient has UTI that is being treated with BACTRIM; no ATB sensitivity yet;

P – When available, monitor urine C & S report for appropriateness of ATB TX;
Assuming BACTRIM is appropriate, its dose may need to be altered due to decreased renal function;
Repeat urinalysis following course of ATB therapy.

Patient Problem 11—Elevated Prothrombin Times

S – Urine has pinkish tinge;

O – Hematest on urine was positive for RBCs;
PT ranges 11.2–34.3 sec from March 28–April 3;
PT ranges 27.6–38.6 sec from April 4–April 13;

A – Patient is not stabilized on COUMADIN; elevated PTs possibly due to COUMADIN and BACTRIM drug interaction; warfarin is being displaced from protein-binding sites;

P – Hold dose of COUMADIN for one day, then begin COUMADIN 1 mg daily;

Monitor daily prothrombin times;

D/C BACTRIM due to very low renal function, and drug inter-action;

Begin amoxicillin 500 mg p.o. every eight hours;

When available, monitor C & S report for effectiveness of amox-icillin therapy; monitor use of drugs that are highly protein bound, or inhibit hepatic microsomal enzymes that could el-evate PT times;

Continue to monitor PTs until stable.

Patient Problem 12—Hiatal Hernia

S — Patient c/o heartburn on April 6; no other reports of heartburn and GI upset;

O — No related patient information available;

A — Hiatal hernia seems to be under control;

P — Reduce use of MYLANTA to prn use only;

Monitor patient for S & Sx of hiatal hernia and GI upset.

Patient Problem 13—Hypertension

S — No related patient information available;

O — BP ranges from 130–146/80–84;

A — Hypertension appears to be under control;

P — Monitor blood pressure on a weekly basis.

Patient Problem 14—Renal Impairment

S — No related patient information available;

O — BUN, 46; SrCr, 2.6 with estimated CrCl of 13 ml/min; I.Phos, 5.1;

A — Estimated CrCl of 13 ml/min; SrCr of 2.6; and BUN of 46 indicate patient has severe renal impairment;

P — Continue to monitor BUN, SrCr, CrCl, I & O, and all drugs that are renally excreted, or cause renal toxicity.

Patient Problem 15—Hypokalemia

S — No related patient information available;

O — Serum potassium was 3.5 mEq/L on April 11;

A — Hypokalemia probably a result of LASIX use;

P — Monitor serum potassium levels closely;

Due to poor renal function, patient may not be excreting much potassium;

Patient may need an oral potassium supplement.

Patient Problem 16—Elevated Uric Acid Level

S — No related patient information available;

O — Serum uric acid level was 9.1 mg/dl on April 11;

A — Uric acid level is elevated, but patient is asymptomatic;

Elevated level may be elevated due to poor renal function;

P – Monitor patient for S & Sx of gout;
Repeat serum uric acid level.

Patient Problem 17—Elevated Lactic Dehydrogenase Level

S – No related patient information available;
O – Serum lactic dehydrogenase level 245 U/L on April 11;
A – LDH is mildly elevated but patient is asymptomatic;
Level may be elevated due to bone atrophy during postmenopause;
P – Monitor serum LDH level with next blood chemistry profile.

Patient Problem 18—Elevated Inorganic Phosphorus Level

S – No related patient information available;
O – Serum inorganic phosphorus level 5.1 mg/dl;
A – Serum inorganic phosphorus is mildly elevated but patient is asymptomatic; the elevated level is probably due to poor renal function; at this point, probably no therapy required;
P – Monitor serum inorganic phosphorus level with next blood chemistry profile.

Patient Problem 19—Low Blood Counts

S – Upon admission, patient eats 75–100% of meals, but later states that she is starved, and the food has no taste;
O – CBC on April 11 was WNL except for low RBCs;
A – Low blood counts may be related to severe renal impairment or poor nutrition;
P – Monitor blood counts with a repeat CBC; at this point therapy is not required.

Patient Problem 20—Elevated Erythrocyte Sedimentation Rate

S – No related patient information available;
O – Erythrocyte sedimentation rate 68 mm/hr;
A – Elevated ESR possible due to inflammatory response from infection and phlebitis;
P – Repeat ESR following UTI course of therapy.

End of Evaluation Answers

Chapter 3
Drug- and Disease-Monitoring Parameters for Therapeutic and Adverse Effects

It is important that the clinical pharmacist approach evaluating a patient's drug therapy by monitoring the patient for both adverse and therapeutic effects. As discussed in Chapter 2, the pharmacist should be concerned with monitoring the patient's response or lack of response to drug therapy by following patient- and disease-monitoring parameters as well as by looking for drug interactions, hypersensitivities, and allergies. Specific drug- and disease-monitoring parameters should be utilized by the pharmacist to help him or her determine therapeutic effectiveness of drug therapy and the occurrence of any drug-related problems (1).

General monitoring parameters for a drug and/or for a disease state may be any of the following: clinical improvements in the patient's medical condition(s); clinical signs and/or symptoms of the onset of an acute medical problem; clinical signs and/or symptoms of a failure to reverse a disease process; clinical signs and/or symptoms of therapeutic success in reversing/controlling a disease process; clinical signs and/or symptoms of a lack of response to appropriate drug therapy; adverse and/or toxic side effects of the drug regimen; and clinical laboratory values or diagnostic tests that indicate serum and/or urine drug levels, blood chemistry, and body and/or organ functions.

Some patients may not need to have every patient-, drug-, and/or disease-monitoring parameter followed at all times, while a few patients may need additional parameters monitored. Therefore, the following list of common drug-and disease-monitoring parameters is to serve only as a guide for the pharmacist to utilize in monitoring drug therapy. Each drug has been grouped by therapeutic class utilizing the *American Hospital Formulary Service Pharmacologic-Ther-*

apeutic Classification. The brand name is listed in all capital letters, while the generic or chemical name is listed in lower case letters.

■ Part 1: Drug-Monitoring Parameters (1–6)

I.   **Antihistamines (4:00)**

Azatadine maleate (OPTIMINE), brompheniramine maleate (DI-METANE), chlorpheniramine maleate (CHLOR-TRIMETON), clemastine fumarate (TAVIST), cyproheptadine HCl (PERIACTIN), diphenhydramine HCl (BENADRYL), hydroxyzine HCl (ATARAX), hydroxyzine pamoate (VISTARIL), meclizine HCl (ANTIVERT and BONINE), terfenadine (SELDANE), astemizole (HISMANAL)

   A.   Central nervous system—Drowsiness (15%), dizziness, and sedation (about 7% with **SELDANE and HISMANAL**, greatest sedation with **BENADRYL**), dry mouth (5%)
   B.   Increased appetite (4%)
   C.   Use alcohol or other CNS depressants cautiously
   D.   Relief of symptoms

II.   **Anti-infective agents (8:00) and antibiotics (8:12)**

   A.   **General drug-monitoring parameters for all antibiotics include**

      1.   White blood cell (WBC) counts

         a.   Elevated WBCs
         b.   Right shift in bands
         c.   Left shift in bands
         d.   Drugs that may increase WBCs

            1)   Steroids (acute)
            2)   Sympathomimetics (acute)

         e.   Drugs that may decrease WBCs

            1)   Cancer chemotherapy
            2)   Immunosuppressive agents

      2.   Body temperature

         a.   Drugs that may elevate body temperature

            1)   Anticholinergics
            2)   Antidepressants
            3)   Antipsychotics
            4)   Antiarrhythmics

         b.   Drugs that may decrease body temperature

            1)   Aspirin

       2) Acetaminophen

       3) Nonsteroidal anti-inflammatory drugs (NSAIDS)

3. Culture and sensitivity (C&S) tests—tissue/blood or urine antibiotic/antibacterial minimum inhibitory concentration (MIC)

4. Subjective patient response to infection and/or drug therapy

5. Factors altering patient response (e.g., patient compliance, long-term steroid therapy, diabetes, leukemia, chemotherapy, alcoholism, aging process in elderly)

6. Allergy (systemic skin rash) or other hypersensitivity reaction to each agent

7. Appropriate drug, dose, dosage form, dosage interval, administration times (e.g., with or without food)

8. Oral/parenteral bioavailability with other drugs/IV solutions

B. Specific drug-monitoring parameters for individual antibiotics/antibacterials

  1. Aminoglycosides (8:12.02)

    a. General drug-monitoring parameters for all aminoglycosides

      1) Renal function tests (e.g., SrCr, CrCl, BUN), fluid intake and output

      2) Audiometric testing—ototoxicity (8th cranial nerve damage)—tinnitus, vertigo, hearing loss

      3) Central nervous system—headache, lethargy

      4) Duration of therapy

      5) Urinalysis—proteinuria, casts, RBCs

    b. Gentamicin (GARAMYCIN), tobramycin (NEBCIN), amikacin (AMIKIN), netimicin (NATROMYCIN)

      1) Serum drug levels (peak and trough levels, pharmacokinetic parameters)

    c. Kanamycin (KANTREX)

    d. Neomycin (oral)—NEOBIOTIC

      1) Blood ammonia (sensorium levels)

      2) Diarrhea, loss of electrolytes

      3) Rash (allergic reaction)

    e. Streptomycin

  2. Antifungal antibiotics (8:12.04)

    a. Amphotericin B (FUNGIZONE)

      1) Renal function tests (e.g., SrCr, CrCl, BUN), fluid intake and output

2) Total daily dose does not exceed 1.5 mg/kg
3) Administration technique (no filter, avoid extravasation)
4) Vehicle or diluent (when given IV, do not use with NaCl or KCl)
5) CBC—causes normochromic, normocytic anemia
6) Expiration time (when given IV)
7) Hypokalemia
8) Central nervous system—fever, shaking, chills, headache, and paresthesia
9) Muscle/joint pain
10) Gastrointestinal—nausea, vomiting, weight loss, diarrhea, dyspepsia

b. Ketoconazole (NIZORAL)

1) Gastrointestinal—nausea, vomiting, diarrhea, and abdominal pain
2) Pruritus
3) Gynecomastia
4) Antacids, anticholinergics, and H_2-antagonists inhibit absorption
5) Liver function tests (e.g., SGOT, SGPT, alkaline phosphatase, bilirubin), jaundice, dark urine, or pale-colored stools
6) Central nervous system—headache, dizziness, nervousness

c. Nystatin (MYCOSTATIN, NILSTAT)

1) Oral suspension should be swished around in mouth and swallowed
2) Gastrointestinal—nausea, vomiting, and diarrhea

3. Cephalosporins (8:12.06)

a. First generation—cefazolin (ANCEF and KEFZOL), cephalothin (KEFLIN), cephapirin (CEFADYL), cefadroxil (DURICEF and ULTRACEF) cephradine (VELOSEF and ANSPOR), cephalexin (KEFLEX)

1) Dermatologic—systemic skin rash, itching (penicillin allergy)
2) Hepatic function (increased SGOT)
3) Renal function tests (e.g., SrCr, CrCl, BUN), fluid intake and output
4) Phlebitis (at injection site), pain at IM injection site
5) Eosinophilia

6) Gastrointestinal—nausea, vomiting, diarrhea
7) Laboratory test interference—false increase in serum creatinine, false positive **CLINITEST**, false positive Coombs' test (**KEFLIN**)

b. **Second generation—cefaclor (CECLOR), cefamandole (MANDOL), cefoxitin (MEFOXIN), cefuroxime (ZINACEF), cefonicid (MONOCID), ceforanide (PRECEF), cefotetan (CEFOTAN)**

1) Dermatologic—systemic skin rash, itching (penicillin allergy)
2) Hepatic function test (SGOT)
3) Phlebitis at injection site, pain on IM injection
4) Eosinophilla
5) False positive Coombs' test (**MANDOL**)
6) Disulfiram-like reaction (**MANDOL**)
7) Laboratory test interference—false positive (**CLINITEST**), false increase in serum creatinine (**CEFOXITIN**)
8) Diarrhea
9) Increased risk of bleeding (**MANDOL**)
10) Renal function tests (e.g., SrCr, CrCl, BUN), fluid intake and output

c. **Third generation—IV or IM administration—cefoperazone (CEFOBID), cefotaxime (CLAFORAN), ceftizoxime (CEFIZOX), ceftazidime (FORTAZ, TAZICEF, and TAZIDIME), cefuroxime (ZINACEF), ceftriaxone (ROCEPHIN), moxalactam (MOXAM)**

Third generation—oral administration—cefuroxime axetil (CEFTIN)

1) Dermatologic—systemic skin rash, itching (penicillin allergy)
2) Phlebitis (at injection site), pain on IM injection
3) Positive Coombs' test (**MOXAM**)
4) Liver function test—increased SGOT
5) Disulfiram-like reaction (**CEFOBID**)
6) Blood dyscrasias (**MOXAM**)
7) Gastrointestinal—diarrhea, pseudomembranous colitis (**CEFOBID**)
8) Renal function tests (e.g., SrCr, CrCl, BUN), fluid intake and output

4. **Miscellaneous—beta-lactam antibiotics (8:12.07)**
   a. **Amdinocillin or mecillinan (COACTIN)**

1) Penicillin allergy, skin rash, SOB, etc.
2) Hematologic—eosinophilia
3) Hepatic function (elevated serum aspartate ami-notransferase and serum alkaline phosphatase)
4) Gastrointestinal—nausea, vomiting, and diarrhea

b. Imipenem/cilastin sodium (PRIMAXIN)

1) Dermatologic—phlebitis/thrombophlebitis, pain at site of injection, skin rash, itching
2) Gastrointestinal—nausea, vomiting, and diarrhea
3) Central nervous system—confusion and seizures
4) Renal function tests (e.g., SrCr, CrCl, BUN), fluid intake and output

5. Chloramphenicol (8:12.08)
Chloramphenicol (CHLOROMYCETIN)

a. CBC (severe blood dyscrasias)
Hemotologic—complete necrosis of bone marrow; aplastic anemia, agranulocytosis, serum iron level, re-ticulocytosis, accumulation of drug and metabolites, slight transient leukopenia, megaloblastic cells in bone mar-row, failure of patient to respond to iron therapy or vitamin B_{12}

b. Accumulation of drug and metabolites

c. Cytochrome P-450 enzyme inhibitor will increase serum drug levels/activity (e.g., dicumoral, phenytoin, phen-obarbital, tolbutamide, chlorpropamide, and cyclo-phosphamide)

6. Erythromycin (8:12.12)
erythromycin stearate (ERYTHROCIN), erythromycin estolate (ILOSONE), erythromycin (E-MYCIN), eryth-romycin ethylsuccinate (EES and PCE), etc.

a. Hepatic function (e.g., cholestatic jaundice from esto-late salt)

b. Gastrointestinal—nausea,vomiting, and diarrhea (loss of electrolytes)

c. Cytochrome P-450 enzyme inhibitor will increase serum drug levels/activity (e.g., theophylline, warfarin, carba-mazepine, phenytoin)

7. Penicillins (8:12.16)

a. Ampicillin (e.g., POLYCILLIN, TOTACILLIN, PRINCIPEN, AMCILL, OMNIPEN), bacampicillin (SPECTROBID), potassium clavulanate (AUG-

MENTIN), sulbactam sodium and ampicillin sodium (UNASYN)

1) Gastrointestinal—nausea, vomiting, diarrhea (loss
of electrolytes)
2) Hepatic function (biliary excretion of drug)
3) Penicillin allergy cross-sensitivity—systemic skin
rash, itching, SOB

b. **Amoxicillin (e.g., AMOXIL, POLYMOX, LARO-
TID)—see ampicillin parameters**

c. **Carbenicillin disodium (GEOPEN, PYOPEN)—oral,
carbenicillin indanyl (GEOCILLIN) and ticarcillin disodium (TICAR)—parenteral, ticarcillin disodium and clavulanate potassium (TIMENTIN)**

1) Penicillin allergy, systemic skin rash, itching, SOB,
etc.
2) Hypokalemia and metabolic alkalosis
3) High sodium content in powder for injection
(**GEOPEN**—4.7 mEq/g, **PYOPEN**—5.3 mEq/g,
TICAR—5.2 mEq/g)
4) Thrombophlebitis (when given as bolus) at injection site
5) IV incompatibilities (especially with aminoglycosides)
6) Renal function tests (e.g., SrCr, CrCl, BUN), fluid
intake and output
7) Hepatic function (elevated liver enzymes with
hepatoxic reaction)

d. **Penicillin G potassium (PENTID, PFIZERPEN)**

1) Take on empty stomach to avoid drug degradation by stomach acid
2) Renal function tests (e.g., SrCr, CrCl, BUN), fluid
intake and output
3) Sodium content of intravenous preparations
4) Potassium content of intravenous preparations
5) Intravenous incompatibilities
6) Penicillin allergy, systemic skin rash, itching, SOB
7) Gastrointestinal—nausea, vomiting, diarrhea (loss
of electrolytes)

e. **Methicillin (STAPHCILLIN)**

1) Renal function tests (e.g., SrCr, CrCl, BUN), fluid
intake and output

2) Gastrointestinal—nausea, vomiting, and diarrhea (loss of electrolytes)
3) Granulocytopenia (bone marrow depression)
4) Hypocalcemia
5) Penicillin allergy, systemic skin rash, itching, SOB, etc.
6) Interstitial nephritis

f. **Nafcillin (UNIPEN), oxacillin (PROSTAPHLIN), dicloxacillin (DYNAPEN), cloxacillin (TEGOPEN)**

1) Gastrointestinal—nausea, vomiting, diarrhea (loss of electrolytes)
2) Renal function tests (e.g., SrCr, CrCl, BUN), fluid intake and output
3) Hepatic function tests
4) Penicillin allergy—systemic skin rash, itching, SOB, etc.

8. **Tetracyclines (8:12.24)**
Tetracycline HCl (ACHROMYCIN-V, SUMYCIN, PANMYCIN, ROBITET), doxycycline (VIBRAMYCIN), minocycline (MINOCIN), oxytetracycline (TERRAMYCIN)

a. Photosensitivity (especially with **DECLOMYCIN**)
b. Renal function tests (e.g., SrCr, CrCl, BUN), fluid intake and output
c. Hepatic function (fatty infiltration with IV administration)
d. Gastrointestinal—nausea, vomiting, and diarrhea
e. Hematologic—blood counts (WBCs, retics)—black stools, easy bruising, mouth lesions, sore throat, etc.
f. Drug interactions and bioavailability (Al, Fe, Mg, and Ca salts)
g. Patient age (do not use this drug if under 8 years of age)
h. Fungal infections
i. Should not use during pregnancy
j. Take on empty stomach

9. **Miscellaneous antibiotics (8:12.28)**

a. **Aztreonam (AZACTAM)**

1) Gastrointestinal—nausea, vomiting, diarrhea
2) Hepatic function tests (transient elevated SGOT and SGPT levels)
3) Local—thrombophlebitis at IV site, discomfort and swelling at IM injection site

4) Renal function tests (e.g., SrCr, CrCl, BUN), fluid intake and output
5) Penicillin or cephalosporin allergy

b. Clindamycin (CLEOCIN) and lincomycin (LINCOCIN)

1) Gastrointestinal—abdominal or stomach cramps, pain, bloating, nausea or vomiting, electrolytes (pseudomembranous colitis)—check stool culture especially for *Clostridium difficile*
2) Hepatic function tests
3) Skin rash
4) Force fluids
5) Take on empty stomach

c. Trimethoprim (PROLOPRIM, TRIMPEX)

1) CBC—thrombocytopenia, leukopenia
2) Gastrointestinal—nausea, vomiting
3) Systemic skin rash

d. Vancomycin HCl (VANCOCIN)

1) Central nervous system—chills, tinnitus, fever
2) Renal function tests (e.g., SrCr, CrCl, BUN), fluid intake and output—nephrotoxic and ototoxic
3) Transient systolic hypotension
4) Extravasation causes local tissue necrosis
5) Gastrointestinal—nausea and vomiting with oral dosing
6) Serum drug levels recommended if given IV
7) Allergic reaction—"Red-neck syndrome" due to too rapid parenteral administration, urticarial rash

10. Antituberculosis agents (8:16)

a. Ethambutol (MYAMBUTOL)

1) Decreased visual acuity and loss of ability to perceive the colors of red and green—vision testing suggested
2) Dosing pattern (single or divided)
3) Renal function tests (e.g., SrCr, CrCl, BUN), fluid intake and output
4) Decreased absorption with aluminum salt compounds
5) Gastrointestinal—nausea, vomiting, diarrhea (take with food), weight loss, abdominal pain
6) Elevates uric acid level
7) Hepatic function tests (jaundice, hepatitis)

    b.   **Isoniazid (isonicotinic acid hydride—INH)**

        1)   Ophthalmic—optic neuritis, peripheral neuropathy, dizziness, burning, tingling or numbness in extremities

        2)   Causes pyridoxine (vitamin B_6) deficiency—pellagra

        3)   Hepatic function tests (SGOT, SGPT, bilirubin and alkaline phosphatase)

        4)   Drug interactions with phenytoin, rifampin (slow acetylators)

        5)   Avoid alcohol use

        6)   Avoid tyramine-containing foods

        7)   Cytochrome P-450 metabolic enzyme inhibitor (will increase serum drug levels of phenytoin, warfarin, carbamazepine, benzodiazepines, etc.

        8)   Hematologic—agranulocytosis, hemolytic anemia, eosinophilia, neutropenia, thrombocytopenia

    c.   **para-Aminosalicylate sodium (PAS)**

        1)   Hepatic function (slow acetylators)

        2)   Vitamin B_{12} deficiency may be induced

        3)   Sodium content of PAS

        4)   Gastrointestinal—do not administer with alkaline compounds (e.g., milk, antacids), nausea, vomiting, diarrhea, and abdominal pain may result

        5)   Renal function tests (e.g., SrCr, CrCl, BUN), fluid intake and output

        6)   Hepatic function tests (jaundice)

    d.   **Rifampin (RIFADIN and RIMACTANE)**

        1)   Gastrointestinal disturbances, "flu-like syndrome," diarrhea, vomiting, abdominal pain

        2)   Hepatic function tests (SGOT, SGPT, bilirubin, and alkaline phosphatase)

        3)   Red-orange coloring of body secretions—sweat, urine, etc.

        4)   Cytochrome P-450 metabolic enzyme inducer (will increase serum drug levels of many drugs)

        5)   Take on empty stomach

        6)   Skin—pruritus, urticaria, rash

11.   **Antivirals (8:18)**

    a.   **Acycloguanosine (ACYCLOVIR)**

        1)   Gastrointestinal—nausea, vomiting, diarrhea

      2)   Central nervous system—headache, vertigo, insomnia, fatigue, irritability, and depression

      3)   Musculoskeletal—arthralgia

      4)   When used with probenecid, the half-life of ACYCLOVIR increases

b.   Amantadine HCl (SYMMETREL)

      1)   Central nervous system—depression, fatigue, confusion, dizziness, hallucinations, anxiety, headache

      2)   Cardiovascular—peripheral edema, orthostatic hypotension

      3)   Gastrointestinal—anorexia, nausea, constipation, vomiting, dry mouth

      4)   Genitourinary—urinary retention

      5)   Renal function tests (e.g., SrCr, CrCl, BUN), fluid intake and output

c.   Vidarabine (VIRA-A)

      1)   Hematologic—bone marrow suppression

      2)   Renal function tests (e.g., SrCr, CrCl, BUN), fluid intake and output

      3)   Hepatic function tests

      4)   Gastrointestinal—nausea, vomiting, diarrhea, anorexia

      5)   Central nervous system—tremors, dizziness, malaise, confusion, ataxia

d.   Zidovadine (RETROVIR and AZT)

      1)   Hematologic—severe bone marrow depression (anemia) granulocytopenia, thrombocytopenia

      2)   Central nervous system—headache, agitation, restlessness, insomnia, confusion, anxiety

      3)   Dermatological—skin rash

12.   Sulfonamides (8:24)

Sulfisoxazole (GANTRISIN), sulfamethoxazole (GANTANOL), sulfamethoxazole and trimethoprim (BACTRIM, SEPTRA)

a.   Sulfa allergy, systemic skin rash, itching, SOB, etc.

b.   Drug interactions producing elevated serum drug levels of warfarin, phenytoin, and many other highly protein-bound drugs

c.   Gastrointestinal—nausea, vomiting, diarrhea, abdominal pain

d.   Hematologic—magaloblastic anemia may develop with long term use (folic acid deficiency)

> e. Renal function tests (e.g., SrCr, CrCl, BUN), fluid intake and output
> f. Encourage fluid intake
> g. Urinary acidifiers (e.g., ascorbic acid, ammonium chloride)
> h. Stevens-Johnson syndrome

13. **Urinary anti-infectives (8:36)**

a. **First generation(4–quinolone synthetic antibacterials)**
Nalidixic acid (NEGGRAM) and cinoxacin (CINOBAC)

1) Hematologic—eosinophilia
2) Gastrointestinal—nausea and vomiting
3) Photosensitivity
4) Use with caution in patients with history of seizures
5) Central nervous system—drowsiness, weakness, headache, dizziness, vertigo, seizures/convulsions
6) Renal function tests (e.g., SrCr, CrCl, BUN), fluid intake and output
7) Hepatic function tests

b. **Second generation (fluorinated 4-quinolone derivative)**
norfloxacin (NOROXIN), ciprofloxin (CIPRO)

1) Take 1 hour before meals or 2 hours after meals
2) Do not take with antacids (take 2 hours before or after an antacid)
3) Renal function tests (e.g., SrCr, CrCl, BUN), fluid intake, and output
4) Force fluids
5) Gastrointestinal—nausea, vomiting, and diarrhea (4%)
6) Central nervous system—headache and dizziness
7) Liver function tests (e.g., elevates SGPT, SGOT, and alkaline phosphatase)
8) Hematologic—decreased neutrophil count
9) Seizures (especially inpatients predisposed to seizures)
10) May cause elevated serum theophylline and phenytoin levels when used concurrently

c. **Nitrofurantoin (FURADANTIN and MACRODANTIN)**

1) Gastrointestinal—anorexia, nausea, and vomiting
2) Renal function tests (e.g., SrCr, CrCl, BUN), fluid intake, and output; may not be effective if CrCl is <30 ml/min
3) Take with milk or food
4) Central nervous system—headache, dizziness, drowsiness
5) Hepatic function tests—hepatitis

d. **Methenamine mandelate (MANDELAMINE) and methenamine hippurate (HIPREX)**

1) Urine pH (5.5 best)
2) Ammonia production in urine caused by infecting organism increases urine pH and decreases effectiveness of drug
3) Gastrointestinal—nausea, vomiting, and diarrhea, GI upset (premature drug release), take with food (1 hour before meals or 2 hours after meals)
4) Force fluids
5) Avoid taking with antacids or alkalinizing foods and/or drugs
6) Renal function tests (e.g., SrCr, CrCl, BUN), fluid intake and output
7) Not effective in patients with indwelling urinary catheters

14. **Miscellaneous anti-infectives (8:40)**

Pentamidine isothionate (PENTAM-300)

a. Elevates serum creatinine levels (23%), and liver function tests (9%)
b. Hemotologic—leukopenia (7.5%), thrombocytopenia (2%)
c. Gastrointestinal—nausea and anorexia (6%)
d. Hypotension (4%)
e. Hypoglycemia (3.5%)
f. Fever (3.5%)
g. Rash (3%)
h. Abscess, pain, or induration at IM injection site
i. May be administered by oral inhalation

III. **Antineoplastic agents (10:00)**

A. Combination Treatment Abbreviations

1. **ABVD (BVDS)—doxorubicin, bleomycin, vincristine, dacarbazine**
2. **BACOP—bleomycin, doxorubicin, cyclophosphamide, vincristine, prednisone**

3. CHOP—cyclophosphamide, doxorubicin, vincristine, prednisone
4. CMFOP—cyclophosphamide, methotrexate, fluorouracil, vincristine, prednisone
5. COMA—cyclophosphamide, vincristine, methotrexate, cytarabine
6. COMLA—cyclophosphamide, ONCOVIN (vincristine), methotrexate, leucovorin, Ara C (cytarabine)
7. COP—cyclophosphamide, ONCOVIN (vincristine), prednisone
8. C-MOPP—cyclophosphamide, ONCOVIN (vincristine), procarbazine, prednisone
9. CVP—cyclophosphamide, vincristine, prednisone
10. MACOP-B—methotrexate, ADRIAMYCIN, cyclophosphamide, ONCOVIN, prednisone, bleomycin—SMX/TMP is usually administered during course of therapy
11. M-BACOD—methotrexate, bleomycin, adriamycin, cyclophosphamide, ONCOVIN, dexamethasone
12. MOPP—mechlorethamine, vincristine, procarbazine, prednisone
13. POMP—prednisone, vincristine, methotrexate, mercaptopurine
14. ProMACE-MOPP—prednisone, methotrexate, ADRIAMYCIN, cyclophosphamide, etoposide, followed by MOPP—SMX/TMP is usually administered during course of therapy
15. ProMACE-CytaBOM—prednisone, ADRIAMYCIN, cyclophosphamide, etoposide, cytarabine, bleomycin, methotrexate. SMX/TMP is usually administered during course of therapy.

B. General drug-monitoring parameters for antineoplastic agents

1. Response of neoplastic process
2. Hematologic—CBC, absolute granulocyte count, bone marrow depression
3. Body temperature, sore throat, and other signs of opportunistic infections
4. Patient knowledge of adverse effects of chemotherapy
5. Extravasation with IV administration
6. Elevated serum uric acid levels
7. Alopecia
8. Oral thrush
9. Mouth ulcers

C. Specific drug-monitoring parameters for individual antineoplastic agents

1. **Azathioprine (IMURAN)**

   a. Decrease dose by ¼ to ⅓ with liver dysfunction or with concomitant allopurinol therapy
   b. Hematologic—bone marrow depression—similar to 6-MP but delayed for 3 to 6 weeks, monitor CBC
   c. Hemorrhagic cystitis—force fluids and take doses before 6 PM to avoid high concentrations in bladder
   d. Take with food
   e. Gastrointestinal—anorexia, nausea, and vomiting
   f. Hepatic function tests

2. **Bleomycin (BLENOXANE)**

   a. Pulmonary fibrosis
   b. Mucosal ulcerations
   c. Fever
   d. Allergic reactions, skin rash (erythema, hyperkeratosis)

3. **Busulfan (MYLERAN)**

   a. Hematologic—bone marrow depression—leukopenia, thrombocytopenia, agranulocytosis (CBC recommended weekly), bruising
   b. Dermatologic—skin hyperpigmentation
   c. Amenorrhea
   d. Interstitial pulmonary fibrosis
   e. Force fluids
   f. Take medication same time each day
   g. Elevated serum uric acid levels

4. **Carmustine (BICNU)**

   a. Hematologic—bone marrow depression—leukopenia and thrombocytopenia (4 to 6 weeks after starting doses), phlebitis
   b. Gastrointestinal—nausea and vomiting
   c. Hepatic function tests
   d. Flushing with rapid IV infusion
   e. Pulmonary fibrosis
   f. Delayed renal damage, monitor renal function tests (e.g., SrCr, CrCl, BUN), fluid intake and output

5. **Chlorambucil (LEUKERAN)**

   a. Hematologic—bone marrow suppression—monitor CBC—granulocytes, platelets, RBCs—effect may be delayed for 3 to 4 weeks
   b. Gastrointestinal—nausea, vomiting
   c. Pulmonary function (fibrosis)

    d.   Force fluids

    e.   Bruising

6. Cisplatin (CDDP, PLATINOL)

    a.   Renal function tests (e.g., SrCr, CrCl, BUN), fluid intake and output

    b.   Ototoxicity

    c.   Gastrointestinal—nausea and vomiting

    d.   Electrolyte abnormalities (hypomagnesemia, hypocalcemia, hypokalemia, and hypophosphatemia)

    e.   Tetany due to hypocalcemia and hypomagnesemia

    f.   Hematologic—minimal bone marrow depression

    g.   Fever

7. Cyclophosphamide (CYTOXAN)

    a.   Hematologic—bone marrow depression—leukopenia with oral therapy, will occur sooner with IV therapy

    b.   Bladder toxicity (urinary frequency, then dysuria, then hematuria); high fluid intake required to keep urine in bladder diluted

    c.   Other drugs affecting liver enzymes (dose adjustment required)

    d.   Alopecia (high IV dose or prolonged oral dose)

    e.   Gastrointestinal—nausea and vomiting (when IV over 4 mg/kg)

8. Cytarabine (CYTOSAR, ARA-C)

    a.   Hematologic—bone marrow depression—monitor CBC—leukopenia, thrombocytopenia, bruising

    b.   Gastrointestinal—nausea, vomiting, diarrhea

    c.   Oral and anal ulcerations

    d.   Hepatic and renal function tests

    e.   Fever

    f.   Rash

9. Dacarbazene (DTIC)

    a.   Hematologic—bone marrow depression—monitor CBC—leukopenia and thrombocytopenia

    b.   Gastrointestinal—anorexia, nausea, vomiting, diarrhea

    c.   Alopecia

    d.   Facial paresthesia and flushing

10. Dactinomycin (COSMEGEN)

    a.   Hematologic—bone marrow depression—monitor CBC—leukopenia, thrombocytopenia

    b.   Gastrointestinal—nausea, vomiting, anorexia, ulcerations of mucosa

    c.   Dermatologic—skin eruptions, acne, erythema, and increased pigmentation of previously irradiated skin

    d.   Alopecia

    e.   Extravasation into tissues

    f.   Toxic effects may appear 2 to 4 days after course of therapy and may not be maximal before 1 to 2 weeks

11.   Doxorubicin (ADRIAMYCIN)
Daunorubicin (CERUBIDINE)

    a.   Gastrointestinal—nausea and vomiting, diarrhea

    b.   Extravasation into tissues

    c.   Alopecia

    d.   Oral and GI ulcerations

    e.   Cardiovascular—monitor ECG, decreased cardiac ejection fraction

    f.   Hematuria

    g.   Hyperpigmentation of nailbeds

    h.   Myelosuppression, monitor CBC

12.   Etoposide ((VP-16)—VEPSEID)
Teniposide ((VM-26)—VURMON)

    a.   Hematologic—bone marrow depression, monitor CBC, phlebitis

    b.   Gastrointestinal—nausea, vomiting, diarrhea

    c.   Peripheral neuropathies

    d.   Central nervous system—fever, chills, bronchospasm, dyspnea, and hypotension

    e.   Alopecia

    f.   Cardiovascular—monitor ECG, tachycardia

13.   Fluorouracil (5–FU) and floxuradine (FUDR)—pyrimidine analog

    a.   Hematologic—bone marrow depression—monitor CBC—leukopenia, thrombocytopenia

    b.   Alopecia

    c.   Gastrointestinal—nausea, diarrhea, anorexia, oral and GI ulcerations

    d.   Dermatologic—hyperpigmentation and scarring (topical use), dermatitis

    e.   Cardiovascular—myocardial ischemia, angina

    f.   Photophobia

14.   Hydroxyurea (HYDREA)

    a.   Hematologic—bone marrow depression—monitor CBC—leukopenia and anemia mainly

    b.   Renal function tests (e.g.,SrCr, CrCl, BUN), fluid intake and output

    c.   Force fluids

    d.   Gastrointestinal—nausea, vomiting, anorexia, and constipation

    e.   Oral ulcerations

    f.   Hyperpigmentation

15. Lomustine (CCNU) (CEE NU)

    a.   Hematologic—bone marrow depression—monitor CBC—leukopenia and thrombocytopenia; bone marrow suppression may be delayed up to 6 weeks after last dose; dose adjustment based on WBCs and platelet counts

    b.   Gastrointestinal—nausea and vomiting (3 to 6 hours after dose)

    c.   Stomatitis, alopecia, hepatic toxicity

    d.   Lethargy, ataxia

16. Mechlorethamine (MUSTARGEN)

    a.   Central nervous system—fever, chills

    b.   Gastrointestinal—nausea, vomiting, diarrhea

    c.   Hematologic—bone marrow depression—monitor CBC—immediate decrease in peripheral lymphocytes and monocytes reaching peak at 6 to 8 days

    d.   Extravasation into tissues

    e.   Alopecia

    f.   Oral ulcerations

17. Melphalan (ALKERAN)

    a.   Hematologic—bone marrow depression—monitor CBC—thrombocytopenia, leukopenia

    b.   Gastrointestinal—nausea (oral doses over 20 mg)

    c.   Pulmonary fibrosis

18. 6-mercaptopurine (6-MP) (PURINETHOL)

    a.   Renal function tests (e.g., SrCr, CrCl, BUN), fluid intake and output

    b.   Dose adjustment (decrease dose by ¼ to ⅓) when used with allopurinol or with hepatic dysfunction

    c.   Hematologic—bone marrow depression—monitor CBC—granulocytes mainly, monitor WBCs, platelets, RBCs

    d.   Hepatotoxicity (SGOT, jaundice)

    e.   Oral and GI ulcerations

19.   Methotrexate (MEXATE, FOLEX)

    a.   Hematologic—bone marrow depression—monitor CBC—WBC, platelets

    b.   Oral and GI ulceration—stomatitis

    c.   Hepatic function tests (SGOT, SGPT, LDH)

    d.   Alopecia

    e.   Dose adjustment when taking drugs highly bound to plasma proteins

    f.   Renal function tests (e.g., SrCr, CrCl, BUN), fluid intake and output

    g.   Urine pH

    h.   Gastrointestinal—nausea, vomiting, and abdominal distress

    i.   Methotrexate serum drug levels

20.   Plicamycin/Mithramycin (MITHRACIN)

    a.   Hematologic—severe bleeding disorders—exercise caution when used with all drugs that decrease platelet aggregation; monitor CBC and platelet count

    b.   Renal function tests (e.g., SrCr, CrCl, BUN), fluid intake and output

    c.   Hypocalcemia

    d.   Stomatitis

    e.   Hepatotoxicity monitor SGOT and LDH

    f.   Central nervous system—fever, weakness, lethargy, malaise, headache, and fever

    g.   Gastrointestinal—nausea, vomiting, and anorexia

    h.   Hypokalemia

21.   Procarbazine (MATULANE)

    a.   Hepatic function tests

    b.   Gastrointestinal—nausea, vomiting

    c.   Hematologic—bone marrow depression—monitor CBC—leukopenia mainly, anemia, thrombocytopenia

    d.   Central nervous system—restlessness, drowsiness, confusion, paresthesias

    e.   Avoid alcohol (disulfiram-like reaction)

    f.   Avoid tyramine-containing foods

22.   Tamoxifen (NOLVADEX)

    a.   Gastrointestinal—nausea and vomiting

    b.   Hot flashes

    c.   Transient increase in bone and tumor pain

    d.   Edema

    e.   Vaginal bleeding

> f.   Ophthalmic—corneal changes, retinopathy
> g.   False elevation in serum calcium levels

23.   Thioguanine (6-Thioguanine)

> a.   Renal function tests (e.g., SrCr, CrCl, BUN), fluid intake and output
> b.   Hematologic—bone marrow depression (similar to 6-MP), monitor CBC
> c.   Gastrointestinal—nausea, vomiting, and stomatitis
> d.   Hepatic function tests
> e.   Elevates uric acid levels

24.   Vinblastine (VELBAN)

> a.   Hematologic—bone marrow depression—monitor CBC—leukopenia, granulocytic depression
> b.   Neurological signs (paresthesia, loss of tendon reflex)
> c.   Alopecia
> d.   Extravasation into tissues
> e.   Gastrointestinal—nausea and vomiting
> f.   Jaw pain

25.   Vincristine (ONCOVIN)

> a.   Hepatic function tests
> b.   Neurological signs (e.g., paresthesia, loss of tendon reflexes)
> c.   Constipation
> d.   Alopecia
> e.   Minimal bone marrow depression, monitor CBC
> f.   Jaw pain
> g.   Extravasation into tissues
> h.   Maximum single dose is 2 mg
> i.   Intestinal necrosis

IV.   Autonomic drugs (12:00)

A.   Parasympatholytic (cholinergic blocker) agents (12:08) Antiparkinsonian agents (12:08.04) atropine sulfate, benztropine mesylate (COGENTIN), trihexyphenidyl HCl (ARTANE)

1.   Narrow angle glaucoma (contraindicated)
2.   Gastrointestinal—dry mouth, constipation
3.   Genitourinary—urinary retention, decreased urinary bladder contractility
4.   Cardiovascular—tachycardia
5.   May mask drug-induced extrapyramidal symptoms (EPS)
6.   Blurred vision

7.   Decreased sweat secretions

B.   Sympathomimetic (adrenergic) agents (12:12)—*intravenous administration*

1.   Dobutamine HCl (DOBUTREX)

a.   Cardiovascular—tachycardia, ventricular arrhythmias, blood pressure, angina, pulmonary artery wedge pressure, cardiac index, and shortness of breath
b.   Gastrointestinal—nausea
c.   Hepatic function tests
d.   Does not release stored catecholamine
e.   Fluid intake and output
f.   Acid-base balance
g.   Central nervous system—headaches

2.   **Dopamine (INTROPIN)**

a.   Same as dobutamine HCl except dopamine releases norepinephrine from synaptic nerve stores

3.   **Isoproterenol (ISOPREL)—similar to dobutamine**

C.   Sympathomimetics (adrenergic) agents (12:12)—*subcutaneous administration*
Epinephrine (ADRENALIN and SUS-PHRINE)

1.   Cardiovascular—blood pressure, tachycardia, angina pain
2.   Relief of symptoms (allergic reaction, asthmatic symptoms, etc.)
3.   Restlessness
4.   Do not use product if solution is brown colored
5.   Respiratory—arterial blood gases, respiration rate, shortness of breath

D.   Beta-2 adrenergic agonists—sympathomimetics—*oral inhalation administration*
isoproterenol HCl (ISUPREL, METAHALER-ISO), albuterol (PROVENTIL), metaproterenol (ALUPENT and METAPREL), isoetharine (BRONKOTAB)

1.   Cardiovascular—heart rate—tachycardia (much less with albuterol), sweating, ECG changes, PVCs, pulmonary artery wedge pressure, cardiac index
2.   Mild tremors
3.   Respiratory—shortness of breath, arterial blood gases, respiration rate
4.   Nervousness

E.   **Pseudoephedrine HCl (SUDAFED and NOVAFED)**

1. Nasal stuffiness
2. Blood pressure
3. CNS stimulation, nervousness, agitated
4. Hyperthyroidism
5. Apical heart rate

V. **Antianemia drugs (20:04)**

A. General drug-monitoring parameters for all antianemia drugs

1. Hematologic—complete blood count (CBC) with indices, reticulocyte count (retic), pallor
2. Gastrointestinal—check for GI bleeding, hematest stools
3. Level of activity (e.g., lethargy, weakness)
4. Dietary intake
5. Duration of therapy

B. Drug-monitoring parameters for specific antianemia drugs

1. **Iron preparations (20:04.04)**
    Ferrous sulfate (FEOSOL and MOL-IRON), ferrous gluconate (FERGON), ferrous fumarate (FUMERIN), polysaccharide-iron complex (NIFEREX)—*oral administration*, **and iron dextran (IMFERON)**—*IM/IV administration*

    a. Hematologic—CBC (MCV and MCHC), serum iron and iron-binding capacity tests. If administered IM, use Z-track technique; hypersensitivity test dose (injectable iron) should be given and results monitored
    b. Gastrointestinal—GI upset, constipation, black stools
    c. Drug interactions and bioavailability of other drugs
    d. Dose and dosage interval
    e. Elemental iron content of preparation
    f. Avoid taking iron with antacids
    g. Vitamin C increases absorption
    h. Duration of therapy 6 to 12 months

2. **Vitamin B$_{12}$ (cyanocobalamine) injectable (BETALIN 12)**

    a. Hematologic—serum B$_{12}$ level, CBC (MCV is elevated)
    b. Peripheral neuropathy
    c. Diet
    d. Duration of therapy for pernicious anemia—lifetime
    e. Duration of therapy for vitamin B$_{12}$ deficiency anemia—treat until body stores are normal and CBC is normal

3. **Folic acid (FOLVITE)**

    a. Hematologic—serum folacin level and CBC (MCV is elevated)

      b.   Folic acid antagonists (e.g., methotrexate, phenytoin, sulfonamides)—primarily with long-term therapy

      c.   Diet

      d.   Duration of therapy—6 to 8 weeks or until CBC returns to normal

VI. Anticoagulants (20:12)

A. General drug-monitoring parameters for all anticoagulants

1. Bruising
2. Concurrent antibiotic use
3. Prolonged bleeding, hematuria
4. Diet—high in vitamin K content will decrease clotting times
5. Hematologic—hematocrit, platelet count
6. Serum albumin
7. Drug therapy with antiplatelet aggregation activity
8. Drug therapy that promotes bleeding

B. Drug-monitoring parameters for specific anticoagulants

1. Warfarin sodium (COUMADIN), bishydroxycoumarin (DICOUMAROL)

      a.   Laboratory tests—prothrombin times (PT)

      b.   Drug interactions with highly protein-bound drugs

      c.   Drugs with cytochrome P-450 metabolic enzyme inducer and/or inhibitor activity

      d.   Dietary pattern

2. Heparin

      a.   Laboratory—Lee-White clotting times, partial thromboplastin times, activated (APPT or PTT), prothrombin times (PT)

3. Recombinant tissue plasminogen activator (rt-PA)—alteplase, recombinant (ACTIVASE)

      a.   Internal bleeding

      b.   Gastrointestinal (5%)

      c.   Genitourinary (4%)

4. Streptokinase (KABIKINASE)

      a.   Phlebitis at injection site

      b.   Hypersensitivity to drug

5. Urokinase (ABBOKINASE)

      a.   Internal bleeding

      b.   Gastrointestinal (5%)

      c.   Genitourinary (4%)

VII.   Cardiovascular drugs (24:00)

Cardiac drugs (24:04)

A.   General drug-monitoring parameters for all cardiac drugs

1. Cardiovascular—apical heart rate, serum electrolytes, ECG, monitor for arrhythmias, blood pressure, fluid retention, edema
2. Respiratory—respiration rate, lung sounds, SOB, DOE
3. Pallor, cyanosis
4. Dietary intake of sodium and potassium
5. Clinical improvement of medical problem
6. Serum drug levels
7. Renal function tests (e.g., SrCr, CrCl, BUN), fluid intake and output

B.   Specific drug-monitoring parameters for cardiac drugs.

1. **Amiodarone (CORDARONE)**
   a. Cardiovascular—apical heart rate—sinus bradycardia or AV block
   b. Pulmonary infiltrate
   c. Gastrointestinal—nausea and vomiting
   d. Hypothyroidism
   e. Ophthalmic—visual disturbances, corneal microdeposits
   f. Central nervous system—tremors, ataxia, anorexia, insomnia
   g. Dermatologic—skin discoloration (blue-gray), photosensitivity
   h. Drug interactions with highly protein-bound drugs (e.g., warfarin), digoxin, and quinidine
   i. Half-life of drug increases with continued use of drug
   j. Liver function tests

2. **Digoxin (LANOXIN and LANOXICAP)**
   Digitoxin (CRYSTODIGIN) and other digitalis glycosides
   a. Renal function tests (e.g., SrCr, CrCl, BUN), fluid intake and output
   b. Liver function tests
   c. Cardiovascular—ECG signs (PVCs, bigeminy of LVH, prolonged PR-interval); toxicity—lethargy, nausea, vomiting, diarrhea, anorexia, normal–low apical pulse, increased mental confusion, agitation, visual disturbances (e.g., white halos, yellow spots, green haze)

    d.   Drug interactions with beta blockers and disopyramide, nifedipine and verapamil (decrease positive inotropic effects)

    e.   Bioavailability of dosage forms

    f.   Concomitant use of antacids, antidiarrheal suspension, and bulk laxatives decrease absorption

    g.   Serum drug levels, increase about two times when used concurrently with quinidine or verapamil

3.   Quinidine sulfate (QUINIDEX EXTENTABS), quinidine glutamate (QUINAGLUTE)

    a.   Cardiovascular—ECG (arrhythmias, A-V block, prolonged PR interval), apical heart rate, conversion of atrial fibrillation to normal sinus rhythm, hypertension, cinchonism

    b.   Central nervous system—tinnitus (2%), fever or headaches (7%), dizziness (14%), fatigue (6%)

    c.   Bioavailability with other drugs

    d.   Drug interaction—about a twofold elevation in serum digoxin level when used concurrently

    e.   Gastrointestinal—nausea, vomiting or diarrhea (5%), constipation (33%), heartburn (21%), anorexia (2%)

    f.   Lupus syndrome—rash (4%)

    g.   Quinidine content in products

    h.   Serum drug level

4.   Procainamide (PRONESTYL and PROCAN-SR)

    a.   Cardiovascular—ECG (arrhythmia conversion to NSR, decrease in PVCs etc.), apical heart rate, hypertension (especially with IV procainamide)

    b.   NAPA and PCA serum drug level concentrations

    c.   Renal function tests (e.g., SrCr, CrCl, BUN), fluid intake and output

    d.   Gastrointestinal—nausea, vomiting, diarrhea, anorexia

    e.   Central nervous system—dizziness/lightheadedness (14%), tremor (4%), changes in sleep habits (12%), weakness (8%), nervousness (6%), fatigue (5%), confusion (4%)

    f.   Lupus syndrome—rash (10%)

    g.   Other—blurred vision (5%), headache (8%), dyspnea (5%), dry mouth (5%), arthralgia (5%)

5.   Disopyramide phosphate (NORPACE)

    a.   Cardiovascular—ECG (arrhythmia conversion, heart block, decrease in PVCs, etc.), tachycardia, CHF signs/symptoms (negative inotropic effect), hypotension

b. Anticholinergic side effects (e.g., urinary retention, constipation, dry mouth, blurred vision)
c. Liver function tests
d. Renal function tests (e.g., SrCr, CrCl, BUN), fluid intake and output
f. CHF signs/symptoms (negative inotropic effect)
g. Gastrointestinal—nausea/vomiting/heartburn (15%), constipation (12%), diarrhea (9%)
h. Central nervous system—dizziness (3%), sleep disturbances (4%), weakness (3%), nervousness (6%)
i. Other—blurred vision (7%), headache (4%), dyspnea (3%), dry mouth (14.5%)

6. **Lidocaine (XYLOCAINE), tocainide HCl (TONOCARD), mexiletine HCl (MEXITIL), flecainide (TAMBOCOR), encainide (ENKAID)**

a. Liver function tests (elevates SGOT)
b. Cardiovascular—palpitations, hypotension, all are negative inotropes (except for encainide), edema
c. Central nervous system—mental status, drowsiness, dizziness/lightheadedness, paresthesia/numbness, hand tremors, ataxia, restlessness, headache, blurred vision
d. Gastrointestinal—nausea, vomiting, anorexia, heartburn, dry mouth, constipation

7. **Calcium channel blockers (24.04)**
Verapamil (CALAN, CALAN SR, ISOPTIN, and ISOPTIN SR), diltiazem (CARDIZEM and CARDIZEM SR), nicardipine (CARDENE), nimodopine (NIMOTOP)

a. Cardiovascular—apical heart rate (decrease), AV block, signs of CHF (negative inotropic effect)—verapamil and nifedapine, transient hypotension, peripheral edema (7–10%)
b. Drug interaction with digoxin (increases digoxin level about twofold, verapamil increases levels the most)
c. Central nervous system—dizziness/lightheadedness (7–10%), flushing, heat sensation, headache, lethargy/weakness
d. Gastrointestinal—nausea, constipation (greatest with verapamil), dyspepsia

8. **Beta adrenergic blockers**

a. **Selective beta-1 blocking agents—Metoprolol (LOPRESSOR), atenolol (TENORMIN), acebutolol (SECTRAL), betaxolol (BETOPTIC)**

    1)   In low doses, less bronchospasm

    2)   Antinuclear antibodies (ANA) with acebutolol

    3)   See section 8.b. below

b.   **Non-selective beta (1 & 2) adrenergic-blocking agents—propranolol (INDERAL), nadolol (COR-GARD), pindolol (VISKEN), acebutolol (SECTRAL), timolol maleate (BLOCADREN and TIMOPTIC)**

    1)   Respiratory—asthma or COPD contraindication (bronchospasm)

    2)   Cardiovascular—symptoms of CHF (decreased myocardial contractility), apical heart rate (monitor closely when less than 60), AV conduction defects, hypotension

    3)   Gastrointestinal—nausea/vomiting/dyspepsia (4%), cramps

    4)   Central nervous system—fatigue (11%), dizziness (6%), headache (6%), mental status (depression and sleep disturbances 2%), masks some signs of hypoglycemia

    5)   Liver function tests

    6)   Discontinue therapy gradually

    7)   Eye drops (e.g., **TIMOPTIC and BETOPTIC**) may cause mild burning/stinging and redness of eyes; if systemic absorption occurs, general effects of beta blockers may also occur

    8)   Sexual dysfunction

VIII.   Antilipemic agents (24:06)

A.   Cholestyramine resin (QUESTRAN), colestipol (COLESTID)

   1.   Gastrointestinal—constipation (34%), nausea and vomiting (9%), diarrhea (8%), flatulence (21%), dyspepsia (13%), heartburn (8%), abdominal pain/cramps (6%); take all other medication 4 to 6 hours before or after taking this drug to avoid absorption problems; decreases absorption of all acidic and lipid soluble drugs

   2.   Always mix drug with applesauce, crushed pineapple, or 4 to 6 ounces of water, fruit juice, soup or non-carbonated beverage

   3.   Special senses—tinnitus, decreased hearing ability, blurred vision

   4.   Laboratory tests—hypoprothrombinemia, hyperchloremia, decreases in LDL levels and may increase VLDL levels, plasma cholesterol levels

   5.   Diet—low fat, cholesterol, etc.

B. Clofibrate (ATROMID-S)

1. Gastrointestinal—nausea, diarrhea and GI distress, peptic ulcer reactivation
2. Central nervous system—headache, dizziness
3. Laboratory tests—CBC, plasma lipid levels
4. Liver function tests—SGOT and SGPT
5. Renal function tests (e.g., SrCr, CrCl, BUN), fluid intake and output
6. Diet—low fat, cholesterol, etc.

C. Niacin, nicotinic acid (NICOBID)

1. Dermatologic—flushing and pruritus initially
2. Central nervous system—headache, hypotension
3. Gastrointestinal—nausea, vomiting, and diarrhea; contraindicated in active peptic ulcer and hepatic dysfunction
4. Laboratory test—serum lipid levels
5. Diet—low fat, cholesterol, etc.

D. Gemfibrozil (LOPID)

1. Laboratory tests—hepatic function, prothrombin times, fasting blood glucose, plasma lipid levels
2. Gastrointestinal—epigastric pain, nausea, vomiting, diarrhea, and flatulence
3. Diet—low fat, cholesterol, etc.

E. Probucol (LORELCO)

1. Laboratory tests—drug accumulates in adipose tissue, serum cholesterol level
2. Gastrointestinal—diarrhea (10%), nausea (6%), abdominal pain/cramps (5%)
3. Headaches (8%)

F. Lovastatin or mevinolin (MEVACOR)

1. Central nervous system—headaches (9%)
2. Gastrointestinal—flatulence (6%), diarrhea (6%), nausea (5%), dyspepsia (4%), constipation (5%), abdominal pain/cramps (6%)
3. Skin—rash/pruritus (5%)
4. Special senses—blurred vision
5. Laboratory tests—serum lipid levels

IX. Hypotensive agents/antihypertensive agents (24:08)

A. General drug-monitoring parameters for all antihypertensive agents

1.   Renal function (e.g., SrCr, CrCl, BUN), fluid intake and output
2.   Cardiovascular—blood pressure, apical heart rate
3.   Drug interactions altering patient response to therapy
4.   Central nervous system—dizziness/drowsiness, impotence or decreased sexual interest, headaches, lethargy/weakness, nosebleeds
5.   Dietary sodium content
6.   Gastrointestinal—nausea
7.   Electrolyte (Na, K, Cl) loss, especially when using a potassium-depleting diuretic

B.   **Specific drug-monitoring parameters for individual antihypertensive agents**

1.   Reserpine (SERPASIL) and rauwolfia alkaloids (RAUDIXIN)

   a.   Cardiovascular—parasympathetic dominance (bradycardia, nausea, vomiting, diarrhea, nasal stuffiness, excess salivation, excess gastric acid leading to ulcers), CNS depression (may last weeks or months)—psychotic patients, nightmares, orthostatic hypotension, edema, CHF

   b.   Increased appetite

   c.   Central nervous system—dry mouth, nervousness or anxiety, headache

   d.   Gastrointestinal—nausea, vomiting, diarrhea

   e.   Slow onset of action (peak about 3 weeks)

2.   **Centrally (CNS) acting alpha$_2$ sympathomimetic**

   a.   **Methyldopa (ALDOMET)**

      1)   Cardiovascular—drug fever, somnolence (transient), sodium retention, orthostatic hypotension, drowsiness, and lightheadedness
      2)   Sexual impotence
      3)   Dry mouth
      4)   Positive direct Coombs' test
      5)   "Influenza" associated with liver damage
      6)   Anemia

   b.   **Clonidine tablets and patches (CATAPRES and CATAPRES-TTS, respectively), guanabenz (WYTENSIN), guanfacine HCl (TENEX)**

      1)   Dry mouth (30%),
      2)   Drowsiness and sedation (21–30%) may enhance the effects of alcohol, barbiturates
      3)   Dizziness (11%)
      4)   Constipation (10%)

5) Discontinuation of therapy gradually (over 2 to 4 days to avoid possible hypertensive crisis)
6) Fatigue (9%)
7) Rotate sites (patches)
8) Rashes (patches)

3. Hydralazine (APRESOLINE)

a. Apical heart rate (rapid or irregular heart beat)
b. Signs of CHF, angina
c. Headaches, palpitation
d. Lupus syndrome with prolonged high doses
e. Anorexia
f. Nausea, vomiting, or diarrhea

4. Guanethidine (ISMELIN)

a. Orthostatic hypotension
b. Parasympathetic predominance (see section IX.B.1.a.)
c. CHF signs
d. Renal function tests (e.g., SrCr, CrCl, BUN), input and output
e. Sexual dysfunction

5. Beta adrenegic blocker agents (see section VII.B.8.)

a. Black patients do not respond as well as white patients

6. Prazosin (MINIPRESS), terazosin (HYTRIN)

a. Syncope and sudden loss of consciousness may occur 30–90 minutes after first dose, after increasing the dose too fast, or after the addition of another antihypertensive drug
b. Dizziness (19%), headache, drowsiness, lethargy, palpitations, nausea
c. Black patients do not respond as well as white patients

7. Minoxidil (LONITEN)

a. Dermatologic—unusual hair growth (hirsutism)
b. Cardiovascular—pericardial effusion, sodium and water retention

8. Diazoxide (HYPERSTAT)—IV administration

a. Sodium and water retention
b. Drug interactions
c. Blood glucose

9. Sodium nitroprusside (NIPRIDE)—IV administration

a. Cyanide toxicity (large amounts)

    b.   Methemoglobin

    c.   Liver function (cyanide metabolism)

    d.   Renal function tests (e.g., SrCr, CrCl, BUN), fluid intake and output

    e.   Serum thiocyanate (long-term use—should not exceed 10 mg/100 ml)

    f.   Gastrointestinal—nausea, retching, diaphoresis

    g.   Apprehension (too rapid reduction in blood pressure)

10. Captopril (CAPOTEN), captopril and hydrochlorthiazide (CAPOZIDE), enalapril maleate (VASOTEC), enalapril and hydrochlorthiazide (VASORETIC), lisinopril (PRINIVIL and ZESTRIL), lisinopril and hydrochlorthiazide (PRINZIDE and ZESTORETIC)

    a.   Dysgeusia—diminution of taste

    b.   Renal function (elevates BUN and SrCr)

    c.   Proteinuria

    d.   Skin rash (2%)

    e.   Hyperkalemia

    f.   Central nervous system—dizziness (7.5%), headache (5%), fatigue (3%), hypotension (2%), cough (4%)

    g.   Gastrointestinal—diarrhea (3%)

    h.   Angioedema (**PRINIVIL AND ZESTRIL**)

    i.   Once daily dosing (**PRINIVIL AND ZESTRIL**)

    j.   Black patients do not respond as well as white patients

11. Labetalol (TRANDATE and NORMODYNE)—nonselective beta (1 & 2) adrenergic and selective alpha-1 receptor blocker, labetalol and hydrochlorthiazide (NORMOZIDE and TRANDATE-HCT)

    a.   Renal function

    b.   Asthma—may cause bronchospasm

    c.   Contraindicated in patients with heart blocks greater than first degree or bradycardia (AP less than 60)

    d.   May mask premonitory signs and symptoms of hypoglycemia

X. Anti-anginal agents (24:12)—vasodilators/beta blockers/calcium antagonists

A. General drug-monitoring parameters for all anti-anginal agents

    1.   Frequency and duration of anginal attacks

    2.   Physical exertion

    3.   Severe, crushing, chest pain that radiates down the left arm

    4.   Severe SOB

5.   Respiratory function
6.   CBC

B.   **Specific drug-monitoring parameters for individual anti-anginal agents**

1.   **Nitroglycerin sublingual tablets (NITROSTAT), nitroglycerin long-acting capsules, (NITRO-BID), nitroglycerin ointment (NITRO-BID), nitroglycerin patch (NITRO-DUR, NITRODISC, and TRANSDERM-NITRO), nitroglycerin transmucosal tablets (NITROGARD)**

Isosorbide dinitrate (ISORDIL, DILATRATE—SR) tablets, and controlled release tablets and capsules

a.   Frequency and duration of attacks and number of NTG SL tablets used (take 1 NTG SL tablets and if needed, repeat every 5 minutes × 3. If no relief, go directly to the hospital emergency room, STAT!)
b.   Onset of action, relief of severe chest pain
c.   Headaches, flushing, dizziness, or hypotension
d.   Proper storage of NTG SL tablets in glass containers
e.   Proper administration technique

2.   **Propranolol (see section VII.B.8.b.)**

3.   **Calcium channel blockers (24:04)—verapamil (CALAN and ISOPTIN), diltiazem (CARDIZEM), and nifedapine (PROCARDIA), also see section VII.B.7.**

XI.   **Central nervous system drugs—(28:00)**
Analgesic and antipyretic—(28:08)

A.   **General drug-monitoring parameters for all analgesics and antipyretics**

1.   Relief of pain
2.   Lowering of body temperature
3.   Frequency of use

B.   **Specific drug-monitoring parameters for analgesics and antipyretics**

1.   **Acetominophen (e.g., TYLENOL, DATRIL, ANACIN-3, PANADOL)**

a.   Liver function tests
b.   Gastric upset (rare)
c.   Toxicity

2.   **Aspirin (includes salsalate [DISALCID], choline magnesium trisalicylate)**

a. Relief of pain, possibly due to swelling and inflammation
b. Gastrointestinal—GI upset, GI bleeding (hematest stool)
c. Central nervous system—salicylism (tinnitus)
d. Frequency of use
e. Drug interactions with highly protein-bound drugs (greatest problem is with aspirin)
f. Renal function
g. Hepatic function
h. Antiplatelet aggregation activity greatest with aspirin
i. Toxicity
j. Serum salicylic acid levels
k. Half-life of serum salicylic acid level increases with dose, frequency, and duration of therapy

3. **Nonsteroidal anti-inflammatory agents (28:08.04)**

   a. **General drug-monitoring parameters for all non-steroidal anti-inflammatory drugs (NSAIDS)**

      1) GI upset, burning in stomach (20%)
      2) Renal function
      3) Hepatic function
      4) Stomach mucosal ulcerations (6%), GI bleeding, CBC, hematest stools for occult blood
      5) Fluid retention, edema (3–9%)
      6) Relief of arthritis, gout symptoms
      7) Allergy or cross-sensitivity to aspirin
      8) Avoid concurrent use with aspirin
      9) Discontinue NSAID 7 to 10 days prior to any surgery
      10) NSAIDS must be taken regularly to achieve and maintain anti-inflammatory activity

   b. **Specific drug-monitoring parameters for nonsteroidal anti-inflammatory drugs**

      Ibuprofen (MOTRIN), tolmetin (TOLECTIN), naproxen (NAPROSYN), piroxicam (FELDENE), fenoprofen (NALFON), sulindac (CLINORIL), meclofenamate (MECLOMEN), ketoprofen (ORUDIS), carprofen (RIMADYL), diclofenac (VOLTAREN), flurbiprofen (ANSAID)

      1) Dose, especially with rheumatoid arthritis
      2) Visual disturbances
      3) Edema (3–9%)
      4) Tinnitus, headaches (3–9%)
      5) Renal function
      6) Hepatic function

7) Antiplatelet aggregation activity
8) Take with food
9) **RIMADYL** reports a stomach mucosal ulceration rate of 1% which is much less than other NSAIDS (6%) and is due to its prostacyclin-sparing gastric prostaglandin E_2

c. **Indomethacin (INDOCIN)**

1) GI upset, stomach pain, etc.
2) GI bleeding, hematest stools
3) Dizziness or lightheadedness
4) Headaches, giddiness, flatulence
5) CBC

d. **Phenylbutazone (BUTAZOLIDIN, AZOLID)**

1) CBC, (WBC, platelets, retic count)
2) GI bleeding (hematest stools)
3) Dose and duration of therapy
4) Diarrhea
5) Infections (sore throat or fever, URIs, etc.)
6) Pedal edema
7) Take with food

4. **Opiate agonists (28:08.08)**
Opium, morphine (MS CONTIN), hydromorphine, oxymorphone, levorphanol, methadone (DOLOPHINE), meperidine (DEMEROL), codeine, oxycodone, hydrocodone, propoxyphene (DARVON and DARVOCET-N)

a. Central nervous system—relief of pain, sedation—potentiated by other CNS depressants, dizziness, lightheadedness, sweaty/clammy feeling, euphoria, constipation, dry mouth, blood pressure
b. Respiratory depression—hold dose if respiration rate less than 10 per minute
c. Gastrointestinal—nausea, vomiting, constipation
d. Cardiovascular—cardiac arrest
e. Drug dependence

5. **Opiate partial agonists (28:08.12)**
Butorphanol (STADOL), nalbuphine (NUBAIN)—SC, IM, or IV administration; **pentazocine (TALWIN)**—SC, IM, IV, and oral administration

a. Central nervous system—relief of pain, sedation potentiated by other CNS depressants, sweaty/clammy skin, dizziness, vertigo, dry mouth
b. Respiratory depression—hold dose if respiration rate is less than 10 beats per minute

  c. Hepatic function tests
  d. Renal function tests
  e. Drug dependence
  f. Gastrointestinal—nausea, vomiting, constipation

6. **Opiate antagonists (28:10)**
 Naloxone (NARCAN), naltrexone (TREXAN), and leval-lorphan tartrate (LORFAN)—administered SC, IM, or IV only

  a. Gastrointestinal—nausea, vomiting, abdominal pain or cramps
  b. Cardiovascular—diaphoresis, tachycardia, increased blood pressure, tremulousness, nervousness, respiration rate
  c. Avoid heroin use—death may result
  d. Gastrointestinal—anorexia

XII. Anticonvulsants (28:12)

A. General drug-monitoring parameters for all anticonvulsants

 1. Central nervous system—seizure activity, lethargy, daytime sedation, slurred speech, monitor EEG for abnormal brain waves
 2. Serum drug levels
 3. Dosage interval
 4. Hepatic function tests
 5. Drug interactions with highly protein bound drugs

B. Specific drug-monitoring parameters for all anticonvulsants

 1. **Phenytoin (DILANTIN)**

  a. Central nervous system—somnolence when achieving proper maintenance dose, ataxia, falling, hyperactive, DTRs, lethargy, nystagmus, vertigo, diplopia, blurred vision, ECG (when used as antiarrhythmic agent)
  b. Gastrointestinal—nausea, vomiting, diarrhea
  c. Dermatologic—skin rash, acne, hirsutism
  d. Hyperplasia of gums
  e. Hepatic function tests
  f. Serum albumin level
  g. CBC (megaloblastic anemia may develop with long-term use)
  h. Drug interactions with highly protein-bound drugs (increases phenytoin levels), cytochrome P-450 metabolicenzyme inhibitors and stimulants
  i. Bioavailability of generic brands varies, try to avoid changing brands or switching dosage forms

2. **Primidone (MYSOLINE)**

   a. Serum drug levels (primidone and phenobarbital)
   b. Central nervous system—drowsiness, ataxia, dizziness
   c. Gastrointestinal—nausea
   d. CBC—monitor for megaloblastic anemia (folic acid deficiency)
   e. Psychotic activation
   f. False positive test for ketones in urine
   g. Drug interactions with highly protein-bound drugs
   h. Acidic urine cause reabsorption of phenobarbital elevating serum levels

3. **Valproic acid (DEPAKENE, DEPAKOTE)**

   a. Central nervous system—drowsiness, anorexia
   b. Hepatic function tests
   c. Pancreatic function tests
   d. Gastrointestinal—GI upset
   e. Monitor bleeding times and platelet counts
   f. Concurrent use with phenytoin (increases phenytoin levels)
   g. False positive test for ketones in urine
   h. Drug interactions with highly protein-bound drugs

4. **Carbamazepine (TEGRETOL)**

   a. Central nervous system—drowsiness, ataxia, dizziness, nystagmus
   b. Gastrointestinal—nausea, vomiting, and diarrhea
   c. CBC—blood dyscrasias
   d. Sore throat

5. **Ethosuximide (ZARONTIN)**

   a. Gastrointestinal—nausea and vomiting
   b. Central nervous system—fatigue, lethargy, dizziness, headache, euphoria
   c. Photophobia

6. **Clonazepam (KLONOPIN)**

   a. Central nervous system—drowsiness, behavior changes, ataxia
   b. Contraindicated in patients with liver disease and narrow angle glaucoma

XIII. Barbiturates (28:12.04)

   A. Central nervous system—drowsiness, lethargy, paradoxical stimulation (rare)

B. Dermatologic—skin rash
C. Drug interactions with other drugs that are metabolized by the cytochrome P-450 metabolic enzymes (stimulates metabolism)
D. Acidic urine increases reabsorption of phenobarbital

XIV. Antidepressants (28:16.04)

A. General drug-monitoring parameters for all antidepressants

1. Patient compliance—must take medication regularly
2. Central nervous system—sedation, dry mouth, blurred vision, constipation, mood improvement, lethargy, lowers seizure threshold
3. Onset of action varies from 1 to 3 weeks
4. Genitourinary—urinary retention, priapism (DESYREL)

B. Specific drug-monitoring parameters for individual antidepressants

1. **Polycyclic antidepressants**
   Amitriptyline (ELAVIL), maprotiline (LUDIOMIL), nortriptyline (PAMELOR), amoxapine (ASENDIN), imipramine (TOFRANIL), desipramine (NORPRAMIN), doxepin (SINEQUAN and ADAPIN), trazodone (DESYREL)

   a. Onset of action varies with drug from 1 to 3 weeks
   b. Duration of therapy
   c. Hepatic function tests
   d. Drug interactions with antihypertensives and CNS depressants
   e. Central nervous system—insomnia, agitation, orthostatic hypotension, extrapyramidal symptoms
   f. Contraindicated in narrow angle glaucoma
   g. Cardiovascular—cardiac arrhythmias

2. **Lithium carbonate (LITHOBID and ESKALITH), lithium citrate (LITHOTAB):** see section XVI for drug-monitoring parameters

3. **Fluoxetine HCl (PROZAC)**

   a. Central nervous system—headaches (20%), nervousness (15%), insomnia (14%), drowsiness (12%), anxiety (9%), tremors (8%), and dizziness (6%)
   b. Gastrointestinal—nausea (21%), diarrhea (12%), dry mouth (10%), anorexia (9%), and dyspepsia (6%)
   c. Skin and appendages—excessive sweating (8%)

XV.   Psychotherapeutic agents (28:16.12)
Chlorpromazine (THORAZINE), thioridazine (MELLARIL), trifluo-
perazine (STELAZINE), thiothixene (NAVANE), haloperidol (HAL-
DOL), dibenzoxazepine (LOXAPINE)

A.   Patient responsiveness and behavior
B.   Central nervous system—sedation, anticholinergic side effects, orthostatic hypotension, extrapyramidal effects (e.g., akinesia, par-
kinsonism, akathisia, dyskinesia; incidences vary with each drug),
seizure activity (decreased seizure threshold), paradoxical exac-
erbation of psychotic symptoms (elderly), phenothiazines block
action of antiparkinsonism therapy (dopamine), hypothermia
C.   Renal function tests (e.g., SrCr, CrCl, BUN), fluid intake and output
D.   Hepatic function tests (may cause cholestatic jaundice)
E.   Pigmentation (**THORAZINE and MELLARIL mainly**)
F.   Lithium serum levels
G.   Serum sodium and dietary sodium content

XVI.   Other psychotherapeutic agents (28:16.12)

Lithium carbonate (LITHOBID, ESKALITH), lithium citrate (LITH-
OTAB)

A.   Central nervous system—signs and symptoms of manic-depressive
affective disorder, mental confusion, drowsiness, lethargy, slurred
speech, tremors, muscle weakness, ataxia
B.   Gastrointestinal—nausea, vomiting, diarrhea
C.   Renal function tests (e.g. SrCr, CrCl, BUN), fluid intake and output;
increased urination and thirst
D.   Thyroid function tests should be run prior to lithium therapy
E.   Complete blood count
F.   Serum lithium level
G.   Serum sodium and dietary sodium content

XVII.   Sedatives and hypnotics (28:24)
Chloral hydrate (NOCTEC), flurazepam (DALMANE), temazepam
(RESTORIL), triazolam (HALCION)

A.   Frequency of use and effectiveness
B.   Central nervous system—sleep patterns, hangover, daytime seda-
tion/drowsiness (especially with flurazepam), drug interactions with
other CNS depressants
C.   Renal function tests (e.g., SrCr, CrCl, BUN), fluid intake and output
D.   Hepatic function tests
E.   Drug interactions with chloral hydrate (stimulates cytochrome P-
450 metabolic enzyme system)

XVIII.   Benzodiazepines (28:24.08)
Prazepam (CENTRAX), clorazepate (TRANXENE), diazepam (VAL-IUM), chlordiazepoxide (LIBRIUM), halazepam (PAXIPAN), oxazepam (SERAX), lorazepam (ATIVAN), alprazolam (XANAX), buspirone (BUSPAR)

A.   Prior use, frequency of use
B.   Central nervous system—drowsiness/sedation, calming effect, effects on sleep, withdrawal symptoms may follow abrupt discontinuation, paradoxical excitation (rare)
C.   Parasympatholytic effects of LIBRIUM and VALIUM
D.   Renal function tests (e.g., SrCr, CrCl, BUN), fluid intake and output
E.   **BUSPAR** has a slow onset of action (1 to 2 weeks)
F.   Hepatic function tests
G.   It elevates serum digoxin levels

XIX.   Electrolytic, caloric, and water balance (40.00)
Potassium supplement solutions (40.12)

A.   General drug-monitoring parameters for all potassium supplements

1.   GI upset, bleeding, obstruction, etc.
2.   Dosing time(s)
3.   Dosage preparation (dilution, icing, mix with water or juice, etc. to help improve taste)
4.   Serum potassium level
5.   Serum chloride level
6.   Renal function tests (e.g., SrCr, CrCl, BUN), fluid intake and output; when CrCl is less than 20 ml/min, little potassium is lost in urine with or without a loop diuretic
7.   Potassium salt being utilized (chloride best)
8.   Concurrent use of salt substitutes
9.   Concurrent use of potassium-sparing diuretics
10.   Concurrent use of antiarrhythmic agents
11.   Diuretic type (e.g., loop, potassium-sparing, thiazide)
12.   Signs and symptoms of hypokalemia

a.   Muscle cramps or weakness
b.   Lethargy
c.   ECG changes
d.   Increases negative chronotropic effects of digitalis therapy—constipation
e.   confusion

13.   Cardiac evaluation
14.   Acid-base balance

B.   Specific drug-monitoring parameters for individual diuretics/potassium supplements

1. **Potassium chloride tablets** (e.g., K-DUR, K-TAB, K-LYTE-CL, K-NORM, SLOW-K, MICRO-K, KAON-CL, TEN-K, and **Potassium chloride solutions** KAOCHLOR, KLOR, KAY-CIEL

2. **Potassium gluconate (KAON)**

    a. Serum potassium level
    b. Serum chloride level

3. **Potassium citrate/bicarbonate (K-LYTE)**

    a. Serum potassium level
    b. Serum chloride level
    c. Serum bicarbonate level

XX. Potassium—removing resins (40:18) Sodium polystyrene sulfonate (KAYEXALATE)

A. Gastrointestinal—constipation, anorexia, nausea, vomiting, and diarrhea

B. Drug interactions—do not use with antacids (decreases potassium exchange)

C. Sodium and fluid retention

XXI. Diuretics (40:28)

A. General drug-monitoring parameters for diuretics

1. Body weight gain or loss
2. Increased urine output
3. Serum electrolytes (Na, K, Cl, CO_2)

    a. Hypokalemia or hyperkalemia
    b. Hypochloremia
    c. Hyponatremia
    d. Hypochloremic alkalosis

4. Blood pressure, dizziness (10%), headache (9%), lethargy/fatigue (4%)
5. Dehydration
6. Skin turgor
7. Muscle cramps (6%), joint pain and swelling (3%)
8. Renal function tests (e.g., SrCr, CrCl, BUN), fluid intake and output; when CrCl is less than 20–25 ml/min, effectiveness of thiazide diuretics significantly decreases
9. Renal function—when CrCl is less than 20–25 ml/min, only a small amount of potassium is excreted in the urine even with loop diuretics
10. Dietary intake of sodium
11. Sodium content of drugs

B. **Specific drug-monitoring parameters for individual diuretic**

1. **Thiazide-type diuretics**
Hydrocholorothiazide (HYDRODIURIL and ESIDREX), chlorthalidone (HYGROTON), metolazone (ZAROXO-LYN, MICROX and DIULO), indapamide (LOZOL), meth-yclothiazide (ENDURON), chlorothiazide (DIURIL)

   a. Potassium supplement
   b. Serum potassium levels
   c. Serum uric acid level
   d. Serum blood glucose levels
   e. BUN (azotemia, sensorium changes)
   f. Renal function tests (e.g., SrCr, CrCl, BUN), fluid intake and output
   g. Blood pressure
   h. Signs/symptoms of hypokalemia

2. **Loop diuretics**
Furosemide (LASIX), ethacrynic acid (EDECRIN), and bumetanide (BUMEX)

   a. Same as above for thiazide-type diuretics
   b. Orthostatic hypotension
   c. Ototoxicity, especially when used with other ototoxic agents

3. **Potassium-sparing diuretics**
Spironolactone (ALDACTONE), triamterene (DIUREN-IUM) and amiloride (MIDAMOR)

   a. Renal function (e.g., SrCr, CrCl, BUN), fluid intake and output; when CrCl is less than 20–25 ml/min, effectiveness of potassium-sparing diuretics decreases significantly
   b. Monitor use of potassium supplements/foods
   c. Serum potassium level
   d. Gynecomastia (spironolactone)
   e. Serum digoxin level (falsely elevated with spironolactone)
   f. Blood pressure
   g. Edema

4. **Potassium-sparing combination diuretics**
Hydrochlorothiazide and triamterene (DYAZIDE, MAXZIDE, and MAXZIDE-25), hydrocholorthiazide and spironolactone (ALDACTAZIDE), hydrochlorothiazide and amiloride (MODURETIC)

   a. Monitor use of potassium supplements, foods, etc.
   b. Serum potassium level usually normal/high

    c.   Low serum potassium levels may occur in one-third of the patients taking potassium-sparing diuretics

    d.   Renal function tests (e.g., SrCr, CrCl, BUN), fluid intake and output

    e.   Gynecomastia (spironolactone)

    f.   Serum digoxin level (falsely elevated when used concurrently with spironolactone)

    g.   Edema

5. Potassium-depleting combination diuretics
Chlorthalidone and atenolol (TENORETIC), chlorthalidone and clonidine (COMBIPRES), hydrochlorothiazide and methyldopa (ALDORIL), hydrochlorothiazide and reserpine (SERPASIL-ESIDREX), hydrochlorothiazide, reserpine, and hydralazine (SER-AP-ES), hydrochlorothiazide and propranalol (INDERIDE), hydrochlorothiazide and labetalol (NORMOZIDE), hydrochlorothiazide and metoprolol (LOPRESSOR-HCT, hydrochlorothiazide and hydralazine (APRESAZIDE)

    a.   General drug-monitoring parameters for diuretics

    b.   Same as thiazide diuretics

    c.   See drug-monitoring parameters for beta adrenergic blockers

XXII. Antigout/uricosuric agents (40:40)

A. Allopurinol (ZYLOPRIM)

1. Renal function tests (e.g., SrCr, CrCl, BUN), fluid intake and output; reduce dose of allopurinol when renal function is low
2. Serum uric acid levels
3. Signs and symptoms of gout or gouty arthritis
4. Urine pH
5. Hypersensitivity rash (discontinue drug immediately if systemic rash hives appears)
6. Diet

B. Colchicine

1. Gout attacks
2. Nausea, vomiting, diarrhea (initiation of therapy and signs of toxicity)
3. Duration and frequency of acute gout attacks
4. Serum uric acid level
5. Relief of pain
6. Diet (limit red meats in diet)

C. Probenecid (BENEMID) and sulfinpyrazone (ANTURANE)

1. Serum uric acid level
2. Gout attacks
3. Renal function tests (e.g., SrCr, CrCl, BUN), fluid intake and output
4. Drug interaction with ASA
5. Nausea, vomiting, or diarrhea
6. Diet (limit red meat intake)
7. Probenecid decreases renal tubule secretion of many drugs leading to elevated serum drug levels
8. Sulfinpyrazone has antiplatelet aggregation activity

  D. **Indomethacin (INDOCIN)—see section XII.B.2.**

XXIII. **Miscellaneous gastrointestinal drugs (56:00)**

  A. **Belladonna preparations (tincture of belladonna, DONNA-TAL, BELLADENAL)**

1. Antispasmodic effects (relief of symptoms)
2. Anticholinergic effects—dry mouth, blurred vision, urinary retention, and constipation
3. Narrow angle glaucoma (contraindicated)
4. Bioavailability with other drugs (e.g., antacids)
5. Drowsiness or lethargy (with **DONNATAL and BELLAD-ENAL**) due to phenobarbital effects
6. Dosing schedule (give dose one-half hour before meals)

  B. **Propantheline (PRO-BANTHINE)**

1. Antispasmodic effects (relief of symptoms)
2. Anticholinergic—dry mouth, blurred vision, urinary retention, and constipation
3. Narrow angle glaucoma (contraindicated)
4. Dosing schedule (give one-half hour before meals)
5. Bioavailability with other drugs (e.g., antacids)

  C. **Clidinium bromide and chlordiazepoxide (LIBRAX)**

1. Same as section XXIII.A. and B. above
2. Drowsiness from chlordiazepoxide

  D. **Histamine H$_2$-antagonists and acid pump inhibitors Cimetidine (TAGAMET), ranitidine (ZANTAC), famotidine (PEPCID), nizatidine (AXID), omeprazole (LOSEC)**

1. Gastrointestinal—relief of GI symptoms and pain in stomach, diarrhea
2. Central nervous system—muscular pain, headache, dizziness, and mental confusion
3. Rash

4. May increase serum creatinine and serum transaminase levels
5. Gynecomastia (rare)
6. Drug interactions (cimetidine inhibits C-P450 hepatic enzyme system resulting in an increase in some drug levels)
7. Avoid use of cimetidine with antacids
8. Hepatic function tests
9. Renal function tests (e.g., SrCr, CrCl, BUN), and decrease dose with impaired renal function
10. Duration of therapy 6 to 8 week for acute cases, then reduce dose to nighttime maintenance dose only

E. Metoclopramide (REGLAN)

1. Central nervous system—drowsiness, fatigue, extrapyramidal side effects (tremors)
2. Gastrointestinal—diarrhea, decreased nausea and vomiting, dopamine-blocking activity similar to phenothiazine, contraindicated with use of MAO inhibitors, tricyclic antidepressants, or anticholinergics (sympathomimetics)

F. Sucralfate (CARAFATE)

1. Duration of therapy—the drug has little if any clinical effects after ulcer heals (6 to 8 weeks typical)
2. Constipation
3. Do not use with tetracycline antibiotics (decreased absorption of tetracycline)
4. Take drug 1 hour before meals not with food
5. When given concurrently, may bind up drugs and decrease/delay absorption (e.g., phenytoin)

G. Misoprostol (CYTOTEC)

1. Gastrointestinal—diarrhea (13–40%), abdominal pain (7–20%), nausea (3%), flatulence, (3%), dyspepsia (2%)
2. Central nervous system—headaches (2.4%)
3. Contraindication—pregnancy

XXIV. Antacids (56:04)
Aluminum hydroxide gel (ALU-CAP, DIALUME, AMPHOJEL, ALTERNAGEL), aluminum and magnesium hydroxide (MAALOX, MYLANTA, GELUSIL, DIGEL, WINGEL, RIOPAN), calcium carbonate (TUMS)

A. Antacid effects
B. Diarrhea or constipation
C. Drug interactions—decreases absorption of many drugs

XXV. Antidiarrheal agents (56:08)
Diphenoxylate and atropine (LOMOTIL), loperamide (IMODIUM)

    A.   Central nervous system—drowsiness, dizziness

    B.   Gastrointestinal—constipation, instestinal obstruction

    C.   Urinary retention

    D.   Not recommended for children under two years of age

XXVI. Antiemetics (56:22)
Promethazine (PHENERGAN)

    A.   Anticholinergic effects

    B.   Antihistamine effects

    C.   Urinary retention

    D.   Extrapyramidal effects

XXVII. Gold compounds (60:00)

A. Auranofin (RIDAURA)—oral dosage form

    1.   Complete blood count

    2.   Urinalysis—monitor for proteinuria and hematuria

    3.   Platelet count

    4.   Renal function tests (e.g., SrCr, CrCl, BUN), fluid intake and output

    5.   Hepatic function tests

    6.   Dermatologic—rash stomatitis

    7.   Gastrointestinal—diarrhea, abdominal pain, nausea, and vomiting

    8.   Onset of action takes 2 to 4 months

B. Myochrysine and solganol (gold sodium thiomaleate)—injectable form

    1.   Onset of action takes 2 to 3 months

    2.   Hypersensitivity—test dose should be given (nitroid or allergic reaction)

    3.   Dermatological—range from pruritis to exfoliative dermatitis

    4.   Renal function (e.g., SrCr, CrCl, BUN), fluid intake and output

    5.   Urinalysis—monitor for proteinuria and hematuria

    6.   Complete blood count

    7.   Toxicity may not occur until 2 to 3 months after therapy has been discontinued

XXVIII. Hormone and synthetic substitutes (68:00)

A. Androgens (68:08)
Fluoxymesterone (HALOTESTIN)

    1.   Masculinization

    2.   Sodium, potassium, and chloride retention

    3.   Hypercalcemia

    4.   Acne

       5.   Cholestatic jaundice

       6.   Gynecomastia

B.   **Estrogens (68:16)**
Diethylstilbestrol or DES, conjugated estrogens (PRE-MARIN), estrone (OGEN), ethinyl estradiol (ESTINYL AND ESTRACE)

       1.   Gastrointestinal—nausea and vomiting

       2.   Central nervous system—headaches, hot flashes

       3.   Feminization and breast tenderness

       4.   Hypercalcemia

       5.   Thrombophlebitis

       6.   Causes false elevation of serum T_3 and depression of T_4

       7.   Hepatic function tests

C.   **Progestins (68:32)**
Progestins (PROVERA and MEGACE)

       1.   Nausea

       2.   Fluid retention

       3.   Hypercalcemia

XXIX.   **Adrenals (68:04)**

    A.   Corticosteroids
       Cortisone, hydrocortisone, prednisone (DELTASONE and METI-CORTEN), dexamethasone (DECADRON)

       1.   Anti-inflammatory effects

       2.   Central nervous system—mental status, depression, elevated blood glucose, duration of therapy, method of discontinuance of therapy, signs of withdrawal (aching joints, lethargy, etc.), blood pressure

       3.   Sodium and water retention, moon face, buffalo hump

       4.   Hypokalemia

       5.   Dosing and dose interval (single dose daily, divided doses daily, alternate days); take dose same time each day (best in AM)

       6.   WBC and platelets (leukemias, Hodgkin's disease)

       7.   Gastric irritation, ulcers

       8.   Potassium loss (varies with preparation)

       9.   Osteoporosis with long-term use

     10.   Infections (opportunistic organisms)

     11.   Increased body weight

XX.   **Insulins and antidiabetic agents (68:20)**

    A.   **Insulins**
       Regular (R), isophane insulin suspension (NPH), lente (L),

semi-lente (S), protamine zinc insulin (PZI), HUMULIN-R, HUMULIN-N, and HUMULIN-L, NOVOLIN

1. Allergies (fewer allergies with all pork and more purified insulins—e.g., **HUMULIN**)
2. Type of insulin and dose, onset, peak and duration of action, route of administration; hyperglycemia (e.g., drowsiness, flushed, dry skin, fruit-like breath odor, polyuria, loss of appetite, excessive thirst, lethargy)
3. Blood glucose (FBS and 4 PMBS), finger-stick (home glucose monitor)
4. **CLINITEST/ACETEST** urine glucose and ketone test
5. Central nervous system—hypoglycemia (e.g., confusion, anxiety, nausea and vomiting, tachycardia, chills, sweating, hunger, pale skin color, nightmares, lethargy)
6. Somogyi effects
7. Patient knowledge of disease, drugs, urine tests, hygiene, insulin administration techniques, aseptic technique, etc.
8. Diet—American Diabetes Association (ADA)
9. Rotation of injection sites
10. HbA_{1C} (glycosolated hemoglobin) laboratory test
11. Restrict alcohol use
12. Body weight
13. Increased risk of infections
14. All pork, beef, and combination of beef and pork insulins are available
15. Retinopathy and neuropathy likely with long-term elevated blood glucose

B. **Oral hypoglycemics—sulfonylureas**
   Tolbutamide (ORINASE), tolazamide (TOLINASE), chlorpropamide (DIABINESE), acetohexamide (DYMELOR), glipizide (GLUCOTROL), glyburide (DIABETA and MICRONASE)

1. Fasting blood glucose (FBS)
2. **CLINITEST/ACETEST** of urine
3. Hypoglycemia/hyperglycemia (see section XXVI.A.5. and 2., respectively)
4. Skin rash
5. Body weight
6. Disulfiram reaction
7. Sulfa allergy (cross-sensitivity)
8. Maximum dosage
9. Liver function tests
10. Renal function tests (e.g., SrCr, CrCl, BUN), fluid intake and output

11. Diet—ADA
12. Alcohol use
13. HbA$_{1C}$ (glycosolated hemoglobin) laboratory test
14. Increased risk of infections
15. Patient knowledge of disease and role of drug therapy
16. Urinalysis—urine glucose, ketones, bacteria

XXXI. Thyroid and antithyroid agents (68:36)

A. Thyroid replacements
Levothyroxine sodium (LEVOTHROID and SYNTHROID), liothyronine sodium (CYTOMEL), thyroid USP (ARMOUR THYROID), thyroglobulin (PROLOID), liotrix (EUTHROID and THYROLAR)

1. Patient compliance, dose must be taken regularly at the same time each day, do not double up doses if one dose is missed
2. Serum T$_4$ level—levothyroxine
3. Serum T$_3$ level—liothyronine
4. Thyroid-stimulating hormone (TSH)
5. Drug interactions with highly protein-bound drugs
6. Signs of hypothyroidism—fatigue, weakness, dry skin, dry and brittle hair, cold intolerance, bradycardia, weight gain, goiter, hypothermia, hoarseness, baggy eyes, anemia, and menstrual problems
7. Signs of hyperthyroidism—headache, palpitations, tachycardia (>100), atrial fibrillation, chest pain, heat intolerance, increased to profuse sweating, leg cramps, weight loss, diarrhea, vomiting, nervousness, depression or apathy, anorexia, exophthalmos (bulging eyes), and cardiomegaly
8. Bioavailability of thyroid extract products varies in ratio of T$_3$ and T$_4$ present

B. Antithyroid agents
Potassium iodide (SSKI), methimazole (TAPAZOLE), propylthiouracil (PTU)

1. Skin eruptions and yellowing of sclera of eyes
2. Patient compliance—do not double up dose if one is missed
3. CBC with differential (if fever, sore throat, or malaise symptoms occur); agranulocytosis may occur with PTU use
4. Serum T$_4$, T$_3$, and TSH levels
5. Prothrombin time prior to surgery, dental extraction, or when taking anticoagulant with PTU use
6. Central nervous system—headaches, dizziness
7. GI upset (SSKI)

XXXII. Spastolytic agents respiratory smooth muscle relaxants (86:00)

A. Aminophylline, anhydrous theophylline (THEO-DUR, THEO-SPRINKLES, THEO-24, SLO-PHYLLIN, RESPBID, THEOLAIR-SR, etc.)

1. Relief of bronchospasm and SOB, wheezing
2. Theophylline levels
3. Central nervous system—nausea, vomiting, seizures, nervousness/agitation, insomnia, respiration rate, improvement in breathing
4. Smoking history
5. Drug interactions with cytochrome P-450 metabolic enzyme inhibitors (e.g., erythromycin, cimetidine) increase theophylline levels
6. Tachycardia
7. Ethylenediamine hypersensitivity
8. Arterial blood gases
9. Lung sounds
10. Do not take **THEO-24** with food (dosage form dumps theophylline when given with food)
11. Dyphilline products are not theophylline salts and are not equivalent to theophylline
12. Anhydrous theophylline content of products varies greatly

B. Beta-2 adrenergic agonists—sympathomimetic amines—*inhalation*
Terbutaline (BRETHINE, BRICANYL), albuterol (VENTOLIN, PROVENTIL), isoproterenol (ISUPREL), isoetharine HCl (BRONKOMETER, BRONKOSOL) metaproterenol (METAPREL, ALUPENT), bitolterol mesylate (TORNALATE)

1. Respiratory—relief of bronchospasm, arterial blood gases, shortness of breath, wheezing, need for O_2 supplement
2. Administration technique
3. Dose limit 12 puffs/day
4. Central nervous system—tremor, nervousness
5. Cardiovascular—arrhythmias, tachycardia, blood pressure

C. Beclomethasone (BECLOVENT, BECONASE, BECONASE-AQ, VANCENASE)

1. Relief of symptoms
2. Administration technique
3. Oral thrush (*Candida* infection), patient should rinse out mouth immediately after each inhalation dose
4. Adrenal suppression
5. Hoarseness or sore throat
6. Nasal burning and stinging (**BECONASE and VANCENASE**)

    D.   **Cromolyn (INTAL, NASALCROME)**

        1.   Relief of asthma symptoms—chronic prophylaxis use only
        2.   Administration technique
        3.   Nose or throat irritation
        4.   Frequency of asthma attacks

    E.   **Atropine sulfate and ipratroprium (ATROVENT)**

        1.   Cardiovascular—tachycardia
        2.   Administration technique
        3.   Nervousness, agitation (3%)
        4.   Give 1 hour before beta agonist (if utilized)
        5.   Cough (6%) and dry throat (3–5%)

XXXIII. Antiparkinson agents—drug induced parkinsonism (92:00)

Benztropine mesylate (COGENTIN), trihexphenidyl HCl (ARTANE), diphenhydramine HCl (BENADRYL)

    A.   Narrow angle glaucoma (contraindicated)
    B.   Central nervous system—drowsiness, constipation, urinary retention, dry mouth, tremors, improvement in drug-induced tremors or EPS; may mask EPS signs when given with phenothiazine antipsychotics

XXXIV. Antiparkinson agents (92:00)

    A.   **Amantadine HCl (SYMMETREL)**

        1.   Central nervous system—restlessness, confusion, decreased mental alertness, hallucinations, orthostatic hypotension
        2.   Renal function tests (e.g., SrCr, CrCl, BUN), fluid intake and output
        3.   Improvement in symptoms of Parkinson's disease

    B.   **Levodopa (DOPAR, LARODOPA)**

        1.   Central nervous system—anorexia, orthostatic hypotension, nausea and vomiting
        2.   Improvement in symptoms of Parkinson's disease
        3.   Avoid use with MAO inhibitors
        4.   Avoid use if patient has narrow angle glaucoma
        5.   Renal function tests (e.g., SrCr, CrCl, BUN), fluid intake and output
        6.   Liver function tests (SGOT, SGPT)
        7.   Avoid vitamin formulas with pyridoxine HCl (B_6)
        8.   Avoid concominant use of neuroleptic drugs (e.g., phenothiazines) or chemically related drugs (e.g., metaclopropamide)
        9.   Drug-free holiday
      10.   On-off effect

C. Carbidopa/levodopa (SINEMET)

1. Fewer GI upset than with levodopa alone
2. Frequency of orthostatic hypotension similar to levodopa
3. Psychic disturbances similar levodopa
4. Cardiac arrhythmias
5. Pyridoxine use appears to have no antagonistic effects
6. Other adverse effects less than that of levodopa
7. Improvement of Parkinson's symptoms

D. **Bromocriptine (PARLODEL)**

1. Adverse effects similar to levodopa, except nausea, vomiting, dizziness, orthostatic hypotension, and mental changes are more frequent; decreasing the dose will decrease adverse effects
2. On-off effect less than levodopa

■ Part II. Disease-monitoring parameters (7–11)

A. **Congestive heart failure (CHF)**

1. General patient-monitoring parameters
2. CHF signs and symptoms include heart and lung sounds, apical heart rate, SOB, orthopnea, exertional fatigue, weakness, sacral and/or pedal edema, chest congestion, nonproductive cough, nocturia, increased respirations, etc.
3. Laboratory tests: serum digitoxin, serum digoxin level, serum electrolytes, serum creatinine, creatinine clearance, ECG, chest x-ray
4. Concurrent diseases and drug therapy
5. CHF therapy includes; digoxin, digitoxin, diet (low Na^+), diuretic, potassium supplement if potassium-depleting diuretic used, and stool softener; to monitor drug therapy, refer to specific drug-monitoring parameters for each drug or combination of drugs

B. **Diabetes mellitus (DM)**

1. General patient-monitoring parameters
2. DM signs and symptoms include;

    a. **Hypoglycemia**—loss of body weight, confusion, anxiety, nausea and vomiting, chills, sweating, hunger, pale skin color, lethargy, etc.
    b. **Hyperglycemia**—drowsiness, flushed, dry skin, fruit-like breath odor, polyuria, loss of appetite, excessive thirst, lethargy, etc.

3. Laboratory tests: glucose tolerance test, fasting blood sugar, 4PMBG, random blood sugar, **urine glucose/ketone tests Clinitest/Acetest, Diastix/Acestix**, HbA_{1C}, finger stick (home glucose monitoring), renal and hepatic function tests
4. Concurrent diseases and drug therapy
5. DM therapy includes insulin, oral hypoglycemic agent, diet and alcohol limitations; to monitor drug therapy, refer to specific drug-monitoring parameters for each drug or combination of drugs

C. Hypertension (HT, HPT, or HTN)

1. General patient-monitoring parameters
2. HTN signs and symptoms include BP with a diastolic pressure >95–100 mm Hg, early morning headache, nosebleeds, orthostatic hypotension, edema, lethargy, easy·fatigability, lightheadedness, palpitations, etc.
3. Laboratory tests: serum electrolytes (Na^+, K^+, Cl^-), renal function
4. Concurrent diseases and drug therapy
5. HTN therapy includes thiazide diuretics, vasodilators, adrenergic-blocking drugs, ACE inhibitors, calcium channel blockers, diet, etc.; to monitor drug therapy, refer to specific drug-monitoring parameters for each drug or combination of drugs

D. Angina pectoris (AP)

1. General patient-monitoring parameters
2. AP signs and symptoms include shortness of breath, respiration rate, severe, pressure-like, chest pain, retrosternal (to the left side) orthostatic hypotension, headache, activity level, blood pressure, number and duration of chest pain episodes, weakness and easy fatigability, heart rate
3. Laboratory tests: ECG, CBC, serum electrolytes (Na^+, K^+, Cl^-)
4. Concurrent diseases and drug therapy
5. AP therapy includes nitrates/NTG (SL tablets or LA capsules, oral spray, oral mucosal tablet, ointment and patches) beta blocker or calcium channel blocker, diet and rest; to monitor drug therapy, refer to specific drug-monitoring parameters for each drug or combination of drugs
6. AP pain therapy: when pain not relieved with SL NTG, use morphine SO_4, meperidine or codeine.

E. Seizures

1. General patient-monitoring parameters
2. Seizure signs and symptoms include level of consciousness, twitches or rigidity in limbs, number and duration of seizures,

appearance and frequency, facial grimacing, mental status, urinary incontinence, etc.
3. Laboratory tests: anticonvulsant serum drug level, CBC, liver function tests, and renal function tests
4. Concurrent diseases and drug therapy
5. Seizure therapy includes anticonvulsants of choice and/or phenobarbital; to monitor drug therapy, refer to specific drug-monitoring parameters for each drug or combination of drugs

F. Urinary tract infections (UTI)

1. General patient-monitoring parameters
2. UTI signs and symptoms include increased urinary frequency, pain and burning upon urination, appearance, color and odor of urine, elevated temperature, chills, pain, and tenderness of the kidneys or backside, hematuria, lethargy, etc.
3. Laboratory tests: UA and C & S, SrCr, CBC with differential
4. Concurrent diseases and drug therapy
5. UTI therapy includes antibiotic of choice based on the C & S report; to monitor drug therapy, refer to specific drug-monitoring parameters for each drug or combination of drugs

G. Depression

1. General patient-monitoring parameters
2. Signs and symptoms include fear, anxiety, crying episodes, anorexia, constipation, dysphoric, withdrawn, feeling of helplessness and hopelessness, unsociable, dejection, insomnia, fatigue, chronic headaches/pains, etc.
3. Laboratory tests usually none specific for depression except possibly a dexamethasone suppression test; if drug therapy used includes lithium, then serum lithium and sodium levels are needed
4. Concurrent diseases and drug therapy
5. Depression therapy includes antidepressant of choice, antianxiety agent, and counseling; to monitor drug therapy, refer to specific drug-monitoring parameters for each drug or combination of drugs

H. Chronic obstructive pulmonary disease (COPD)

1. General patient-monitoring parameters
2. COPD signs and symptoms: SOB, "smoker's cough," wheezing, dyspnea, constipation, weakness, weight loss, skin color of face (pink or blue), etc.
3. Laboratory tests: x-ray, spirometric tests, arterial blood gases (ABG) and serum electrolytes, theophylline level, CBC
4. Concurrent diseases and drug therapy
5. COPD therapy includes bronchial dilators, O_2, expectorants;

to monitor drug therapy, refer to specific drug-monitoring parameters for each drug or combination of drugs

I. Anemia (iron, vitamin B_{12}, and folate deficiencies)

1. General patient-monitoring parameters
2. Anemia signs and symptoms

   a. **Iron deficiency anemia:** signs and symptoms include marked tiredness, tires easily, shortness of breath, dyspnea on exertion, palpitations, irritability, headache, paresthesia, lightheadedness, postural hypotension, dementia, angular stomatitis, glossitis, thin, brittle fingernails; and flattened as well as spoon-shaped fingernails; pale conjunctival membranes; nail beds, and complexion, etc.; CBC—decreased MCV

   b. **Vitamin B_{12} deficiency anemia (pernicious anemia):** signs and symptoms include: weakness, sore tongue, irritability, apathy, numbness and tingling peripherally, anorexia, pale/yellow complexion, vertigo, ataxia, shortness of breath, dyspnea on exertion, somnolence, loss of reflexes, etc.; CBC—elevated MCV

   c. **Folate deficiency anemia:** signs and symptoms include irritability, sleeplessness, faintness, palpitations, smooth and waxy appearing skin; CBC—elevated MCV

3. Laboratory tests: CBC with indices, reticulocyte count, serum iron, total iron-binding capacity, serum transferrin, serum folacin, and B_{12} levels
4. Concurrent diseases and drug therapy
5. Anemia therapy includes iron, vitamin B_{12}, and folic acid; to monitor drug therapy, refer to specific drug-monitoring parameters for each drug or combination of drugs

J. Rheumatoid arthritis (RA)

1. General patient-monitoring parameters
2. Signs and symptoms include symmetrical joint involvement of body, morning stiffness in joints, joint mobility, pain, joint swelling and redness, and activity level
3. Laboratory tests: erythrocyte sedimentation rate (ESR), rheumatoid factor (RF), complete blood count (CBC), x-ray
4. Concurrent diseases and drug therapy
5. RA therapy includes ASA, NSAID, steroid, gold, penicillamine, immunosuppressive agents, exercise, diet, and rest; to monitor drug therapy, refer to specific drug-monitoring parameters for each drug or combination of drugs

K. Thyroid disorders

1. General patient-monitoring parameters
2. Signs and symptoms include:

    a. **Hypothyroid**—fatigue, weakness, dry skin, dry and brittle hair, cold intolerance, bradycardia, weight gain, goiter, hypothermia, hoarseness, baggy eyes, anemia, menstrual problems, etc.

    b. **Hyperthyroid**—headache, palpitations, tachycardia (>100), atrial fibrillation, high output heart failure, chest pain, heat intolerance, increased to profuse sweating, leg cramps, weight loss, diarrhea, vomiting, nervousness, depression or apathy, anorexia, exophthalmos (bulging eyes), cardiomegaly, etc.

3. Laboratory tests: serum T_3, T_4, TSH levels, CBC
4. Concurrent diseases and drug therapy
5. Therapy includes

    a. **Hypothyroid**—levothyroxine sodium, liothyronine sodium, thyroid, thyroglobulin, or liotrix

    b. **Hyperthyroid**—methimazole, potassium iodide (SSKI), and propylthiouracil; to monitor drug therapy, refer to specific drug-monitoring parameters for each drug or combination of drugs

L. Upper and lower respiratory infections

1. General patient-monitoring parameters
2. Signs and symptoms: cough, chest congestion, discolored sputum, fever, chills, headache, pain in chest upon inspiration, lethargy, general myalgia, etc.
3. Laboratory tests: culture and sensitivity, CBC with differential, chest x-ray
4. Concurrent diseases and drug therapy
5. Therapy: antibiotic drug of choice based upon culture and sensitivity results or empirical therapy; to monitor drug therapy, refer to specific drug-monitoring parameters for each drug or combination of drugs

M. Parkinson's disease (PD)

1. General patient-monitoring parameters
2. PD signs and symptoms: involuntary hand tremors, mask face, muscle rigidity, fatigue, cogwheel movement of joints, stooped posture, unsteady and shuffling gait, increased salivation, difficulty swallowing, etc.
3. Laboratory test: CBC
4. Concurrent diseases and drug therapy
5. PD therapy includes: levodopa, levodopa and carbidopa,

amantadine and bromocriptine; to monitor drug therapy, refer to specific drug-monitoring parameters for each drug or combination of drugs

N. Asthma

1. General patient-monitoring parameters
2. Asthma signs and symptoms: choking, wheezing, dyspnea, tachypnea, cough, tightness or pressure in chest, fatigue, cyanosis, confusion, and lethargy
3. Laboratory tests: arterial blood gases, pulmonary function tests, CBC, serum drug levels (primarily theophylline), sputum evaluation, chest x-ray and serum electrolytes
4. Concurrent diseases and drug therapy
5. Asthma therapy includes:

   a. **Acute asthma attack:** epinephrine, aminophylline, adrenal cortical steroids, O_2, inhalation therapy of a bronchodilator (e.g., albuterol, terbutaline, metaproterenol, isoproterenol, isoetharine), and hydration (IV D_5W with or without sodium bicarbonate)

   b. **Chronic asthma:** O_2, theophylline, adrenal cortical steroids, albuterol, bitolterol, cromolyn sodium, ipratropium, and atropine sulfate; to monitor drug therapy, refer to specific drug-monitoring parameters for each drug or combination of drugs.

References

1. Fletcher HP, Bennett RW. The use of parameters—following in a therapeutics course. *J Clin Pharmacol* 1974; 14:9–12.
2. Knoben JE, Anderson PO, eds. *Handbook of Clinical Drug Data*, 6th ed., Drug Intelligence Publications, Inc., Hamilton, IL, 1988.
3. Kastrup EK, Boud JR., eds. *Facts and Comparisons*, JB Lippincott Co., Philadelphia, 1989.
4. Drug Information for the Health Care Provider, vol 1, *USP DI*, 5th ed, 1985. United States Pharmacopeial Convention, Inc., Mack Printing Co., Easton, PA, 1988.
5. McEvoy GK. *American Hospital Formulary Service*. American Society of Hospital Pharmacists, Bethesda, MD, 1989.
6. Mittman M, Best M, eds. *Compendium of Drug Therapy*. Biomedical Information, New York, 1989.
7. Wyngaarden JB, Smith LH Jr., eds. *Cecil Textbook of Medicine*, 16th ed. WB Saunders, Philadelphia, 1985.
8. Katcher BS, Young LY, Koda-Kimble MA. *Applied Therapeutics: The Clinical Use of Drugs*, 4th ed. Applied Therapeutics, Inc., San Francisco, 1988.
9. Herfindal ET, Hirschman JL, eds. *Clinical Pharmacy and Therapeutics*, 3rd ed. Williams & Wilkins, Baltimore, 1988.
10. Gilman AG, Goodman LS, Gilman A, eds. *Goodman and Gilman's The Pharmacologic Basis of Therapeutics*, 6th ed. Macmillan, New York, 1985.
11. Smith LH Jr, Thier SO, Wyngaarden JB, eds. *Pathophysiology: The Biological Principles of Disease*. WB Saunders, Philadelphia, 1985.

Chapter 4
Clinical Laboratory Diagnostic Tests (1–12)

A patient's serum and/or urine laboratory values may be utilized as direct indicators of medical condition; a guide for the clinician for rapid and thorough understanding of a patient's medical condition; and a diagnostic tool in reviewing vital body systems of metabolism and excretion. In some instances, laboratory tests may be essential in order to monitor and assess properly how well a patient's disease is being controlled or to help prevent drug toxicity when there are no physical signs or clinical symptoms present. In most patients, abnormal laboratory values usually indicate either present or impending complications that may require immediate medical attention. When monitoring drug therapy, the pharmacist always must be concerned with the meaning and significance of both normal and abnormal laboratory values and must be able to correlate the laboratory values with clinical signs and symptoms the patient is exhibiting.

This chapter describes some common clinical laboratory tests and includes the following information: an explanation of each test; normal test values; and disease states or disorders that may alter laboratory test values. Since normal laboratory values may vary between institutions as a result of differences in laboratory equipment and personnel, the pharmacist must be aware of this variation when monitoring a patient's drug therapy.

I.   **Complete blood count (CBC)**
       A complete blood count (CBC) may sometimes be referred to as a hemogram. The test will usually contain the following components in the following order.

       A.   **White blood cell (WBC) count**

1. White blood cells (leukocytes) are necessary for the body to defend itself adequately against invading microorganisms. The WBC count is defined as a measure of leukocytes in the blood. A differential white blood count will specifically identify the types of WBCs.

2. WBCs may be elevated in

   a. Bacterial infections
   b. Malignant disease
   c. Tissue necrosis
   d. Leukemia
   e. Long-term steroid therapy
   f. Chronic respiratory diseases—when inflammation is present
   g. Lithium therapy

3. WBCs may be decreased in

   a. Bone marrow depression
   b. Immunosuppressive drug therapy
   c. Overwhelming infections
   d. Chronic disease

4. Normal values

   a. Males, $4.1-11.0 \times 103/mm^3$
   b. Females, $4.2-12.1 \times 103/mm^3$

B. Red blood cell (RBC) count

1. Red blood cells are often referred to as erythrocytes. Their life expectancy is approximately 120 days. They contain the body's hemoglobin and carry oxygen to various cells in the body. The RBC count is defined as a measurement of the level of red blood cells in the blood.

2. RBCs may be elevated in

   a. Dehydration
   b. Chronic respiratory diseases
   c. Living in high altitudes
   d. Polycythemia vera

3. RBCs may be decreased in

   a. Hemorrhage
   b. Anemias due to decreased RBC production (e.g., iron, vitamin B_{12}, and folate deficiencies)
   c. Anemias due to increased RBC destruction (e.g., hemolytic anemia, etc.)
   d. Anemias due to increased RBC destruction and decreased production

  e. Leukemia
  f. Multiple myeloma

 4. Normal values

  a. Males, $4.6–6.2 \times 10^6/mm^3$
  b. Females, $4.2–5.4 \times 10^6/mm^3$

C. Hemoglobin (Hgb)

 1. Hemoglobin is a protein in the blood and is defined as the oxygen-carrying component of the red blood cell. Hemoglobin gives the blood its rich red color.

 2. Hgb may be elevated (hyperchromic) in

  a. Chronic respiratory diseases
  b. Polycythemia vera
  c. Severe tissue destruction (e.g., resulting from burns)

 3. Hgb may be decreased (hypochromic) in

  a. Anemias due to decreased RBC production (e.g., iron, vitamin B_{12}, folate deficiencies)
  b. Anemias due to increased RBC destruction (e.g. hemolytic anemia, etc.)
  c. Anemias due to increased RBC destruction and decreased production
  d. Severe hemorrhage
  e. Cirrhosis of the liver

 4. Normal values

  a. Males, 14–18 g/dl
  b. Females, 12–16 g/dl

D. Hematocrit (Hct)

 1. The hematocrit is sometimes referred to as the packed cell volume (PCV). The Hct value is determined by measuring the height of the red blood cell column after it has been centrifuged and comparing it to the height of the original whole blood sample. Therefore, the Hct may be defined as the percentage of red blood cell mass in the blood.

 2. Hct may be elevated in

  a. Dehydration, decrease in fluid volume (low fluid intake, diarrhea, excessive vomiting, profuse sweating, severe burns, etc.)
  b. Shock
  c. Polycythemia vera

 3. Hct may be decreased in:

   a. Anemias due to decreased RBC production (e.g., iron, vitamin B_{12}, folate deficiencies)
   b. Anemias due to increased RBC destruction (e.g., hemolytic anemia)
   c. Anemias due to increased RBC destruction and decreased production
   d. Acute massive hemorrhage
   e. Leukemia
   f. Cirrhosis of the liver

4. Normal values

   a. Males, 42–52%
   b. Females, 37–47%

E. Mean corpuscular volume (MCV)

1. The mean corpuscular volume is determined by calculating the effect that RBCs have on the hematocrit. The MCV may be defined as the mean volume (cell size) of the individual red blood cell and is expressed in cubic microns (μm^3). The MCV is useful in classification of anemia. The MCV detects the changes in cell size. The formula is:

   $$Hct \times 10 / RBC \times 10^6 = MCV \text{ in } \mu m^3.$$

2. MCV may be elevated (macrocytic cell) in

   a. Liver disease
   b. Vitamin B_{12} deficiency
   c. Folic acid deficiency
   d. Alcoholism

3. MCV may be decreased (microcytic cell) in

   a. Iron deficiency anemia
   b. Chronic hemorrhage
   c. Pyridoxine deficiency
   d. Copper deficiency

4. Normal value, 82–92 μm^3

F. Mean cell hemoglobin (MCH)

1. The mean cell hemoglobin is determined by calculating the effect Hgb has on RBC count. The MCH may be defined as the weight of hemoglobin in an average red blood cell and is expressed as picograms (pg). The formula is:

   $$Hgb \text{ (in grams)} \times 10 / RBC \times 10^6 = MCH \text{ in pg.}$$

2. MCH may be elevated in

   a. Hyperchromic anemias

b.   Macrocytic anemias

3.   MCH may be decreased in

a.   Normochromic and hypochromic anemias
b.   Microcytic anemias

4.   Normal value is 27–29 pg

G.   Mean corpuscular hemoglobin concentration (MCHC)

1.   The mean corpuscular hemoglobin concentration is determined by calculating the effect hemoglobin has on the hematocrit. The MCHC is a measure of the concentration of hemoglobin in the average red blood cell. The MCHC may be defined as the average hemoglobin concentration in an individual red blood cell and is expressed as a gram percentage (g/dl). The formula is:

Hgb (in grams) $\times$ 100 / Hct = MCHC in g/dl.

2.   MCHC may be elevated in macrocytic anemias
3.   MCHC may be decreased in microcytic anemias
4.   Normal value is 32–36 g/dl

H.   Reticulocyte count (retic count)

1.   The reticulocyte count is an index of the production of mature red blood cells by blood-forming organs. Reticulocytes are immature erythrocytes. The reticulocyte count may be defined as a measure of the number of immature red blood cells and is expressed as a percentage.
2.   Retic count may be elevated in

a.   Three to 4 days following hemorrhage
b.   Hemolytic anemia
c.   Leukemia
d.   Metastatic carcinoma
e.   Increased bone marrow activity due to anemia therapy

3.   Retic count may be decreased in

a.   Iron deficiency
b.   Aplastic anemia
c.   Pernicious anemia
d.   Chronic infection

4.   Normal value is 0.5–1.5%

I.   Platelet count (thrombocytes)

1.   Platelets are cells that are produced by the bone marrow and are necessary for proper clotting of blood. Their life expec-

tancy is approximately 7–10 days. Platelets swell and adhere to the endothelial fibrils as a temporary hemostatic plug. They release adenosine diphosphate (ADP), which is involved in thrombin generation. Bleeding may occur when the platelet count is below 70,000–90,000 platelets/mm^3.

2. Platelet counts may be elevated (thrombocytosis) in

   a. Hemolytic anemia
   b. Polycythemia vera
   c. Thrombocythemia
   d. Cachexia
   e. Acute hemorrhage
   f. Chronic myelogenous leukemia
   g. Splenectomy
   h. Fractures of the neck of the femur
   i. Rheumatoid arthritis
   j. Pregnancy

3. Platelet counts may be decreased (thrombocytopenia) in

   a. Acute and chronic leukemia
   b. Vitamin B_{12} or folic acid deficiency
   c. Septicemia
   d. Bacterial endocarditis
   e. Idiopathic thrombocytopenic purpura
   f. Aplastic anemia
   g. Chronic use of aspirin or NSAIDs

4. Normal value 150,000–400,000 platelets/mm^3

J. Erythrocyte sedimentation rate (ESR or sed rate)

The ESR is a nonspecific indicator of increased acute-phase proteins and is useful for diagnosing infection in children and for monitoring rheumatic disease in adults.

1. This test involves the speed at which RBCs settle in oxalated whole blood. Usually, a column 100 mm (Wintrobe) or 200 mm (Westergren) high by 1 millimeter in diameter is used, and the sample is left undisturbed for 1 hr. The rate of settling depends on the concentration of plasma proteins and on the concentration and changes in the shape of red blood cells. The significance of this test serves to document and monitor an inflammatory process.

2. ESR may be elevated in

   a. Inflammatory or autoimmune disease (e.g., rheumatoid arthritis, COPD, temporal arteritis)
   b. Pregnancy
   c. Infection
   d. Cancer/malignancy

e. Active tuberculosis
f. Kidney disease
g. Thyroid disease

3. ESR may be decreased in

a. Severe liver disease
b. Polycythemia
c. Sickle cell anemia
d. Congestive heart failure

4. Normal values

a. Male, 0–10 mm/hr (Wintrobe) 0–13 mm/hr (Westergren)
b. Female, 0–15 mm/hr (Wintrobe) 0–20 mm/hr (Westergren)

K. Differential white blood cell count (Diff.)

1. White blood cells (leukocytes) are necessary for the body to defend itself adequately against invading microorganisms. However, not all leukocytes help fight infection. For this reason, it is important to know the number of bacteria-fighting leukocytes (neutrophils). The Diff. is determined by counting 100 WBCs of all kinds and calculating the relative percentage for each type of cell.

Type of WBC	Normal value	Area of involvement
Neutrophils	60–70%	Bacterial infections
Bands	0–5%	A significant increase in Bands (immature neutrophils) as in a bacterial infection is called a "left shift"; a decrease to normal is called a "right shift."
Segmented (Segs)	40–60%	Mature neutrophils
Eosinophils	1–4%	Allergic disorders
Basophils	0.5–1%	Blood dyscrasias, infection, inflammation, and polycythemia vera
Lymphocytes	20–40%	Viral infections and other infectious diseases
Monocytes	2–6% / 100%	Severe infections when the infection is becoming controlled 100% (e.g., tuberculosis, subacute bacterial endocarditis) and Hodgkin's disease

2. Types of WBCs

a. **Neutrophils (Polys, Segs, PMNs or granulocytes)**
These cells are neutral staining. They are produced in the bone marrow and are the most common white cell in circulating blood. The classification of neutrophils is based upon the normal maturation sequence of the leukocyte. The stem cells give rise to myeloblasts, which

mature into promyelocytes, neutrophil myelocytes, neutrophil metamyeloytes, band neutrophils, and, finally, into polymorphonuclear segmented neutrophils.

Neutrophils may be increased (leukocytosis) in heart attacks, burns, stress response, bacterial infections, or inflammatory states such as pneumonia and appendicitis.

Neutrophils usually decrease (leukopenia) in acute viral infections, radiation, cancer chemotherapy, lupus erythematosus, and vitamin B_{12} or folic acid deficiencies.

These cells make up pus (pyria) and may ingest bacteria and other foreign material. Neutrophils are a combination of banded neutrophils (bands or immature neutrophils) and segmented neutrophils (segs or mature neutrophils).

b.   Eosinophils (eos)

These are acid-staining cells. They are formed in bone marrow from eosinophilic myelocytes. They are capable of locomotion and phagocytosis. They also contain digestive enzymes that are dispersed with ingestion of foreign material. Their primary importance is somewhat unknown, but it appears that they are attracted to and ingest "antigen-antibody" complexes.

They may be increased in parasitic and allergic reactions (e.g., hay fever, bronchial asthma, drug therapy, hypersensitivity), autoimmune diseases, adrenal insufficiency, some cancers and leukemias, and skin diseases. Eosinophils transport significant amounts of histamine in their granules.

c.   Basophils

These are basic-staining cells that are multinucleated. They are probably produced in bone marrow from myelocytes and are increased in blood dyscrasias and leukemias. Basophils would be increased in myelogenous leukemias, polycythemia vera, and Hodgkin's disease. Basophils would be decreased in hyperthyroidism, or pregnancy, following x- irradiation, chemotherapy, or administration of steroids.

d.   Lymphocytes (lymphs)

These cells are formed in lymphoid tissue of the spleen, intestine, and lymph nodes and are not phagocytic in nature. Lymphocytes constitute the second most common white cell in circulating blood. In early life, they originate from the thymus gland and usually survive about 100 days. Lymphocytes (about 33% of the leukocytes) are important in the process of producing immunity in the body. They are generally increased in number in immune diseases, bacterial infections, viral infections such as mumps, infectious mononucleosis, and German measles, and leukemias. Glucocorticoid (e.g., prednisone) therapy decreases lymphocyte production.

e. **Monocytes (monos)**

These are large mononucleated (lobulated) leukocytes that mature into macrophages. They are the largest corpuscle in the body (2–3 times RBC size). They possess phagocytic function, and are capable of locomotion. The cells contain lipases. They are attracted to the tubercle bacilli and leprosy bacilli. They are increased during chronic infections and during the recovery phase of an acute infection. They are also increased in subacute bacterial endocarditis, malaria, and tuberculosis.

f. **WBC normal values**

1) WBC 4,800–10,800/mm^3
2) Neutrophilia (>8000 cells/mm^3)
3) Neutropenia (<2000 cells/mm^3)
4) Agranulocytosis/severe neutropenia (<500 cells/mm^3)

II. **Serum electrolytes (sodium, potassium, chloride, and bicarbonate)**

A. Normal metabolism

1. Intake—enter the body by ingestion

a. 70–100 mEq daily of potassium
b. 69–208 mEq daily of sodium and chloride
c. 1500–3000 ml of water daily

2. Absorption—Potassium, sodium, chloride, and water are absorbed by an active diffusion process.

3. Normal values—all the major electrolytes and water are transported in the blood and lymphatics. The normal serum concentrations are

a. Sodium, 135–150 mEq/L
b. Potassium, 3.5–5.0 mEq/L
c. Chloride, 100–106 mEq/L
d. Bicarbonate, 24–30 mEq/L

A large amount of carbon dioxide is transported inside the red cells.

4. Production—Carbon dioxide and water are products of body metabolism of carbohydrate, fat, and protein. Approximately 300 ml of water are produced in this manner daily. Sodium, chloride, and potassium, by contrast, are fully exogenous in origin, but potassium and water are released from storage by cellular catabolism.

5. Storage—Sodium and chloride exist primarily in the extracellular and intravascular space in practically equivalent concentrations. In addition, a sizable amount of sodium is deposited in the bone and can be released as a safety device in acidosis.

   Potassium is mainly an intracellular cation. Its concentration here is approximately 160 mEq/liter. Potassium may be released into the extracellular space by catabolism. Potassium moves into the cell with the absorption of glucose with the aid of potassium ATPase.

   Bicarbonate is an extracellular ion, in concentration similar to that of the blood, but a ready supply is constantly pouring in from the catabolism of carbohydrate, protein and fat. Of course, it first appears as carbon dioxide, then carbonic acid, and thereafter much of it is transformed to sodium bicarbonate by the buffers of the plasma and red cells.

   Water in the amount equivalent to 40% of body weight is stored intracellularly, and an amount equivalent to 15–20% of body weight is stored extracellularly.

6. Secretion—Over 8 liters of fluid are secreted and reabsorbed in the gastrointestinal tract each day. The four types of secretions—gastric, biliary, pancreatic, and small intestine—all contain sodium, potassium, chloride, and bicarbonate. The gastric juice contains little or no bicarbonate but large amounts of hydrogen and chloride ions. The pancreatic, biliary, and intestinal fluids contain substantial amounts of bicarbonate but few hydrogen ions.

7. Excretion—The kidney, the major excretory organ, excretes in the urine 80–90% of the sodium, potassium, and chloride that is ingested. This amounts to about 111 mEq of sodium, 119 mEq of chloride, and 25–100 mEq of potassium in 24 hr. Although the kidney can reduce sodium chloride excretion to a bare minimum in deficiency states, significant potassium excretion continues.

   Bicarbonate is excreted by the kidney in varying amounts according to body needs. Carbon dioxide, by contrast, is excreted by lungs.

   The major portion of water is normally excreted by the

kidney. Approximately 400 ml are lost by way of the lungs and the skin by vaporization.

B.   Regulation—Two organs, the kidney and the lung, are primarily responsible for the control of body fluids and electrolytes and acid-base balance. Although variable amounts of fluids and electrolytes may be lost by way of the sweat glands and the gastrointestinal tract, these organs do not adjust their rate of secretion to meet body fluid and electrolyte requirements.

C.   The kidney—The kidney, under the influence of aldosterone hormone from the zona glomerulosa of the adrenal cortex and the antidiuretic hormone (ADH) from the posterior pituitary, plays a major role in the regulation of the tonicity, volume, and acidity of body fluids.

1.   Tonicity—If the plasma is hypertonic, the osmoreceptors in the supra-aortic nucleus are stimulated to release antidiuretic hormone (ADH). This activates the distal tubule to reabsorb more water from the filtrate, diluting the blood and concentrating the urine. If the plasma is hypotonic, then the secretion of ADH is inhibited, and the distal tubule reabsorbs less water from the filtrate, concentrating the blood and diluting the urine.

2.   Volume—If the blood and the extracellular fluid are low in volume, volume receptors, the exact location of which is unknown, are activated to induce aldosterone secretion, and more sodium is reabsorbed from the filtrate in exchange for potassium and hydrogen ions. The resulting hypertonicity of the plasma will lead to ADH secretion and water retention. Thus the volume is returned to normal.

3.   Acidity—The average diet contains substances with acid end-products (e.g., ammonium salts, sulfur-containing amino acids, phosphoric acid compounds). Furthermore, carbon dioxide is constantly being poured into the blood as an end-product of cellular metabolism. To a lesser degree, keto-acids are being produced in fat metabolism. These substances are buffered by the bicarbonate, phosphate, and other buffer systems so that the blood does not change radically from the normal pH range 7.35–7.45. These buffers must be maintained, particularly the sodium bicarbonate. The kidney and lung are primarily responsible for this.

The kidney's task is to recover bicarbonate and sodium from the glomerular filtrate. The kidney accomplishes this by three mechanisms:

a.   By reabsorbing all the sodium bicarbonate from the glomerular filtrate

b.   By acidifying urinary buffer salts such as disodium phosphate

c.   By excreting hydrogen ions as the ammonium salts of strong acids

All three mechanisms are based on one fundamental process: the tubular secretions of hydrogen ion in exchange for sodium in the tubular urine. A readily available source of hydrogen ion is provided by the conversion of water and carbon dioxide to carbonic acid under the influence of carbonic anhydrase in the tubular cell. The hydrogen ion of the carbonic acid is then exchanged for the sodium of sodium bicarbonate, sodium diphosphate, and strong acid salts (e.g., sodium chloride) of the glomerular filtrate in the following manner:

1) $Na\, HCO_3 \underset{\longleftarrow}{\overset{H^+}{\longrightarrow}} H_2CO_3 + Na^+$

2) $Na_2HPO_4 \underset{\longleftarrow}{\overset{H^+}{\longrightarrow}} NaH_2PO_4 + Na^+$

3) $NaCl \underset{NH_3}{\overset{H+}{\rightleftharpoons}} NH_4Cl + Na_+$

(ammonium is added by the renal tubular cells)

The sodium released by these mechanisms combines with the bicarbonate of the tubular cell and enters the blood as sodium bicarbonate.

D.   The lung—Extra carbon dioxide produced by the metabolism of carbohydrate, fat, and protein or the buffering of acids stimulates the respiratory center to increase respirations, so that the extra carbon dioxide is excreted through the lung, and the normal pH range is maintained.

E.   Other mechanisms—Water secretion may be influenced by thyroid hormone. The electrolyte composition of the extracellular fluid may be altered by the pH of the blood through other than renal mechanisms. For example, in acidosis, hydrogen ions move into the cell in exchange for potassium. In alkalosis, sodium ion moves into the cell in exchange for potassium, which is then excreted. Thus, the cell itself becomes an effective buffer.

F.   Clinical significance of electrolytes

1.   **Serum sodium (Na^+)**
Sodium is the chief cation in extracellular fluid and in association with anions; it provides the bulk of the osmotically active solutes in the plasma. Water tends to follow the sodium ion because of its high osmotic activity, and a change in the

sodium concentration will cause a change in the extracellular fluid volume. It is also essential in acid-base balance.

a.   Normal value, 135–150 mEq/L
b.   Hypernatremia, elevated sodium levels

    1)   Dehydration
    2)   Primary aldosteronism
    3)   Nephrotic syndrome
    4)   Drugs (e.g., antihypertensive agents, phenylbutazone and nonsteroidal anti-inflammatory drugs, steroids)
    5)   Diabetes insipidus
    6)   Hyperadrenocorticism
    7)   CNS trauma or disease

c.   Hyponatremia—decreased sodium levels

    1)   Adrenal insufficiency syndromes, including Addison's disease
    2)   Renal tubular acidosis
    3)   Overhydration (dilutional)
    4)   Cirrhosis of liver—especially patients with ascites
    5)   Severe diarrhea or vomiting
    6)   Salt-wasting renal failure
    7)   Over-aggressive diuretic therapy
    8)   Trauma, burns
    9)   Syndrome of inappropriate antidiuretic hormone

2.   Serum potassium (K^+)
Like sodium, potassium is important in cation-anion balance and is the all important intracellular cation. Potassium concentration in the plasma or serum will affect intracellular potassium (equilibrium) and determine the state of neuromuscular and muscular irritability. High extracellular levels can lead to arrhythmias and cardiac standstill.

a.   Normal value—3.5–5.0 mEq/L
b.   Hyperkalemia—elevated K^+ levels:

    1)   Renal disorders: renal insufficiency with excess protein and breakdown of other tissues
    2)   Iatrogenic: inappropriate use of K supplements and/or K-sparing diuretics
    3)   Adrenal insufficiency
    4)   Drugs: potassium-sparing diuretics, angiotensin-converting enzyme inhibitors
    5)   Diabetic ketoacidosis

      6)   Hemolized serum specimen (RBCs lyse) during sample collection or during vigorous exercise

c.   Hypokalemia—decreased K^+ levels:

    1)   Starvation
    2)   Loss due to vomiting and diarrhea
    3)   Unusual urinary loss—in polyuric phase of chronic nephritis
    4)   Unusual urinary loss due to hyperadrenalcorticism and adrenal corticosteroid therapy
    5)   Unusual loss due to intense potassium-wasting diuretic therapy (e.g., thiazides, furosemide, ethacrynic acid, metolazone, bumetanide)

3.   **Serum chloride (Cl^-)**
Chloride is the principle inorganic anion in the extracellular fluid. Shifts in the amounts of this ion usually mean a shift in the acid-base balance. Loss of Cl as HCl or NH_4Cl will lead to alkalosis; retention of Cl will cause acidosis.

a.   Normal value—100–106 mEq/L
b.   Hyperchloremia—elevated Cl levels

    1)   Renal insufficiency when chloride intake exceeds excretion
    2)   Nephrosis, overtreatment with saline infusion, i.e., hypertonic saline IVs
    3)   Hyperparathyroidism
    4)   Dehydration (severe)
    5)   Excessive salt intake

c.   Hypochloremia—decreased Cl levels

    1)   Excess loss of GI fluids: vomiting, diarrhea, severe burns
    2)   Alkalosis—can be induced by diuretic therapy
    3)   Renal insufficiency (with salt deprivation)
    4)   Diabetic ketoacidosis
    5)   Respiratory acidosis
    6)   Excessive diuresis
    7)   Adrenal insufficiency

4.   **Serum bicarbonate (HCO_3^-)**
Bicarbonate-carbonic acid buffer is one of the most important buffer systems maintaining the normal pH of body fluids. Bicarbonate levels indicate the acid-base balance in the body.

a.   Normal value, 24–30 mEq/L
b.   Elevated levels in

1) Metabolic alkalosis
2) Respiratory acidosis associated with emphysema, hypoventilation, sedative overdose, narcotics
3) Protracted vomiting and loss of potassium
4) Excessive intake of antacids
5) Diuretics (thiazides and loop diuretics)

   c. Decreased levels in

1) Metabolic acidosis associated with salicylate intoxication, diabetic ketoacidosis, lactic acidosis, and renal insufficiency.
2) Respiratory alkalosis associated with hyperventilation
3) Starvation
4) Severe diarrhea

III. Kidney function—tests for renal function, glomerular filtration, and tubular reabsorption

A. Blood urea nitrogen (BUN)

1. Physiological basis and function
   Urea is the end-product of protein metabolism and prevents the accumulation of toxic ammonia resulting from protein catabolism. Urea in the body is synthesized primarily in the liver and is excreted by the kidneys. Some urea is reabsorbed from the tubule filtrate.

   a. Characteristics of BUN
      1) Amount filtered—100%
      2) Amount reabsorbed—40%
      3) Amount renally excreted—60%

   b. Interferences with BUN

      1) Gastrointestinal tract bleeding—increase BUN
      2) Hemolytic anemia—increase BUN
      3) Diet—increase or decrease BUN
      4) Deydration will increase BUN concentration
      5) Fluid overload will decrease BUN concentration

2. Normal values, 8–25 mg/dl
3. Clinical significance

   a. Elevated levels

      1) Renal insufficiency or failure
      2) Decreased renal blood flow (shock or very low blood pressure)
      3) Dehydration

　　　　　　　4) Nephritis
　　　　　　　5) Drugs (e.g., diuretics, nephrotoxicity from drugs: aminoglycosides, cephalosporins)
　　　　　　　6) Muscle-wasting diseases
　　　　　　　7) Hyperthyroidism
　　　　　　　8) Increased nitrogen metabolism
　　　　　　　9) Urinary tract obstruction
　　　　　　10) Gastrointestinal bleeding or hemolytic anemia

　　　b. Decreased levels

　　　　　　　1) Hepatic failure (no synthesis)
　　　　　　　2) Dilutional state
　　　　　　　3) Low protein diet or malnutrition
　　　　　　　4) Toxemia of pregnancy

B. Serum creatinine (SrCr)

　　1. Physiological basis
　　　Creatinine is a breakdown product of muscle metabolism. It has a relatively constant hourly and daily production and stable blood levels. Creatinine is transported through the blood to the kidneys where it is excreted almost exclusively by filtration through the renal glomeruli. Since creatinine is excreted solely by the kidney, increased levels of creatinine are normally a reliable index of decreased renal function. However, in elderly patients, the SrCr may be in the normal range in values but, due to decreased muscle mass, may in fact indicate decreased renal function. Individuals with large muscle mass have higher serum creatinine levels than those with less muscle. Normal values for men are usually slightly higher than those for women. Creatinine is excreted through the kidneys in quantities proportional to the serum content. The most common cause of elevated serum creatinine levels is impairment of renal function. As renal function diminishes, serum creatinine levels increase. Factors that may elevate SrCr include muscle-wasting diseases, corticosteroid therapy, urinary tract obstruction, hyperthyroidism, and drug-laboratory interactions (e.g., cephalosporins increase SrCr levels).
　　2. Normal values, 0.7–1.5 mg/dl

C. Creatinine clearance (CrCl)

　　1. Physiological basis
　　　Creatinine clearance is defined as that volume of plasma from which a measured amount of creatinine could be completely eliminated ("cleared") into urine per unit time. For all practical purposes, creatinine clearance parallels glomerular filtration rate. Creatinine clearance indicates the efficiency with

which the kidneys remove creatinine from the blood; thus, declining renal function leads to a decline in creatinine clearance. Creatinine clearance determinations require a 24–hour urine collection. When urine specimen collections are either impractical or cannot be obtained, creatinine clearance may be estimated from the serum creatinine by using the Cockroft-Gault or Jelliffe methods.

2. Normal values, 90–120 ml/min

    a. Cockroft—Gault formula (for males)

$$(140 - \text{age})\ \text{LBW}\ (\text{kg})/72 \times \text{SrCr} = \text{CrCl in ml/min}/1.73\ \text{m}^2$$

    (female CrCl = male CrCl x 0.9)

    b. Jelliffe formula (for males)

$$98 - (0.8)(\text{age-20})/\text{SrCr} = \text{CrCl in ml/min}/70\ \text{kg}$$

    (female CrCl = male CrCl x 0.9).

IV. Serum acid and alkaline phosphatases

Due to measurable changes in their serum concentrations in diseases of the prostate, hepatobiliary, and skeletal systems, the phosphatases are one group of many groups of enzymes that are of clinical significance.

A. Production—The alkaline phosphatases are highly active at pHs of 9 to 10 and are widely distributed in tissue of the intestinal mucosa (where it most active), followed by the kidney, bone, thyroid, and liver. The acid phosphatases are highly active at a pH of 5.0 and are more prevalent in male urine.

B. Physiologically—They are necessary for the hydrolysis of organic phosphates, and in this role they become important in digestion and mucosal absorption. They also function in aiding deposition of $CaPO_4$ in bony tissue.

C. Normal values—Both alkaline and acid phosphatase are found circulating in the blood.

    1. **Acid phosphatase levels**—Normal level is 0.2–0.8 Bodansky units (1–4 King-Armstrong units)/100 ml.

    2. **Alkaline phosphatase levels**—Normal level is 1–4 Bodansky units (8–14 King-Armstrong units)/100 ml or 35–120 U/L.

D. Clinical significance

    1. **Alkaline phosphatase**—This test is very useful in distinguishing hepatocellular obstruction and jaundice. In hepatocellular or biliary tree obstruction, jaundice is infrequently

present, whereas in hepatocellular damage, jaundice is almost always present. Hepatomegaly without jaundice suggests metastatic liver disease, leukemia, tuberculosis, sarcoidosis, amyloidosis, and fibrosis. Values are usually elevated in hyperparathyroidism, rickets, hepatic duct obstruction, hepatitis, and hepatocellular diseases. Slightly elevated concentrations (5–15 Bodansky units) are found in the growth phase of development, pregnancy, and hyperparathyroidism, this being due to increased osteoblastic activity. General debility and hypothyroidism anemia have been associated with somewhat lower values.

2. **Acid phosphatase**—This test is sometimes called the "male PAP test" and is most useful in diagnosing metastatic carcinoma of the prostate that has spread beyond the capsule. Elevated values may be found in cancer of the breast (with skeletal metastasis) and cancer of the prostate (with bone metastasis). When tumors have been successfully treated, enzyme levels decrease within 3–4 days of surgical castration (or after 3–4 weeks of estrogen therapy).

V. **Serum amylase—test for pancreatic function**

A. Physiological basis and function
Amylases are a group of enzymes responsible for the hydrolytic degradation of starch and glycogen. The enzymes are present in the pancreas and salivary glands. Their activity is extracellular, and they are excreted in the urine.

B. Normal values—80–180 Somogyi units/dl or 0.8–3.2 U/L

C. Clinical significance

1. Elevated levels in

   a. Acute pancreatitis
   b. Obstruction of pancreatic ducts
   c. Mumps (parotitis epidemic)
   d. Perforated peptic ulcer
   e. Cirrhosis of liver with pancreatic involvement
   f. Diabetic ketoacidosis
   g. Analgesic narcotics (codeine, morphine, etc.)
   h. Renal insufficiency
   i. Use of drugs (e.g., corticosteroids, indomethacin, salicylates, furosemide, tetracyclines, chlorthalidone, ethacrynic acid, codeine, morphine, meperidine, alcohol, cyproheptadine)

2. Decreased levels in

   a. Hepatitis (acute and chronic)
   b. Pancreatic insufficiency

   c.   Toxemia of pregnancy
   d.   Drug use—barbiturates

VI.   **Serum bilirubin (Bili)**
Serum bilirubin concentration is the foundation of laboratory diagnosis of liver disease. It is also a value that aids understanding of liver physiology.

A.   Production—Bilirubin is a by-product of hemoglobin metabolism and is derived mainly from this substance. However, 25–30% is derived from other substances, such as myoglobin, catalases, and cytochromes. As a result of physiological red cell destruction, 7–8 g of hemoglobin becomes available for disintegration each day. The site of this disintegration lies within the cells of the reticuloendothelial system (liver, spleen, bone marrow, etc.). Unconjugated bilirubin (fat-soluble) binds with plasma albumin and is then cleared by the liver. Bilirubin is conjugated with glucuronide in the liver (water-soluble now) and excreted as bile via the feces. The total bilirubin test value is the sum of the conjugated and unconjugated. If only the conjugated form is increased, this means the bile drainage is obstructed. If the unconjugated form is increased, the liver is not functioning properly.

B.   Normal values

   1.   Direct (conjugated), 0.1–0.4 mg/100 ml
   2.   Indirect (unconjugated), 0.2–0.8 mg/100 ml
   3.   Total, up to 1.0 mg/100 ml (indirect + direct bilirubin)

C.   Metabolism—Serum bilirubin is insoluble in water and is transported in the plasma to the liver parenchymal cells, where it is conjugated with glucuronic acid in the presence of glycuronyl transferase and uridine triphosphate to form bilirubin diglucuronide. The conjugated form is water-soluble and is excreted in the bile.

D.   Excretion—Bilirubin is a waste product and is excreted in the bile, where it accounts for the bile's pigmentation. After bilirubin is transferred into the bile, it passes through the bile canaliculi, cholangioles, the hepatic ducts, the common bile duct, and into the duodenum. Once in the gastrointestinal tract, bilirubin is changed by the colon bacteria to other compounds (i.e., the uro- and the sterco- bilinogens and bilins). It is the stercobilins that give the characteristic brown color to feces. Absence of bilirubin products make feces light brown, gray, or colorless, as in obstructive jaundice. Water soluble bilirubin can be excreted by the kidneys in cases of its accumulation in the blood (e.g., obstructive jaundice).

E.   Clinical significance
      Hyperbilirubinemia—elevated levels

1. Acute or chronic hepatitis (swelling of ducts causes obstruction)
2. Biliary tract obstruction (stones or tumor)
3. Drug reaction (toxic or hypersensitivity, hepatotoxic reactions (e.g., anabolic steroids, isoniazid, phenothiazines, and erythromycin estolate)
4. Increased production of bilirubin due to red blood cell destruction (hemolytic anemia)—indirect
5. Decreased excretion of bilirubin from liver disease (e.g., viral, alcoholic or toxic hepatitis, cirrhosis, infectious mononucleosis).

VII.   Bromsulphalein retention test (BSP)

A. Physiologic basis and function
The BSP is the most sensitive measure of hepatic function. BSP, a dye, is administered intravenously and its degree of clearance from blood is measured. Normally, BSP is completely cleared by the liver. There are two factors involved in the test:

1. Normal hepatic function (metabolism or conjugation)
2. Adequate hepatic circulation
About 80% of the injected dye is cleared by the liver. The remaining 20% is excreted by other organs. The patient is weighed and given an IV dose of 5 mg/kg. After 45 minutes, the dye concentration in the blood is determined and expressed as the amount retained. Normally, individuals have less than 5% retention after 45 minutes. The test is of greatest value in patients with little or no jaundice.

B. Excretion of BSP—This process depends upon three steps:

1. The dye is transported from the blood to a hepatic cell (transportation)
2. It is stored in the cell and conjugated with glutathione (conjugation)
3. The conjugate is excreted by active transport into the liver bile (bile excretion)

C. Elevated BSP retention occurs in the following conditions:

1. Biliary cirrhosis or obstruction
2. Cancer of the liver
3. Chloroform poisoning
4. Chronic congestion of the liver
5. Hepatitis
6. Acute cholestasis (cholecystitis)

VIII. Serum calcium

Disorders of calcium metabolism are associated with alterations in serum phosphates and alkaline phosphatase as well as calcium.

A. Physiological basis and function

In addition to contributing to anion-cation balance, calcium is essential for the formation of bony tissue, for proper muscle activity, and in blood coagulation. Endocrine, renal, gastrointestinal, and nutritional factors are involved in maintaining the serum calcium concentration.

B. Intake

The usual daily requirement of calcium for premenopausal females and males is 1000 mg. Postmenopausal females should take 1500 mg of calcium per day. The daily requirement of phosphorus is about 800 mg.

C. Absorption

Calcium and phosphorus are absorbed by the small intestine with the help of vitamin D and parathyroid hormone. Absorption is assisted by the acid pH in the intestine. Large amounts of phosphorous, fats, or phytic acid in the diet inhibit calcium absorption (decreases 50%).

D. Normal values

Calcium is transported in the blood in two forms. Half is in an unionized protein-bound form, and the other half is ionized with phosphate. The total calcium concentration is normally 8.5–10.5 mg/dl and the ionized fraction is 4.5 to 5.0 mg/dl. The ionizable fraction is distributed throughout the extracellular fluid, but neither the protein-bound nor the ionizable fraction is present in significant quantities in the intracellular fluid. The inorganic phosphate of the plasma ranges from 3 to 4 mg/dl in adults and 4.5 to 6.5 mg/dl in children. Unlike calcium, it is present in large quantities in the cell.

E. Storage

Approximately 1100 g of calcium are stored in the bones (2–3% of body weight). About 80–90% of the total body phosphate is "stored" in bone. The remainder is stored in both intracellular and extracellular fluid. Vitamin D probably exerts a calcemic effect on bone, and parathyroid hormone stimulates resorption of bone.

F. Excretion

Calcium and phosphate are excreted in the urine and feces. Most calcium in the feces is that which has escaped absorption. In 24 hr, 100–150 mg of calcium are excreted in the urine. Of the calcium filtered through the glomerulus, about 99% is reabsorbed. The amount of reabsorption is apparently influenced by vitamin D and parathyroid hormone. Urinary phosphate accounts for about

60% of the total excretion under normal conditions. The rest is excreted in the feces. About 80% is reabsorbed by the renal tubules, the remainder passes into the urine. The amount of urinary phosphate excretion is influenced by parathyroid hormone and vitamin D, as well as by the glomerular filtration rate.

G. Regulation

A fall in serum calcium stimulates the secretion of the parathyroid hormone. As a consequence, calcium is mobilized from bone by reabsorption, calcium absorption from the intestine and the renal tubule is enhanced, and phosphate secretion by renal tubules is increased, or its reabsorption by the renal tubules is inhibited. A rise in serum calcium stimulates the secretion of calcitonin from either the thyroid or parathyroid gland, returning the serum calcium to normal. Vitamin D influences serum calcium by raising the intestinal absorption of calcium. The total serum concentration of calcium varies directly with the concentration of the serum protein. The ionizable fraction varies indirectly with the pH. A high pH (alkalosis) decreases the ionizable calcium fraction and a low pH (acidosis) increases its level.

H. Clinical significance

A disorder of calcium metabolism might be suspected whenever a patient presents with renal calculi, bone disease, convulsions, or tetany.

1. Hypercalcemia—elevated levels

    a. Hyperparathyroidism
    b. Hypervitaminosis D
    c. Invasion of bone by metastatic carcinoma
    d. Multiple myeloma
    e. Paget's disease
    f. Drugs—thiazide diuretics

2. Hypocalcemia—decreased levels

    a. Hypoparathyroidism
    b. Vitamin D deficiency
    c. Cushing's syndrome or long-term corticosteroid therapy
    d. Renal insufficiency
    e. Pancreatitis
    f. Hypoproteinemia (albuminemia)
    g. Drugs—furosemide and phenytoin
    h. Low dietary intake of calcium
        Body deficits of calcium, whether due to the decreased intake or excessive output, induce the compensatory mechanism of secondary hyperparathyroidism.

IX.   **Serum cholesterol (Chol)**

    A.   Physiological basis and function

        Cholesterol concentration is associated with lipid metabolism. It is derived from dietary intake and synthesized by most body tissues. It seems to have an antihemolytic effect, perhaps serving as an insulator in brain tissue and as a precursor for synthesis of steroids and vitamin D. The liver has a prominent role in cholesterol metabolism, and liver function is measured by cholesterol levels. High serum cholesterol levels are thought to increase the risk of atherosclerosis.

    B.   Normal values—150–200 mg/dl

    C.   Clinical significance

        1.   Hypercholesterolemia—elevated levels

            a.   Hereditary defects

            b.   Hypothyroidism

            c.   Chronic hepatitis, obstructive jaundice

            d.   Poorly controlled diabetes

            e.   Nephrotic syndrome

            f.   Biliary cirrhosis

        2.   Hypocholesterolemia—decreased levels

            a.   Acute infections

            b.   Anemia and malnutrition

            c.   Hyperthyroidism

            d.   Acute hepatitis

X.   **Creatine phosphokinase (CPK) or creatine kinase (CK)**

    A.   Physiological basis and function

        This is an enzyme involved in the transfer of the high-energy phosphates between creatine, phosphocreatine, ADP, and ATP. The highest concentrations of this enzyme occur in striated muscle (skeletal and heart) with lesser amounts in heart and cerebral cortex. There is no CPK in red blood cells or liver. Tests to measure levels of this enzyme can help distinguish between acute myocardial infarction and liver diseases.

    B.   Normal values

        1.   Males, 55–170 IU/L

        2.   Females, 30–135 IU/L

    C.   Clinical significance

        1.   CPK elevations occur in the following conditions:

            a.   Progressive muscular dystrophy

            b.   Strenuous exercise

  c. Myocardial infarction: here, CPK increases after 4 h, peaks between 24 and 36 h, and is again normal in 2–4 days.

  d. Electrical cardiac defibrillation

  e. Seizures

  f. IM injections

  g. Muscular inflammation

The levels of CPK appear normal in angina, pericarditis, pulmonary infarction, renal infarction, renal disease, biliary obstruction, pernicious anemia, and malignancies. Thus, this test is useful in ruling out disorders of the pancreas and biliary tract.

D. Creatine kinase isoenzymes—consist of three proteins

 1. Clinical significance

  a. Elevated CK isoenzymes in:

   1) CK-MM (found mainly in skeletal muscle) Injury to skeletal muscle, myocardial muscle, and brain; after severe exercise

   2) CK-MB (found mainly in heart muscle) Elevated (within 2–4 hours) after a myocardial infarction and remains elevated for 72 hours

   3) CK-BB (found mainly in brain tissue) Occasionally elevated in severe shock; oat cell carcinoma, carcinoma of the ovary, breast, or prostate; and biliary atresia

 2. Normal values

CK isoenzymes		Normal levels (% of total)
(Fastest)	Fraction 1, BB	0
	Fraction 2, MB	<4–6
(Slowest)	Fraction 3, MM	>94–96

XI. Blood glucose and normal metabolism

A. Physiological basis and function—Blood sugar is measured to determine the body's insulin production ability.

B. Intake—Glucose enters the body by way of the mouth in the form of starch, dextrin, or other carbohydrates. In the gastrointestinal tract, these substances are broken down by ptyalin, hydrochloric acid, pancreatic amylase, lactase, and other enzymes to glucose, fructose, and other sugars.

C. Absorption—Glucose is absorbed in the small intestine by both an active and a passive diffusion process. It is believed that glucose is phosphorylated by the intestinal cell and then discharged to the blood with the aid of a phosphatase. Absorption seems favorably influenced by thyroid and adrenocortical hormones as well as by vitamin B complex.

D.   Normal value—Glucose is transported by the blood. The concentration is maintained within a relatively narrow range of 70–110 mg/100 ml under fasting conditions.

E.   Storage—Glucose is stored as glycogen, primarily in the liver and muscle. Approximately 300–500 g are stored in this manner in the average adult. Liver glycogen is readily returned to the blood by the action of hepatic phosphorylase and glucose-6-phosphatase, according to body needs. Peripheral stores of glucose may be converted to fat and stored in this form.

F.   Production—The liver is the primary site of glucose production. It may convert lactic acid to glycogen and subsequently convert this to glucose under the influence of epinephrine. The liver may convert fat and protein to glucose (gluconeogenesis) by way of Krebs cycle.

G.   Destruction—When metabolized, glucose forms carbon dioxide, water, and energy. Many enzymes influence the anaerobic and the aerobic catabolism of glucose. Thiamine and pantothenic acid are essential for proper utilization so that glucose may be transferred into the cell. Apparently, insulin is responsible for this process.

H.   Excretion—Glucose is filtered through the glomeruli, but ordinarily almost all of this is reabsorbed by the proximal tubules (similar to intestinal absorption-phosphorylation). If the blood sugar exceeds 180 mg/dl (the renal threshold), increasing amounts of sugar will appear in the urine.

I.   Regulation—In a fasting individual, the liver is the primary source of blood glucose. A decrease in blood sugar will increase liver output of glucose. Increased blood sugar stimulates the islet cells of the pancreas to secrete insulin and inhibits the liver output of glucose. This homeostatic mechanism of the liver is influenced by several hormones—notably insulin, thyroid, adrenocortical hormone, and epinephrine and possibly by glycogen.

1.   Insulin—Facilitates the transfer of extracellular free glucose across the cell membrane. It may also influence the deposition of glycogen in the liver and inhibits gluconeogenesis from protein.

2.   Thyroid—Stimulates the intestinal and renal tubular absorption of glucose. By elevating the metabolic rate, it increases the peripheral utilization of glucose.

3.   Adrenocortical hormone—The glucocorticoids mobilize protein and fat stores and in some way favorably influence hepatic gluconeogenesis. Adrenocortical hormone may also decrease the cells' capacity to utilize glucose.

4.   Epinephrine—Either directly or indirectly, provokes glycogenolysis in both liver and muscle. An increase in blood sugar occurs after its administration.

5. Glucagon—This hormone in the alpha cells of the pancreas promotes glycogenolysis in the liver.
6. Growth hormone—This hormone of the anterior pituitary is believed to reduce the rate of glucose phosphorylation by the cell, to cause insulin resistance, and to lead to destruction of beta cells of the pancreas.

J. Clinical significance

1. Elevated blood glucose by drugs: steroids, diuretics (especially thiazides), phenytoin, and beta blockers. Increased levels are usually found in diabetes mellitus, hyperthyroidism, hyperpituitarism, and adrenal hyperactivity.
2. Decreased blood glucose by drugs: oral hypoglycemic drugs, insulin, and beta blockers. Blood glucose levels are decreased in hyperinsulinism or adrenal insufficiency and hypopituitarism.

K. Glucose tests for diabetes mellitus

1. **Acetone (urine)**
   In a condition such as diabetes, sugar is not utilized properly, and therefore, excessive fat may be metabolized. The fatty acids are metabolized and converted into ketone bodies (acetone), which are then excreted by the kidneys. The Acetest detects ketones and is read as: negative, trace, moderate, or large amounts.
2. **Fasting blood glucose/sugar (FBS)—70–110 mg/dl**
   Elevated in diabetes mellitus, hyperthyroidism, and adrenocortical hyperactivity. It is decreased in hyperinsulinism, adrenal insufficiency, and hypopituitarism.
3. **Glucose tolerance test (GTT)—70–110 mg/dl**
   Purpose—to measure the ability of the body to absorb and metabolize glucose. A measured amount of glucose is administered orally, and, at intervals, blood and urine samples are obtained and analyzed for glucose.

   a. Diabetic curve—A higher than normal peak with a slow return to fasting level.

	FBS	30 min	1 hr	2 hr	3 hr	Clinitest
Normal	100	160	160	110	80–110	neg.
Equivocal	120	130–160	160	110–120	110–120	1+–2+
Diabetes	120	160	160	120	120	2+–4+

   b. Hyperinsulinism—A normal curve with exaggerated fall to the hypoglycemic level.

    c.   Hepatic disease—A higher than normal curve with a rapid return to and below the fasting level in 3–4 hours.

4.   **2-hour postprandial blood glucose/sugar (2HrPPBS)**

In patients who have normal insulin secretion, this value should not increase above 140–160 mg/dl and is usually <120 mg/dl. Patients who are between 140 and 200 mg/dl should probably be tested by a GTT for diabetes. Patients who are above 200 mg/dl on the 2HrPPBS are in all probability diabetics. The 2HrPPBS is also used to determine if a patient's insulin dose is providing adequate coverage for the meal tested.

5.   **4-PM blood glucose/sugar (4PMBS)**

Should be normal (70–110 mg/dl). This test is used to see if an intermediate acting insulin is maintaining proper control of the blood sugar at its peak action (6–8 hours). The 4PMBS should not be too high or too low. It is a very useful test for adjusting the maintenance dose of intermediate insulins.

6.   **CLINITEST**

Urine test for reducing substances. Normally it should be negative. Positive results are read from a color chart and are classified 1+ to 4+, based on the quantitative amount of sugar in the urine.

7.   **Glycohemoglobin (glycosolated hemoglobin or HbA$_{1c}$)**

The glycosolated hemoglobin test measures the percentage of hemoglobin molecules that have sugar molecules attached to them. The percentage of the total hemoglobin that has sugar attached to it reflects the "average" blood sugar levels over the preceding 3–4 months. Elevated values may indicate diabetes in poor control. Highly elevated values almost always indicate diabetes in poor control.

Normal values, 3–6% of total hemoglobin.

XII.   **Serum aspartate aminotransferase (AST)—formerly called glutamic oxaloacetic transaminase (SGOT)—and alanine aminotransferase (ALT)—formerly called serum glutamic pyruvic transaminase (SGPT)**

A.   Physiological basis and function

These enzymes are responsible for biochemical reactions involving the transamination of amide groups according to the body's amino acid requirements. These enzymes are only intracellular and only minute amounts are normally found in the blood. They are released from cells when they are damaged (trauma, ischemia) and undergo necrosis. SGOT and ALT (SGPT) have their highest concentration in heart and liver cells, and ALT (SGPT) is highest in liver cells. SGOT is present in skeletal muscle, brain, and kidney tissue. Therefore, increased levels must be correlated with symptoms to determine the site of their release.

B.   Normal values—vary widely with clinical laboratories

    1.   AST (SGOT), 8–40 U/ml
    2.   ALT (SGPT), 5–35 U/ml

C.   Clinical significance

    1.   Elevated levels

        a.   Myocardial infarction—elevated in first 12 hr, reaches maximum in 24–48 hr, and returns to normal in 4–7 days (mainly SGOT)
        b.   Liver disease (hepatitis) ALT (SGPT) mainly
        c.   Severe burns—tissue damage causes rise of both SGOT and ALT (SGPT)
        d.   Cerebral thrombosis or hemorrhage
        e.   Trauma to muscles (SGOT)
        f.   Drugs that may cause hepatic damage (see bilirubin)
        g.   Hemolytic anemia
        h.   Infectious mononucleosis and polymyositis

XIII.   Serum iron

A.   Physiological basis and function of iron
Iron is an essential mineral for the body. The total amount of iron absorbed from a regular diet is about 10%. Absorption of iron is greatest in the proximal portion of the small intestine. Gastric juice or acidity enhances iron absorption. Iron in the stomach exists as the ferrous or the ferric ion. The ferric ion is reduced to the *ferrous* ion and is then absorbed into the mucosal cell of the GI tract. In the mucosal cell, ferrous ions are oxidized to the ferric state and then become attached to a complex known as *ferritin*. When the iron is liberated to the plasma, it exists in the ferrous state and is picked up by an iron-binding protein (beta-globulin). This combination is known as *transferrin*. This molecule is the transporting mechanism of iron throughout the body and is also known as "serum iron."

B.   Normal values, 50–150 µg/dl

C.   Clinical significance

    1.   Elevated levels

        a.   Sickle cell anemia
        b.   Hemolytic anemia
        c.   Excessive iron intake (oral, IM, or IV)
        d.   Pernicious anemia

2. Decreased levels

    a. Iron deficiency anemia
    b. Hemorrhage
    c. Anemia of chronic disease
    d. Infections
    e. Nephrosis
    f. Chronic renal insufficiency

XIV. Total iron-binding capacity (TIBC)

A. Physiological basis and function
Free iron in the plasma is picked up by iron-binding proteins (beta-globulins) called transferrin. The amount of iron that can bind with transferrin and the amount of transferrin itself can be measured. The ability of transferrin to bind and transport iron in the plasma is the idea of total iron binding capacity.
B. Normal value, 250–410 mcg/dl
C. Clinical significance

1. Elevated values

    a. Acute hemorrhage
    b. Anemia due to pregnancy
    c. Iron deficiency anemia
    d. Use of oral contraceptives
    e. Pyridoxine deficiency

2. Decreased values

    a. Hemolytic anemia
    b. Sickle cell anemia
    c. Anemia of chronic disease
    d. Cirrhosis of the liver
    e. Uremia
    f. High serum iron

XV. Serum lactic dehydrogenase (LDH)

A. Physiological basis and function
LDH is found within most body cells and consists of five proteins. It is an intracellular enzyme and is found in high concentration in the serum if tissue damage and necrosis have occurred. The tissue releasing the enzyme cannot be determined by the test and so must correlate with clinical symptoms. The enzyme is a catalyst for reactions involving lactic acid and pyruvic acid.
B. Clinical Significance

1. Elevated levels

    a. Myocardial infarction—rises within 72 hr and remains high for 1 week

      b.   Pulmonary embolism

      c.   Increased in 50% of patients with malignant advanced tumors and in 90% with acute leukemia

      d.   Infectious mononucleosis

      e.   Acute liver disease

      f.   Patients receiving radiation therapy

      g.   Trauma

      h.   Hemolytic anemia, B_{12} and folate deficiencies

      i.   Osteoporosis

      j.   Polycythemia vera

C.   Normal value (Wacher), 100–225 IU/L

Of more value than the total LDH is the electrophoretic measurement of LDH isoenzymes. LDH has five isoenzymes that are separable through chromatography.

D.   LDH isoenzymes:

    1.   Normal values

LDH isoenzymes		% of total (range)
(Fastest)	1 (alpha$_1$)	28 (15–30)
	2 (alpha$_2$)	36 (22–50)
	3 (beta)	23 (15–30)
	4 (gamma^1)	6 (0–15)
(Slowest)	5 (gamma$_2$)	6 (0–15)

    2.   Clinical significance

      a. $LDH_1(\alpha^1)$ The greatest concentration occurs in heart with a lesser concentration in red blood cells and kidney cortex.

      b. LDH_2 (α_2) Equal concentrations in RBC and heart.

      c. LDH_3 (β) A greater concentration occurring in long and skeletal muscles than in RBCs.

      d. LDH_4 (γ_1) Lung is greater than skeletal muscle concentrations.

      e. LDH_5 ($\gamma2$) Liver is greater than red blood cell concentration, which is greater than lung and skeletal muscle concentrations.

    3.   Interpretation

      a.   In a myocardial infarction, the alpha isoenzymes are elevated to yield a ratio of $LDH_1:LDH_2$ of 1.0.

      b. LDH_5 and LDH_4 are relatively increased in acute hepatitis, acute muscle injury, dermatomyositis, and muscular dystrophies.

XVI.   Total proteins (TP)

A.   Physiological basis and function

1.   Total proteins in the blood include albumin, globulins, and fibrinogen.

    a.   Albumin—the most abundant protein. It is synthesized in the liver and is responsible for 75% of the total colloidal osmotic pressure of plasma. It binds with many drugs.

    b.   Globulins—have an important role in the immune mechanism of the body. The globulins carry drugs as well as sex and thyroid hormones, lipids, and iron.

    c.   Fibrinogen—the soluble precursor of fibrin which forms blood clots.

B.   Normal values

1.   Albumin, 3.5–5.0 g/dl
2.   Globulin, 2.3–3.5 g/dl
3.   Fibrinogen, 0.2–0.4 g/dl
4.   Total protein, 6.0–8.5 g/dl

C.   Clinical significance

1.   Albumin (3.5–5.0 g/dl)

    a.   Elevated in dehydration, shock and anabolic hormones
    b.   Decreased in malnutrition, malabsorption, nephrosis, acute and chronic hepatic insufficiency, neoplastic disease, leukemia, overhydration, and severe burns

2.   Globulin (2.3–3.6 g/dl)

    a.   Elevated in liver and biliary cirrhosis, acute and chronic infections, neoplastic diseases, and malaria
    b.   Decreased in malnutrition, hepatic insufficiency, and lymphatic leukemia

3.   Fibrinogen (0.2–0.4 g/dl)

    a.   Elevated in nephrosis, glomerulonephritis, and infectious diseases
    b.   Decreased in hepatic insufficiency and metastatic prostate cancer

XVII.   Serum uric acid—test for purine metabolism and renal excretion

A.   Physiological basis and function

Uric acid (UA) in humans is derived from three sources: end-product of endogenous purine metabolism, from purine compounds in the diet, and from catabolism of nucleic acids in tissues. It is found in the serum and plasma bound to albumin and also in free form. Total body urate is influenced by dietary intake (meat, liver, legumes, mushrooms, and spinach increase uric acid). In gout, the urate pool may be increased 3–25 times normal along with decreased urate excretion. In persons suffering from gout, high levels of uric acid in the blood (resulting from a hereditary metabolic defect) lead to the deposition of urate crystals in the tissues, (e.g., joints and kidneys).

  B.   Normal value, 2.5–8.0 mg/dl
  C.   Clinical significance

    1.   Hyperuricemia—elevated levels

      a.   Gout
      b.   Leukemias (high purine turnover)
      c.   Renal insufficiency/failure
      d.   Diuretic therapy (e.g., thiazides, LASIX, EDECRIN), cytotoxic agents, aspirin at low doses
      e.   Hemolytic anemia
      f.   Eclampsia
      g.   Polycythemia vera
      h.   Postmenopause—decrease in estrogen production

    2.   Hypouricemia—decreased levels

      a.   Low protein diets
      b.   Liver necrosis
      c.   Steroid therapy
      d.   High doses of aspirin

XVIII. Serum phosphorus (inorganic)

  A.   Physiological basis
    The concentration of inorganic phosphate in circulating plasma is influenced by parathyroid gland function, action of vitamin D, intestinal absorption, renal function, bone metabolism, and nutrition.
  B.   Normal values
    Children, 4–7 mg/dl
    Adults, 3–4.5 mg/dl
  C.   Clinical significance

    1.   Elevated levels

      a.   Renal insufficiency
      b.   Hypothyroidism
      c.   Hypervitaminosis D

    2.   Decreased levels

      a.   Hyperparathyroidism
      b.   Hypovitaminosis D
      c.   Malabsorption

    d.   Chronic alcoholism
    e.   Acid-base disturbances
    f.   Renal tubular defects
    g.   Thiazide diuretics
    h.   Aluminum antacids

XIX. Serum gamma glutamyl transpeptidase or transferase (GGT)

A. Physiological basis

Gamma glutamyl transferase (GGT) is an extremely sensitive indicator of liver damage. Serum GGT levels are often elevated even though transferases and alkaline phosphatase are normal and are generally considered to be more specific for identifying alcohol-induced liver impairment.

The enzyme, induced by alcohol, is present in liver, kidney, and pancreas and transfers C-terminal glutamic acid from a peptide to other peptides or L-amino acids.

B. Normal values

1. Males, 30 mU/ml at 30°C
2. Females, 25 mU/ml at 30°C
3. Adolescents, 50 mU/ml at 30°C

C. Clinical significance

Elevated in acute infections or toxic hepatitis, chronic and subacute hepatitis, cirrhosis of the liver, intrahepatic or extrahepatic obstruction, primary or metastatic liver neoplasm, and liver damage due to alcoholism. Elevated levels may also be seen in congestive heart failure.

XX. Anion gap

The anion gap (representing undetermined plasma anions) is estimated by subtracting the sum of the serum chloride and serum bicarbonate concentrations from the serum sodium concentration. The unmeasured anions usually include anionic protein, sulfates, phosphates, and anionic groups of organic ions.

A. Normal values, 12–15 mEq/L
B. Clinical significance

1. Elevated anion gap

    a. Metabolic acidosis: >30 mEq/L usually indicative of an identifiable organic anion acidosis such as lactic acidosis or ketoacidosis, or ingestion of substances such as ethylene glycol, methanol, or salicylates.
    b. Significant elevations in the anion gap always indicate metabolic acidosis.

2. Respiratory alkalosis—small elevations of >15–16 mEq/L are occasionally seen with respiratory alkalosis.

XXI. Arterial blood gas (ABG)

A. Arterial blood pH

1. Normal values, 7.35–7.45
2. Clinical significance
   The pH reflects regulation of hydrogen ions or the body's principal means of regulating acid-base balance.

   a. A low pH means a high concentration of hydrogen ions, indicating acidity.
   b. An elevated pH means a low hydrogen ion concentration, indicating alkalinity.
   c. Arterial blood usually has a higher pH due to loss of carbon dioxide during respiration.

B. Partial pressure of carbon dioxide (pCO_2)

1. Normal values, 35–45 mm Hg (Torr)
2. Clinical significance
   The partial pressure of carbon dioxide in the blood reflects alveolar ventilation during respiration.

   a. Hypercapnia is an elevation of pCO_2 and indicates acidity. Carbon dioxide is being retained by the lungs through hypoventilation.
   b. Hypocapnia is a decrease in pCO_2 and indicates alkalinity. Carbon dioxide is being blown off through hyperventilation.

C. Partial pressure of oxygen (pO_2)

1. Normal values, 80–100 mm Hg (Torr) in an adult under 60 years of age (on room air)
2. Clinical significance
   The partial pressure of oxygen measures arterial blood oxygenation and usually decreases from normal after the age of 18 years or in patients with acute/chronic respiratory diseases. pO_2 is a more sensitive indicator of hypoxemia than saturated oxygen.

   a. An elevated pO_2 usually results from hyperventilation.
   b. Hypoxemia is represented by less than normal pO_2 and may mean: COPD, chronic respiratory acidosis, asthma, neuromuscular diseases such as amyotrophic lateral sclerosis and multiple sclerosis. A pO_2 of <60 mm Hg that is not corrected represents a potentially life-threat-

ening situation, and body systems begin to fail (e.g., skin, gastrointestinal tract, kidneys, liver, brain).

D. Bicarbonate (HCO_3^-)

   1. Normal values, 21–28 mEq/L
   2. Clinical significance
       Carbon dioxide dissolves in the blood into bicarbonate. The blood bicarbonate level is regulated by the kidneys.

       a. An elevated bicarbonate blood level makes the blood alkaline; therefore, excess bicarbonate will be excreted in the urine. Greater than normal values may mean liver disease, rapid breathing, drug toxicity (e.g., aspirin), kidney disease, severe diarrhea or shock.
       b. A low bicarbonate blood level makes the blood acidic; therefore, the kidneys will reabsorb bicarbonate from the urine. Less than normal values may mean severe vomiting, excessive intake of bicarbonate (e.g., antacids), diuretic or steroid therapy, and difficulty in breathing.

E. Saturated oxygen (SaO_2)

   1. Normal values, 95–100% of capacity
   2. Clinical significance
       The saturated oxygen represents the percentage of oxygen attached to hemoglobin in the red blood cell. SaO_2 is a less sensitive indicator of hypoxemia than pO_2.

F. Base excess (BE)

   1. Values range from 0 to ± 5 mEq of base
   2. Used to titrate acid or base and represents the amount of basic compounds used with 1 liter of blood

G. Fraction of inspired air (FiO_2)
    Normal values, 0.21–1.0 or 21–100%

XXII. Prothrombin time (PT)

A. Normal values or control is 10–13 sec
B. Therapeutic values—strive for 1½–2½ times the control value; in some cases, 1.2–1.5 times the control value is more desirable.
C. Used to monitor warfarin therapy (clotting factors II, VII, IX, and X)
D. Elevated values

   1. Vitamin K deficiency
   2. Liver disease
   3. Leukemias

4. Factor deficiencies
5. Antibiotic therapy
6. Anticoagulant therapy

E. Decreased values

1. Vitamin K excess

XXIII. Partial thromboplastin time (PTT)—activated

A. Normal values or control, approximately 19.5–29.0 sec
B. Therapeutic values—strive for 1 1/2–2 1/2 times the control value
C. Used to monitor heparin therapy (clotting factors)
D. Elevated values

1. Factor deficiencies
2. Heparin therapy

E. Decreased values

1. Hemorrhages
2. Neoplastic disease
3. Protamine sulfate

XXIV. Urinalysis (UA)

A. Characteristics—normally crystal clear
B. Color—normally straw-yellow color
C. Odor—normally little to no odor
D. Specific gravity—indicates the relative proportion of dissolved solid compounds to the total volume of urine

1. Normal values—1.003–1.030
2. General guide—As the color of urine becomes darker, the specific gravity increases, and as the color lightens, the specific gravity decreases.

E. Urine pH

1. Normal pH 4.5–8.0 (average about 6.0)
2. Dependent upon diet and medication
3. Urea splitting organisms will increase urine pH

F. Protein—normally only small amounts of protein are excreted into the urine (0–100 mg/dl/24 hr)

1. Normally negative
2. Proteinuria (positive protein)

    a. 0 (trace), up to 30 mg/100 ml/24 hr
    b. 1+, 30–100 mg/dl/24 hr
    c. 2+, 100–300 mg/dl/24 hr
    d. 3+, 300–1000 mg/dl/24 hr

    e.   4+, >1000 mg/dl/24 hr

    f.   Significant proteinuria most commonly stems from glomerular and tubular damage. It may also indicate glomerulonephritis and impending renal failure.

  3.   Trace proteinuria is normal following exercise

  4.   False-positive proteinuria

    a.   Tolbutamide metabolites

    b.   Penicillin

    c.   Para-aminosalicylic acid

G.   Glucose

  1.   Normally negative

  2.   Positive or glucosuria may occur when blood glucose level exceeds reabsorption capacity of renal tubules (renal threshold >180 mg/dl), as in diabetes mellitus or in renal tubular dysfunction.

  3.   Urine glucose tests

    a.   CLINITEST (Copper reduction-Benedict's) for any reducing sugar: neg., 0%; trace, 1/4%; +1, 1/2%; +2, 3/4%; +3, 1%; +4, 2%.

        If more than 2% sugar, the color will pass through the +4 range and go back to +2 or +3.

    b.   2-drop CLINITEST will measure up to 5% sugar.

    c.   TES-TAPE (glucose oxidase-glucose specific): neg., 0%; +1, 0.1%; +2, 1/4%; +3, 1/2%; +4, 2%; or more.

    d.   DIASTIX (glucose oxidase-glucose specific): neg., 0%; trace, 0.1%; +1, 1/4%; +2, 1/2%; +3, 1%; +4, 2% (large quantities of ketones may alter results).

  4.   False positive glucose may result from use of ascorbic acid.

H.   Ketones (acetoacetic acid, acetone, and betahydroxybutyric acid)

  1.   Normally negative.

  2.   Positive ketones usually result from fatty acid metabolism as an energy source (e.g., starvation or altered carbohydrate metabolism).

  3.   False positives may result from medication (e.g., levodopa, methyldopa).

I.   Bile

  1.   Normally not present.

  2.   When present (yellow-green urine), it suggests biliary obstruction.

J.   Urobilinogen (UBG)

1. Normally not present.
2. When present (dark brown-colored urine), it suggests increased amounts of bilirubin, bleeding, or liver dysfunction that prevents the reabsorption of urobilinogen from the portal circulation.

K. Nitrites

1. Normally not present.
2. A positive nitrite test is usually indicative of a gram-negative infection (bacteria convert nitrates to nitrites).

L. Microscopic examination—helps identify and detect cells, casts, crystals, or bacteria from centrifuged sediment of a urine sample

1. WBCs—Five or more per high-powered field (HPF) indicates inflammation of genitourinary system and tubular injury (i.e., acute pyelonephritis or glomerulonephritis, etc.); 25–50 WBCs present probably indicate a bacterial infection and a culture and sensitivity test should be run.
2. RBCs—The presence of >1 RBC may suggest acute glomerulonephritis, acute renal infarction, collagen disease, or acute interstitial nephritis. Acute nonpathologic bleeding must be ruled out (e.g., bleeding from urethral catheter irritation).
3. Epithelial cells—may be present following renal tubular damage
4. Casts—cylindrical molds of the renal tubular lumen produced by precipitation of protein. (Tamm-Horsfall mucoproteins form the basic matrix of all casts.) When present, they usually represent significant renal disease or damage. Casts are usually classified as follows:
    a. Hyaline—formed in renal tubules in the distal portion of the nephron and readily dissolvable in dilute and alkaline urine.
    b. Epithelial—presence represents normal wear; increased with renal infection.
    c. Granular—usually present during fever or after strenuous exercise.
    d. Fatty—formed by degeneration of cellular casts with the incorporation of fat droplets or cholesterol estrus. They may be present in patients with nephrotic syndrome and in diabetic patients.
    e. Red cell—represent glomerular inflammation.
    f. White cell—leukocytes trapped in the protein matrix of renal tubules.
    g. Waxy—represent the ultimate stage of disintegrated cellular casts and have a "broken off" appearance. When present, they usually indicate prolonged urinary stasis

within the kidneys and are characteristic of chronic renal failure.

5. Bacteria—usually represents the actual count of bacteria seen by the examiner

   a. Normally not present.
   b. When present, may indicate bacterial infection.
   c. When greater than 20–30 (2+ or 3+), a culture and sensitivity test should be performed.

6. Mucus

   a. Normally not present
   b. When present, may indicate bacterial/yeast infection

7. Crystals—a variety of crystals and amorphous compounds may appear in the normal urine as sediment, depending on the pH and osmolality of the urine. In acid urine, crystals become uric acid or calcium oxalate. In alkaline urine they may become phosphates.

   a. Calcium oxalate—a 12–sided crystal, common in acid urine, and associated with renal calculi
   b. Uric acid—a hexagonal crystal (yellow), common in acid urine, and associated with increased uric acid levels (gout)
   c. Triple phosphate—6- to 8-sided crystals (prisms), common in alkaline urine, often accompanies obstructive uropathy or colonic urinary tract infections
   d. Amorphous urates—common in acidic urine
   e. Miscellaneous—sulfonamides, and various Ca, Mg, and Al salt crystals.

■ References

1. Knoben JE, Anderson PO, eds. *Handbook of Clinical Drug Data*, 6th ed, Drug Intelligence Publications, Inc, Hamilton, IL, 1988.
2. Kastrup EK, Olin BR, eds. *Facts and Comparisons*, JB Lippincott, St. Louis, MO, 1989.
3. *Drug Information For The Health Care Provider, vol 1, USP DI*, 5th ed, 1985, United States Pharmacopeial Convention, Inc., Mack Printing Co., Easton, PA, 1988.
4. McEvoy GK. *American Hospital Formulary Service*, American Society of Hospital Pharmacists, Bethesda, MD, 1989.
5. Krupp MA, Chatton MJ, eds. *Current Medical Diagnosis and Treatment*, Lange Medical Publications, Los Altos, CA, 1989, 1085–1103.
6. Wallach J. *Interpretation of Diagnostic Tests*, 3rd ed, Little, Brown & Co., Boston, 1978.
7. Katcher BS, Young LY, Koda-Kimble MA. *Applied Therapeutics*, 3rd ed, Applied Therapeutics, Spokane, WA, 1988, pp 13–30.
8. Widmann FK. *Clinical Interpretation of Laboratory Tests*, 8th ed, FA Davis, Philadelphia, 1980.

9. Sobel DS, Ferguson T. *The People's Book of Medical Tests,* Summit Books, New York, 1985.
10. Wyngaarden JB, Smith LH Jr, eds. *Cecil Textbook of Medicine*, 16th ed, WB Saunders, Philadelphia, 1985.
11. Sonnenwirth AC, Jarett L, eds. *Gradwohl's Clinical Laboratory Methods and Diagnosis,* 8th ed, vol 1 and 2, CV Mosby, St. Louis, 1980.
12. Tresseler KM. *Clinical Laboratory Tests,* Prentice-Hall, Englewood Cliffs, NJ, 1982.

Chapter 5
Monitoring Drug Therapy
with Laboratory Data

In some situations, drug therapy may be monitored effectively only by utilizing clinical laboratory tests to obtain objective data (e.g., serum or urine drug levels, serum or urine electrolytes, enzymes, blood components, organ function/dysfunction). Generally, the results of these tests provide patient and drug information that may not otherwise be obtainable. Many physicians run certain laboratory tests as a standard procedure for screening recently admitted patients or for reevaluating a patient who has no recent clinical laboratory tests. These laboratory tests may also be run in conjunction with changes in clinical signs or symptoms in a patient's medical status or to help make an accurate diagnosis of the medical problem. Data from these tests may be utilized to: (a) establish a baseline chemistry profile for a patient; (b) help confirm a drug's therapeutic effectiveness when the patient does not exhibit any typical subjective patient data (e.g., signs and symptoms); (c) indicate the serum drug concentration at the time the specimen was obtained; (d) show that the serum drug concentration is either subtherapeutic, within normal limits, or toxic, based upon standard laboratory values; (e) help calculate appropriate drug dosages for those medications that have very low therapeutic and toxic serum levels (e.g., aminoglycosides, digoxin); and (f) titrate those drugs whose dosages must be adjusted to the body's ability to metabolize and excrete the drug.

Questions that are often asked by nurses, pharmacists, and physicians about monitoring drug therapy with laboratory data include: (a) What drugs should be monitored by laboratory tests? (b) Which laboratory tests should be conducted for a specific drug? (c) What is the most appropriate time (hour, day, predose, postdose, etc.) to draw the blood specimen to get meaningful drug data? (d)

How often should these laboratory tests be conducted? The following information represents suggested guidelines that may be used when monitoring drug therapy with laboratory data.

TABLE 5.1 DRUGS FOR WHICH LABORATORY TESTS MAY BE HELPFUL (1–36)

DRUG PRODUCT	LABORATORY TESTS	REASON(S) FOR REQUESTING TEST	GENERAL COMMENTS
Acetohexamide (DYMELOR)	1. Glycosolated hemoglobin (HbA_{1C})	1. To evaluate diabetes control over previous 6- to 8-week period	
	2. FBS	2. Medication can cause significant reductions in serum glucose levels.	
	3. Urine glucose	3. Monitor for hyperglycemia	
Allopurinol (ZYLOPRIM)	1. Serum uric acid level	1. To determine medication effectiveness	1. Diuretics (e.g., HCTZ, furosemide, metalozone, bumetamide) may cause increased uric acid levels.
	2. CBC	2. Monitor for blood dyscrasias (rare)	
	3. Liver function tests (SGOT, SGPT, bilirubin, and alk. phos.)	3. Medication may cause hepatotoxicity.	3. Discontinue drug at first sign of systemic allergic reaction (rash).
Amiloride (MIDAMOR), amiloride with HCTZ (MODURETIC)	1. Serum electrolytes (Na, K, Cl)	1. Medication conserves K^+ and an occasional test is needed to monitor for hyperkalemia.	1. Patients with decreased renal function are at greater risk of developing hyperkalemia.
	2. Serum electrolytes (Na, K, Cl)	2. Combination medications usually conserve K^+ but may be K^+ wasting. Periodic test needed to monitor hyperkalemia/hypokalemia.	2. Potassium supplements should be used only when routine electrolytes are monitored.
	3. Serum creatinine level and BUN	3. Medication is generally not effective if the CrCl is <25 ml/min.	
Aminoglycosides amikacin (AMIKIN), gentamicin (GARAMYCIN), tobramycin (NEBCIN)	1. Culture and sensitivity test	1. Determine effectiveness of therapy	
	2. Serum creatinine level and BUN	2. Medications are ototoxic, nephrotoxic, laboratory tests needed to help determine effectiveness and/or possible toxicity of drug.	2. Adjust drug dosages based on renal function (CrCl) and serum drug levels.

TABLE 5.1 *Continued*

DRUG PRODUCT	LABORATORY TESTS	REASON(S) FOR REQUESTING TEST	GENERAL COMMENTS
	3. Serum drug levels (peak and trough)	3. Toxicity associated with peak levels above 10 μg/ml and/or trough levels above 2 μg/ml for gentamicin and tobramycin and 35 and 5 for amikacin.	
Calcium channel blockers verapamil (CALAN, ISOPTIN), nifedipine (PROCARDIA)	1. Serum digoxin level	1. Calcium channel blockers (except for Cardizem) may cause up to 50% increase in serum digoxin levels.	1. Dose of digoxin may need to be reduced by as much as 50%.
	2. Liver function tests (SGOT, SGPT, bilirubin, and alk. phos.)	2. Periodic monitoring of liver function tests is recommended.	2. Bradycardia may develop when used in combination with digoxin or beta blockers.
Captopril (CAPOTEN), enalapril (VASOTEC), lisinopril (PRINIVIL and ZESTIL)	1. Urine protein (dipstick)	1. Medication may cause proteinuria, leading to nephrotic syndrome.	1. Elderly patients are more sensitive to initial dose of medication and marked hypotension and syncope may result.
	2. Urinary acetone	2. False-positive reaction	
	3. White blood cell count from CBC	3. Medication may cause neutropenia.	
	4. Serum potassium level	4. Serum potassium levels increase in patients taking an ACE inhibitor.	4. Elderly and renally impaired patients at higher risk of hyperkalemia. Concurrent use of a K^+- sparing diuretic or a K^+ supplement should be closely monitored.
	5. Serum creatinine level and BUN	5. Dosage reduction needed with renal impairment.	
Carbamazepine (TEGRETOL)	1. Serum drug levels	1. Therapeutic range 3–14 μg/ml. Range 3–8 μg/ml when used in conjunction with other anticonvulsants.	
	2. Liver function tests (SGOT, SGPT, bilirubin, and alk. phos.)	2. Monitor for hepatotoxicity	

TABLE 5.1 *Continued*

DRUG PRODUCT	LABORATORY TESTS	REASON(S) FOR REQUESTING TEST	GENERAL COMMENTS
	3. CBC	3. Monitor for bone marrow depression (rare).	
Cephalosporins (KEFLIN, KEFLEX, MANDOL, others)	1. Culture and sensitivity test	1. Determine effectiveness of therapy.	
	2. Serum creatinine level and BUN	2. Serum creatinine may be falsely elevated.	2. Decrease usual adult dose in patients with impairment of renal function.
	3. Coombs' test	3. False-positive results	
	4. Urine glucose	4. False-positive reaction with CLINITEST copper reduction tests	4. Use TES-TAPE for urine glucose determinations or switch to fingertip blood glucose level testing.
	5. Urine protein	5. False-positive reaction with cefamandole only.	
Chloramphenicol (CHLOROMY-CETIN)	1. CBC	1. Medication may cause blood dyscrasias, including aplastic anemia and agranulocytosis.	1. Elderly patients at greater risk of developing blood dyscrasias.
	2. Urine glucose	2. False-positive reaction with CLINITEST copper reduction tests	2. Use TES-TAPE for urine glucose testing or switch to fingertip blood glucose level determinations.
Chlorpropamide (DIABINESE)	1. Glycosolated hemnoglobin (HbA$_{1C}$)	1. To evaluate diabetes control over previous 6 to 8 week period	
	2. FBS	2. Medication can cause significant reductions in serum glucose levels.	2. Elderly patients show increased sensitivity to medication, because of the medication's long half-life.
	3. Urine glucose	3. Monitor for hyperglycemia.	
	4. Serum creatinine level and BUN	4. Dosage reduction needed with renal impairment.	
Clofibrate (ATROMID-S)	1. Serum cholesterol and triglyceride levels	1. To evaluate effectiveness of therapy	
	2. CBC	2. Blood dyscrasias (rare)	
	3. Liver function tests (SGOT, SGPT, bilirubin, and alk. phos.)	3. Hepatotoxicity (rare)	
	4. Serum creatinine level, BUN, and urinalysis	4. Renal damage proteinuria (rare)	

TABLE 5.1 *Continued*

DRUG PRODUCT	LABORATORY TESTS	REASON(S) FOR REQUESTING TEST	GENERAL COMMENTS
Colestipol (COLESTID)	1. Bleeding times (PT or PTT)	1. Medication may reduce absorption of vitamin K, leading to prolonged bleeding.	1. If patient on digoxin, serum levels should be done routinely as colestipol can inhibit digoxin absorption.
	2. Cholesterol levels	2. To help monitor effectiveness of therapy	
Corticosteroids (cortisone, prednisone, hydrocortisone)	1. Serum electrolytes (Na, K, Cl)	1. May cause K^+ loss, Na^+ and water retention	1. Laboratory tests may be needed routinely with long-term therapy.
	2. FBS	2. Steroids have intrisic hyperglycemic activity.	
	3. Thyroid function tests (T_3, T_4, and TSH)	3. Medication may cause decrease in protein-bound iodine.	
	4. Stool for occult blood (Hematest), CBC	4. May cause chronic blood loss; anemia may result.	4. False-positive test may result if patient is currently taking an iron product.
	5. Glaucoma testing	5. May increase intraocular pressure	
	6. ESR	6. To monitor therapeutic effects of drug in anti-inflammatory diseases	
Dantrolene (DANTRIUM)	1. Liver function tests (SGOT, SGPT, bilirubin, and alk. phos.)	1. Hepatotoxicity	1. Hepatotoxicity appears to be more common in older women, especially those receiving concurrent therapy with estrogens.
Desmopressin (DDAVP), Lypressin (DIAPID)	1. Serum electrolytes (Na, K, Cl)	1. To assess effectiveness of therapy; electrolytes may be high or low depending on effectiveness of therapy.	1. Elderly patients are prone to developing water intoxication and hyponatremia, so intake and output must be closely monitored.
Digitoxin (CRYSTODIGIN)	1. Serum digitoxin level	1. To monitor for therapeutic effects and toxicity	1. If patient taking digitoxin, serum digitoxin levels must be specified.
	2. Liver function tests (SGOT, SGPT, bilirubin, and alk. phos.)	2. Digitoxin is hepatically metabolized and has a very long half-life. Hepatic dysfunction may lead to prolonged drug levels.	

TABLE 5.1 *Continued*

DRUG PRODUCT	LABORATORY TESTS	REASON(S) FOR REQUESTING TEST	GENERAL COMMENTS
	3. Serum electrolytes (when patient also on a K^+-depleting diuretic)	3. Low serum potassium level potentiates effects of digitoxin.	
Digoxin (LANOXIN)	1. Serum digoxin level (especially when taking quinidine, verapamil or nifedipine—see calcium channel blockers)	1. To monitor for therapeutic effect and/or toxicity. For CHF, a level of 1.0 ng/ml is needed, and for antiarrhythmia activity, levels of 1.5–2.0 ng/ml may be needed.	1. Serum digoxin levels are especially important in geriatrics as these patients often may not exhibit classic signs and symptoms of digoxin toxicity.
	2. Serum creatinine level and BUN	2. Digoxin is renally eliminated and a decrease in renal function can lead to drug accumulation.	2. Concurrent use of spironolactone will interfere with lab assay and gives a falsely elevated digoxin level.
	3. Serum electrolytes (when patient also on a K^+-depleting diuretic)	3. Low serum potassium levels potentiate effects of digoxin.	
Disopyramide (NORPACE)	1. Serum drug levels	1. To monitor therapeutic effect range 2–4 µg/ml and toxicity (above 4 µg/ml)	
	2. Serum creatinine level and BUN	2. Dosage reduction needed with renal impairment.	2. Accumulation of drug may occur in renal impairment.
Diuretics—potassium wasting (HCTZ-HYDRODIURIL, furosemide—LASIX, bumetamide—BUMEX, metalozone—ZAROXOLYN)	1. Serum electrolytes (Na, K, Cl)	1. To monitor for electrolyte loss, especially potassium	1. In most patients (especially elderly), a dose of 50–100 mg/day HCTZ or 40–80 mg/day furosemide will usually cause significant electrolyte loss.
	2. Serum uric acid level	2. In patients with gout, drug may increase frequency and severity of gout episodes due to increased uric acid levels.	
	3. Serum creatinine level and BUN	3. HCTZ effectiveness decreases significantly with renal impairment (CrCl <25 ml/min).	

TABLE 5.1 *Continued*

DRUG PRODUCT	LABORATORY TESTS	REASON(S) FOR REQUESTING TEST	GENERAL COMMENTS
Diuretics— potassium sparing (amiloride— MIDAMOR, spironolactone— ALDACTONE, triamterene— DYRENIUM, others— DYAZIDE, MAXZIDE, ALDACTAZIDE, MODURETIC)	1. Serum electrolytes (Na, K, Cl)	1. Monitor for hypokalemia/hyperkalemia (elderly are more susceptible). Medication usually K^+ sparing, may be K^+ wasting. Periodic electrolytes needed to monitor hyperkalemia/hypokalemia.	1. When the combination diuretics (K^+ sparing and wasting) are used, periodic electrolytes are needed as potassium-sparing effect may not be adequate.
	2. Serum creatinine level and BUN	2. Serum K^+ will increase in renal impairment. Effectiveness of therapy decreases significantly with renal impairment (CrCl <25 ml/min).	
Ergocalciferol and other vitamin D analogs	1. Serum calcium level	1. Calcium levels should be maintained at 9 to 10 mg/dl.	1. Toxicity may occur with vitamin D doses of 50,000 units/day over prolonged periods. Death may occur due to renal or cardiovascular failure.
	2. Serum phosphorus level 3. Serum magnesium level 4. Serum creatinine level and BUN	2. Serum levels >15 mg/dl may be fatal.	
Ethosuximide (ZARONTIN)	1. Serum drug level	1. Serum level of 40–100 μg/ml therapeutic range. Serum level must be interpreted in conjunction with patient's clinical status.	
	2. CBC	2. CBCs may be needed periodically as drug has potential to cause blood dyscrasias.	
Ferrous sulfate and other iron preparations	1. CBC with indices	1. CBC should indicate iron deficiency anemia (low MCV).	1. In the elderly, TIBC may be an unreliable test and should not be used alone for determining iron deficiency anemia.

TABLE 5.1 *Continued*

DRUG PRODUCT	LABORATORY TESTS	REASON(S) FOR REQUESTING TEST	GENERAL COMMENTS
	2. Serum iron level and TIBC	2. Decreased serum iron and elevated TIBC usually indicate iron deficiency anemia.	2. Laboratory tests should return to normal within weeks, but iron therapy should continue 6–12 months to replace body stores of iron. While patient is on iron therapy, hematest of stools may test false-positive.
	3. Reticulocytre count	3. Once therapy started, retic count should be increased to show development of new red blood cells.	
	4. Urine glucose	4. False-negative reaction with TES-TAPE glucose oxidose tests.	4. Use CLINITEST for urine glucose testing or switch to finger-tip blood glucose level determinations.
Fludrocortisone (FLORINEF)	1. Serum electrolytes (Na, K, Cl)	1. Drug retains sodium and water and increases excretion of potassium.	1. Hypernatremia and hypokalemia should be monitored, especially in the elderly patient.
Folic acid (FOLVITE)	1. CBC with indices	1. With folic acid or vitamin B_{12} deficiencies, the CBC will usually show a megaloblastic or macrocytic anemia (elevated MCV) before therapy.	
	2. Serum folacin and vitamin B_{12} levels	2. Decreased folic acid levels should return to normal within 6 weeks after initiating therapy.	2. Vitamin B_{12} levels need to be checked also as B_{12} therapy may be needed to correct the macrocytic anemia.
Gold compounds aurothioglucose, gold sodium thiomalate, auranofin (SOLGANOL, MYOCHRYSINE, RIDAURA)	1. CBC 2. Platelet count 3. Urinalysis	1. Drug may cause blood dyscrasias. 2. Drug may cause thrombocytopenia. 3. Proteinuria may indicate that nephrotic syndrome is developing.	1. There are many serious adverse effects from therapy with gold compounds

TABLE 5.1 *Continued*

DRUG PRODUCT	LABORATORY TESTS	REASON(S) FOR REQUESTING TEST	GENERAL COMMENTS
Heparin sodium (various)	1. PTT	1. To evaluate therapeutic effect	1. Elderly patients must be observed closely for bleeding episodes.
	2. Platelet count	2. To monitor for thrombocytopenia	
	3. Hemastix	3. To test urine for blood	
Indomethacin (INDOCIN)	1. CBC	1. Drug may cause blood dyscrasias.	
	2. ESR	2. To monitor drug's effectiveness in gout therapy	
	3. Serum creatinine level and BUN	3. Drug may cause renal impairment.	
Insulin (various)	1. FBS, 4PMBS, random blood glucose levels	1. To monitor for glucose status and control of diabetes	1. In most patients, the finger stick method is recommended over urine glucose determinations as there may be little correlation between urine glucose and blood glucose.
	2. Glycosolated hemoglobin (HgA_{1C})	2. To monitor diabetes control over the previous 6- to 8-week period	
	3. Finger stick blood glucose	3. Most accurate nonlaboratory monitoring test	
Isoniazid (INH, others)	1. Liver function tests (SGOT, SGPT, bilirubin, and alk. phos.)	1. Drug may cause drug-induced hepatitis, hepatotoxicity. Risk is higher in the elderly and alcoholics.	1. Patients also taking phenytoin (DILANTIN) should have serum phenytoin levels done as INH can cause significant increases serum levels. 2. Vitamin B_6 therapy should be initiated along with INH.
	3. Urine glucose	3. False-positive reaction with CLINITEST copper reduction tests.	3. Use TES-TAPE for urine glucose testing or switch to fingertip blood glucose level determination.
Ketoconazole (NIZORAL)	1. Liver function tests (SGOT, SGPT, bilirubin, and alk. phos.)	1. Drug may cause drug-induced hepatitis, hepatotoxicity.	
Lactulose (CEPHULAC, CHRONULAC)	1. Blood ammonia levels	1. To monitor therapeutic effect when used for hepatic encephalopathy	1. Drug acts to acidify the colonic contents and decreases ammonia production.

TABLE 5.1 *Continued*

DRUG PRODUCT	LABORATORY TESTS	REASON(S) FOR REQUESTING TEST	GENERAL COMMENTS
	2. Serum electrolytes (Na, K, Cl)	2. When used as chronic laxative, hypokalemia may develop.	2. Drug acts as a laxative, and electrolyes may be lost with long-term use.
Levodopa (L-DOPA, DOPAR)	1. Urine glucose	1. May cause false-positive reaction with Tes-Tape and a false-negative with glucose oxidose tests (e.g., DIASTIX) 2. May cause false positive reaction for urine ketones	1. May wish to switch to fingertip blood glucose level determination 3. Vitamin B_6 increases metabolism of dopamine.
Lithium (ESKALITH, LITHOBID)	1. Serum lithium levels	1. Usual therapeutic range is 0.5–1.5 mEq/liter	1. Toxicity may occur with serum levels in the therapeutic range.
	2. WBC with differential	2. Drug may cause leukocytosis.	
	3. Serum creatinine level and BUN	3. Renal impairment can lead to toxicity.	
	4. Serum electrolytes (Na, K, Cl)	4. Salt-restricted diets greatly increase risk of toxicity; lithium will be retained and sodium excreted.	
	5. Thyroid function tests	5. Hypothyroid may occur; therefore, thyroid supplement may be needed.	
Meclofenamate (MECLOMEN)	1. CBC and occult blood in stool	1. To monitor for chronic blood loss and possible blood dyscrasias	
	2. Serum electrolytes (Na, K, Cl)	2. Drug can cause severe diarrhea. Prolonged use may lead to significant electrolyte loss.	
Methenamine (MANDELAMINE, HIPREX)	1. Urinary pH	1. Urine pH must be kept below 6 to allow the formation of formaldehyde (active drug).	1. As the reaction to formaldehyde takes 1–2 hr, depending on pH of urine, the use of the drug in catheterized patients may not be effective. 2. Concurrent use with sulfonamides increases the risk of an insoluble precipitate and crystalluria.

TABLE 5.1 *Continued*

DRUG PRODUCT	LABORATORY TESTS	REASON(S) FOR REQUESTING TEST	GENERAL COMMENTS
	3. Serum creatinine level and BUN	3. Effectiveness is significantly decreased in renal impairment.	
Methyldopa (ALDOMET)	1. CBC	1. Drug may cause hemolytic anemia.	
	2. Liver function tests (SGOT, SGPT, bilirubin and alk. phos.)	2. May cause drug-induced hepatitis	
	3. Urine glucose	3. False-positive reaction with CLINITEST copper reduction tests	3. Use TES-TAPE for urine glucose testing or switch to fingertip blood glucose level testing.
Metronidazole (FLAGYL)	1. CBC	1. Drug may cause leukopenia.	
Nalidixic acid (NEGRAM)	1. Culture and sensitivity test	1. To determine appropriateness and effectiveness of therapy	
	2. CBC (if treatment longer than 2 weeks)	2. Drug may cause blood dyscrasias.	2. Long-term use in the geriatric is not recommended.
	3. Serum creatinine level, BUN, liver function tests—SGOT, SGPT, and alk. phos.	3. To monitor for possible accumulation of drug if used for more than 2 weeks	3. May cause false-positive results with Clinitest. Use Clinistix.
	4. Urine glucose	4. False-positive reaction with CLINITEST copper reduction tests	4. Use TES-TAPE for urine glucose testing or switch to fingertip blood glucose level testing.
Nitrofurantoin (FURADANTIN, MACRODANTIN)	1. Culture and sensitivity test	1. Determine effectiveness of therapy	
	2. Serum creatinine level, BUN	2. Patients with creatinine clearance <40 ml/min are at high risk of developing toxicity due to decreased clearance; therefore, the drug should not be used in these patients.	2. Drug may cause false positive urine determinations with Clinitest (copper sulfate method).
NSAIDS (ibuprofen, indomethacin, fenoprofen, ketoprofen, mechofenamate, naproxen, piroxicam, and sulindac)	1. Serum creatinine and BUN	1. All NSAIDs decrease renal function and may cause renal impairment.	
	2. Liver function tests (SGPT, SGOT, bilirubin, and alk. phos.)	2. All NSAIDs are primarily hepatically metabolized and renally excreted. Elevated liver enzymes may lead to withdrawal of the drug.	

TABLE 5.1 *Continued*

DRUG PRODUCT	LABORATORY TESTS	REASON(S) FOR REQUESTING TEST	GENERAL COMMENTS
Penicillamine (CUPRIMINE)	1. CBC	1. Blood dyscrasias (agranulocytosis and aplastic anemia)	1. Risk of developing blood dyscrasias is significantly greater in elderly patients. Concurrent iron therapy will cause a decrease in effect of both drugs through complexation (insoluble) in the gut. Patients should also avoid using dietary supplements containing high concentrations of other heavy metals (zinc, calcium, or aluminum).
	2. Platelet counts	2. Thrombocytopenia may develop.	
	3. Urinalysis	3. Proteinuria and hematuria may develop, and, if unchecked, may progress to nephrotic syndrome. Proteinuria may resolve with continued therapy. Progressively increasing proteinuria or urine protein more than 1 g/day requires dosage reduction or cessation of therapy.	
Phenobarbital (various)	1. Serum phenobarbital level	1. To help monitor effects of drug	1. Acidic urine increases renal tubule absorption of phenobarbital and increases blood levels.
Phenylbutazone (BUTAZOLIDIN)	1. CBC	1. May cause blood dyscrasias, with aplastic anemia. Chronic blood loss may also be significant problem with long-term therapy.	1. In most patients, therapy should not exceed 1 week due to significantly increased risk of serious and potentially fatal toxic reactions.
	2. Liver function tests (SGOT, SGPT, bilirubin, and alk. phos.)	2. Hepatotoxicity may occur with chronic therapy.	

TABLE 5.1 *Continued*

DRUG PRODUCT	LABORATORY TESTS	REASON(S) FOR REQUESTING TEST	GENERAL COMMENTS
Phenytoin (DILANTIN)	1. Serum phenytoin levels	1. Therapeutic range 10–20 μg/ml. Since it may take up to 1 month to reach steady state levels in many patients, weekly levels for the first month of therapy are suggested, then periodic determinations based on clinical status.	1. Phenytoin suspension and chewable tablets are not appropriate for daily dosing due to rapid absorption. When stable, do not change phenytoin dosage forms or brands.
	2. Folate levels and CBC	2. Many patients on phenytoin will show decreased folate levels and macrocytosis.	2. Folic acid therapy may cause variations in phenytoin blood levels.
Primidone (MYSOLINE)	1. Serum primidone and phenobarbital levels	1. To help monitoring for therapeutic effect	1. Acidic urine increases renal tubule absorption of phenobarbital and increases blood levels.
Procainamide (PRONESTYL, PROCAN-SR)	1. Serum procainamide levels	2. A level of 4–10 μg/ml is considered the therapeutic range. Toxicity is usually at levels greater than 12 μg/ml.	1. Interpretation of procainamide levels and NAPA levels should be based on several determinations while on the same dose.
	2. Serum *N*-acetylprocainamide (NAPA) level	2. Levels of 15–25 μg/ml are considered effective levels.	
	3. Antinuclear antibodies (ANA)	3. Gives an indication of the potential for procainamide to cause drug-induced SLE	
	4. Serum creatinine level and BUN	4. Dose must be adjusted when renal function decreases.	4. Adjust dosage to serum levels and renal function.
Propranolol (INDERAL) and other nonselective β-blockers	1. FBS (for diabetic patients only)	1. β-blockers have the potential to alter glucose homeostasis which can result in either an increase or decrease in blood glucose levels. β-blockers with more β₁ specificity are less likely to cause this effect.	1. β-blockers also tend to mask the symptoms of hypoglycemia (except sweating).

TABLE 5.1 *Continued*

DRUG PRODUCT	LABORATORY TESTS	REASON(S) FOR REQUESTING TEST	GENERAL COMMENTS
			2. FBS should be done when patient is initiated on β-blocker therapy and with each dosage adjustment.
Quinidine (various)	1. Serum quinidine level	1. Therapeutic serum quinidine levels range from 2–5 µg/ml.	
	2. Serum creatinine level and BUN	2. Dosage must be reduced in the patient with significantly decreased renal function.	
	3. ECG	3. Prolongation of the QRS complex by more than 25% or 0.14 sec indicate patient is approaching toxic levels.	3. Concurrent use with digoxin may increase serum digoxin levels (about 2×) and decrease quinidine levels.
		4. Quinidine content of product	
Rifampin (RIFADIN)	1. Liver function tests (SGPT, SGPT, bilirubin, and alk. phos.)	1. Drug may produce drug-induced hepatitis	1. Elevated liver enzymes alone should be considered indicative of hepatitis as elevated enzymes may return to normal even with continued use of the drug. Clinical evidence of hepatitis should also be present.
	2. CBC including platelet count	2. Drug may cause blood dyscrasias (thrombocytopenia).	
	3. Serum creatinine level and BUN	3. Drug may cause renal failure due to a hypersensitivity reaction.	
	4. Culture and sensitivity test	4. Bacterial resistance can quickly develop.	
Sodium fluoride (various)	1. Serum acid phosphatase	1. May cause falsely decreased levels	
	2. SGOT	2. May cause falsely increased levels	
	3. CBC	3. High doses of fluoride may cause chronic blood loss and anemia.	

TABLE 5.1 *Continued*

DRUG PRODUCT	LABORATORY TESTS	REASON(S) FOR REQUESTING TEST	GENERAL COMMENTS
	4. Urine glucose	4. False-negative reaction with CLINITEST copper reduction tests	4. Use TES-TAPE for urine glucose testing or switch to finger-tip blood glucose level testing.
Spironolactone (ALDACTONE)	1. Serum creatinine level and BUN	1. Medication is generally not effective if CrCl is <25 ml/min.	
	2. Serum potassium	2. With excess dietary potassium intake, hyperkalamia may develop, especially with renal impairment.	
	3. Digoxin levels	3. Drug may cause a reduction in clearance of digoxin from the body. Also spironolactone interference with digoxin radioimmunoassay may give falsely elevated digoxin levels.	3. Since spironolactone may interfere with digoxin assays, close attention must be paid to monitoring of digoxin toxicity in patients receiving both drugs.
Sulfinpyrazone (ANTURANE)	1. Serum uric acid	1. To help monitor therapeutic effect	
	2. Serum creatinine level and BUN	2. As sulfinpyrazone is more than 90% renally excreted, reduced renal function will necessitate reduced dosage.	
	3. CBC	3. May cause blood dyscrasias and/or chronic blood loss.	3. A high fluid intake is recommended to help prevent urate stone formation.
Sulindac (CLINORIL)	1. Liver function tests (SGOT, SGPT, bilirubin, and alk. phos.)	1. Transient rise in liver values may occur, returning to normal with discontinued drug use. If values continue to rise or are grossly abnormal, drug should be discontinued.	
	2. CBC	2. Elevated eosinophil (24+), skin rash and pruritis may indicate hypersensitivity reaction.	

TABLE 5.1 *Continued*

DRUG PRODUCT	LABORATORY TESTS	REASON(S) FOR REQUESTING TEST	GENERAL COMMENTS
Testosterone (various)	1. Liver function tests—SGOT and SGPT	1. Drug may cause hepatocellular damage with prolonged use.	1. Sodium and water retention may be a problem exacerbating CHF and hypertension.
	2. Serum and urinary calcium levels	2. Levels may be increased, especially in female patients with breast cancer and in bedridden patients.	
Theophylline (various; % theophylline in parentheses) Oxtriphyllin (64%) (CHOLEDYL) Aminophyllin (86%) Theophylline glycinate (49%) (SYNOPHYLATE) Theophylline olamine (75%) Theophylline calcium salicylate (50%) (QUADRINAL)	1. Serum theophylline levels	1. To help monitor therapeutic effect Therapeutic levels are 10–20 μg/ml. Dyphylline (Lufyllin) cannot be accurately monitored by theophylline levels as it is a separate entity.	1. Since nausea and vomiting may precede life-threatening arrhythmias in only 50% of toxic patients, empirical dosing is dangerous. Patients with hepatic disease, CHF, alcoholism, and COPD exhibit reduced theophylline and, therefore, require reduced dosages. 2. Smokers may require increased dosages due to microsomal enzymes induction. 3. Cimetadine and erythromycin can cause increased theophylline levels due to microsomal enzyme inhibition.
Thyroid (ARMOUR THYROID)	1. Thyroid function tests (T_4, T_3, FTI, and TSH)	1. To help monitor therapeutic or toxic effects of the drug	1. The TSH level is the most useful test for long-term monitoring (provided the problem is not at the pituitary level). When patient is stabilized, do not change brands of thyroid.
Tolazamide (TOLINASE)	1. Glycosolated hemoglobin (HgA_{1C})	1. To evaluate diabetes control over previous 6- to 8-week period	1. There is great interpatient variation in absorption of tolazamide which will determine the frequency of administration.

TABLE 5.1 *Continued*

DRUG PRODUCT	LABORATORY TESTS	REASON(S) FOR REQUESTING TEST	GENERAL COMMENTS
	2. FBS and urine glucose	2. To help monitor therapeutic effect of the drug	
	3. Serum creatinine level and BUN	3. Patients with reduced renal and hepatic function require reduced dosages.	
Tolbutamide (ORINASE, others)	1. Glycosolated hemoglobin (HgA$_{1C}$)	1. To evaluate diabetes control over previous 6- to 8-week period	
	2. FBS and urine glucose	2. To monitor therapeutic effect of the drug	
Triamterene (DYRENIUM)	1. Serum creatinine and BUN	1. Medication is generally not effective when the CrCl is <25 ml/min.	
	2. Serum potassium level	2. To monitor for hyperkalemia	2. Hyperkalemia may result in decreased renal function. Potassium supplement is generally not needed.
	3. CBC with indices	3. May cause blood dyscrasias, risk is increased with liver disease	3. Triamterene antagonizes the conversion of inactive folate to active folate.
Valproic acid (DEPAKENE)	1. Serum drug level	1. To monitor effectiveness of therapy	
	2. CBC including platelets	2. May cause blood dyscrasias and thrombocytopenia	
	3. Liver function tests (SGOT, SGPT, bilirubin, and alk. phos.)	3. Drug may cause hepatotoxicity	
Warfarin (COUMADIN)	1. Prothrombin time (PT)	1. To monitor therapeutic effect of the drug	1. Prothrombin time should be about 1.5 to 2 times the control value.
		2. Many drugs can increase prothrombin times.	

■ References

1. Benett W, Aronoff GR, Morrison G, Golper TA, Pulliam J, Wolfson M, Singer I. Drug prescribing in renal failure: Dosing guidelines for adults. *Am J Kidney Dis* 1983; 3:155–193.

2. Friedman H, Greenblatt DJ. Rational therapeutic drug monitoring. *JAMA* 1986; 256:2227–2233.

3. Perrca E, Grimaldi R, Crema A. Interpretation of drug levels in acute and chronic disease states. *Clin Pharmacokinet* 1985; 10:498–513.

4. Roch RC. Monitoring therapeutic drug levels in older patients. *Geriatrics* 1985; 40:75–86.

5. Aronson JK. Clinical pharmacokinetics of digoxin. *Clin Pharmacokinet* 1980; 5:137–149.

6. Bassey HI, Hoffman EW. A prospective evaluation of therapeutic drug monitoring. *Ther Drug Monit* 1983; 5:245–248.

7. Billing B, Dahlquist R, et al. Separate and combined use of theophylline in asthmatics. *Eur J Respir Dis* 1982; 63:399–409.

8. Clague HW, Twum-Barima Y, Carruthers G. An audit of requests for therapeutic drug monitoring of digoxin: Problems and pitfalls. *Therap Drug Monit* 1983; 5:249–254.

9. Elin RJ. Discrepant results for the determination of theophylline in serum from a patient with renal failure. *Clin Chem* 1983; 29:1275.

10. Elin RJ, Ruddell M. Discrepant results for determination of theophylline in serum of uremic patients. *Clin Chem* 1983; 29:1670.

11. Giacomini KM, Blaschke TF. Effect of concentration-dependent binding to plasma proteins on the pharmacokinetics and pharmacodynamics of disopyramide. *Clin Pharmacokinet* 1984, 9(suppl 1):42–48.

12. Gibson TP, Nelson AH. The question of digoxin metabolites in renal failure. *Clin Pharmacol Therap* 1980; 27:219–223.

13. Graves S, Brown B, Valdes R. Digoxin-like substance in uremic patients: False positive effects on digoxin assays. *Clin Chem* 1983; 29:1166.

14. Jusko WJ, Weintraub M. Myocardial distribution of digoxin in renal failure. *Clin Pharmacol Therap* 1974; 16:449–454.

15. Koch-Weser J. Serum drug concentrations as therapeutic guides. *N Engl J Med* 1972; 287:227–231.

16. Nandedkar A, Williamson R, et al. A comparison of plasma phenytoin level determinations by EMIT and gas-liquid chromatography in patients with renal insufficiency. *Ther Drug Monit* 1980; 4:181–184.

17. Richens A, Warrington S. When should plasma drug levels be monitored? *Drugs* 1979; 17:488–500.

18. Weintraub M. Interpretation of the serum digoxin concentration. *Clin Pharmacokinet* 1977; 2:205–219.

19. Yosselson-Superstine S. Drug interferences with plasma assays in therapeutic drug monitoring. *Clin Pharmacokinet* 1984; 9:67–87.

20. Greenblatt DJ, Shader RI. *Pharmacokinetics in Clinical Practice*. WB Saunders, Philadelphia, 1985.

21. Ochs HR, Greenblatt DJ, Bodem G, Smith TW. Serum digoxin concentrations and subjective manifestations of toxicity. *Pharmacology* 1980; 20:149–154.

22. Blaschke TF, Rubin PC. Hepatic first-pass metabolism in liver disease. *Clin Pharmacokinet* 1979; 4:423–432.

23. Levy RH, Moreland TA. Rationale for monitoring free drug levels. *Clin Pharmacokinet* 1984; 9(suppl 1):1–9.

24. Greenblatt DJ, Sellers EM, Koch-Weser J. Importance of protein binding for the interpretation of serum or plasma drug concentration. *J Clin Pharmacol* 1982; 22:259–263.

25. Froscher W, Burr W, et al. Free level monitoring of carbamazepine and valproic acid: Clinical significance. *Clin Neuropharmacol* 1985; 8:362–371.

26. Piafsky KM. Disease-induced changes in the plasma binding of basic drugs. *Clin Pharmacokinet* 1980; 5:246–262.

27. Caranasos GJ, Stewart RB, Cluff LE. Drug-induced illness leading to hospitalization. *JAMA* 1974; 228–7137.

28. Greenblatt DJ, Sellers EM, Shader RI. Drug disposition in old age. *N Engl J Med* 1982; 306:1081–8.

29. Wilkinson GR. Drug disposition and renal excretion in the elderly. *J Chronic Dis* 1983; 36:91–102.

30. Williams RL. Drug administration in hepatic disease. *N Engl J Med* 1983; 309:1616–22.

31. Bennett WM, Muther RS, Parker RA, et al. Drug therapy in renal failure: Dosing guidelines for adults. *Ann Intern Med* 1980; 93:62–89; 286–325.

32. Lee TH, Smith TW. Serum digoxin concentration and diagnosis of digitalis toxicity: current concepts. *Clin Pharmacokinet* 1983; 8:279–285.

33. Barza M, Lauermann M. Why monitor serum levels of gentamicin? *Clin Pharmacokinet* 1978; 3:202–215.

34. Brown JE, Shand DG. Therapeutic drug monitoring of antiarrhythmic agents. *Clin Pharmacokinet* 1982; 7:125–48.

35. Ochs HR, Greenblatt DJ, Woo E. Clinical pharmacokinetics of quinidine. *Clin Pharmacokinet* 1980; 5:150–68.

36. Powell JR, Dunn KH. Histamine H2–antagonist drug interactions in perspective: Mechanistic concepts and clinical implications. *Am J Med* 1984; 77(suppl 56):57–84.

Chapter 6
Medical Terminology

■ Origin of Medical Terminology

Medical terminology is the language utilized by health care professionals involved in the delivery of health care. Modern medicine owes the inception of its terminology to the Greek culture dating back to the time of Hippocrates (460–375 B.C.) and to the fall of the Roman empire in the sixth century A.D. Greek medical terminology was so completely accepted by the Romans that only a few Latin terms have survived through the ages (1–3).

Aristotle (384–322 B.C.) and Galen (130–200 A.D.) were very influential in the development of medical terminology. In the writings of Aristotle, baldness and certain eye conditions are mentioned. Galen's writings describe the human anatomy, physiology, and theories of disease processes.

Several animal names also have become the origin of medical terms. For example, *carcinoma* derives from the Greek word for *crab* (*karkinos*), the Latin word for *crab* is *cancer* and the Latin word *lupus* means *wolf*. Other medical terms that reflect the warlike spirit of the Hellenistic Age include *xiphoid, thyroid,* and *thorax*—derived from the Greek words for *sword, shield,* and *breastplate,* respectively (1–3). The os sacrum (*sacred bone*) was named by the Romans (about 330 B.C.) as a direct translation from Greek (*hieron osteon*). The sacrum was believed to be the last bone in the body to disintegrate after death. Jews believed that the sacrum was a sacred bone and necessary for resurrection of the body after death (4).

Since the Greek and Latin languages are not commonly used in our daily conversation today, Greek and Latin words have almost the same meaning in every country and provide a universal language. However, some medical terms are hybrids and may be a combination of a Greek prefix along with a Latin root word. Sometimes, medical terms may have more than one acceptable pronunciation and/or spelling. In these situations, both Greek and Latin spellings of the term have been accepted and utilized.

■ Medical Term Components (1–3)

Most medical terms are composed of root words that have been derived from either Greek or Latin and may be used in combination with prefixes and/or suffixes. It is important to remember that the root word is the main body of the word and may indicate either an organ or a body part which is modified by a prefix and/or suffix. Prefixes are attached to the beginning of a root word and are frequently used in the formation of medical terms. Suffixes are attached to the end of a root word to indicate the type of disease or abnormality. Therefore, in analyzing a medical term it is usually best first to determine the meaning of the suffix and then to proceed to the root word and the prefix.

■ Anatomical Terminology

Anatomical terms refer to the body in what is called the anatomical position. In this position, the body is erect, eyes looking forward, upper limbs hanging at the sides with palms of hands facing forward, and the lower limbs are parallel with toes pointing forward. Medical terms frequently used to describe a patient always relate to the anatomical position as a point of reference (see Figure 6.1).

The body is divided into a series of planes so that specific references to an organ and/or structure may relate to each other as follows (5):

(*a*)　Frontal or coronal plane—vertical plane which divides the body or structure into the anterior and posterior portions.

(*b*)　Horizontal/transverse or oblique plane—a plane running across the body parallel to the ground and dividing the body or structure into upper and lower portions.

(*c*)　Sagittal plane/median plane—divides the body or structure into a lengthwise plane and divides the body into symmetrical right and left halves or portions.

(*d*)　Inferior or caudal—refers to away from the head and below other structures.

(*e*)　Superior or cephalic—refers to toward the head and situated above other structures.

(*f*)　Anterior or ventral—refers to the front of the body.

(*g*)　Posterior or dorsal—refers to the back of the body.

(*h*)　Abduction—refers to movement away from the body midline.

(*i*)　Adduction—refers to movement toward the midline or back of the body.

The following tables contain some commonly used medical terms, prefixes, suffixes, and medical abbreviations. A basic understanding of the origin of medical terminology along with the use of these reference tables should help the clinical pharmacist better interpret and understand patient data.

FIGURE 6.1   ANATOMICAL POSITION OF THE BODY

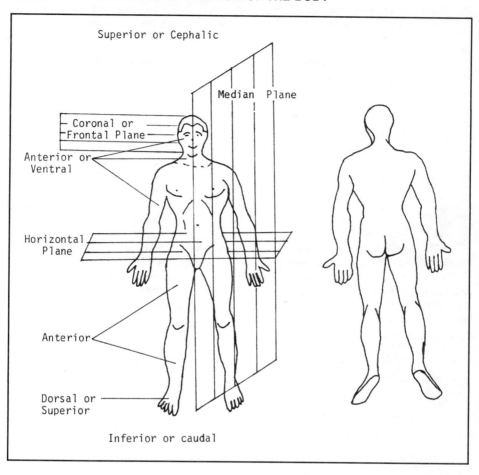

Medical Abbreviations

A	Assessment; artery; ambulatory
A_2	Aortic second sound
$A_2 > P_2$	Aortic second sound greater than second pulmonary sound

AA	Alcoholics Anonymous; amino acid
AAA	Abdominal aortic aneurysmectomy
Ab	Abortion; antibody
ABD	Abdomen; abdominal

ABE	Acute bacterial endocarditis
ABG	Arterial blood gases
ABS	At bedside; admitting blood sugar
AC	Acute; before meals; antecubital; acetate
ACB	Antibody-coated bacteria
ACE	Angiotensin-converting enzyme
ACh	Acetylcholine
ACT	Activated clotting time
ACTH	Corticotropin (adrenocorticotrophic)
ADA	American Diabetes Association; adenosine deaminase
ADD	Attention deficit disorder
add.	Adduction
ADH	Antidiuretic hormone
ADL	Activities of daily living
ad lib	As desired/at liberty
ADM	Admission; doxorubicin
ADP	Adenosine diphosphate
AF	Atrial fibrillation; acid fast
AFB	Acid-fast bacilli
A.fib	Atrial fibrillation
A/G	Albumin to globulin ratio
aggl.	Agglutination
AGL	Acute granulocytic leukemia
AGN	Acute glomerulonephritis
AHA	Autoimmune hemolytic anemia, American Hospital Association
AHF	Antihemophilic factor
AHFS	American Hospital Formulary service
AI	Aortic insufficiency
AIDS	Acquired immune deficiency syndrome
AK	Above knee
AKA	Above-knee amputation
ALA	Aminolevulinic acid
ALAT	Alanine transaminase (alanine aminotransferase: SGPT)
Alb	Albumin
ALD	Alcohol liver disease; aldolase
ALG	Antilymphocyte globulin
alk	Alkaline
ALL	Acute lymphocytic leukemia

ALP	Alkaline phosphatase
ALS	Amyotrophic lateral sclerosis; acute lateral sclerosis
ALT	Alanine transaminase (liver heart enzyme), formerly SGPT
AMA	Against medical advice
Amb	Ambulate; ambulatory
AMI	Acute myocardial infarction
AML	Acute myelogenous leukemia
AMP	Amputation; ampul; ampicillin; adenosine monophosphate
ANA	Antinuclear antibody
ANF	Antinuclear factor
ANS	Autonomic nervous system
ant.	Anterior
ante	Before
AODM	Adult onset diabetes mellitus
A & P	Anterior and posterior; ausculation and percussion; assessment and plans
AP	Anterior and posterior; ausculation antepartum; apical pulse; appendicitis; assessment and plans
APAP	Acetaminophen
APC	Aspirin, phenacetin and caffeine; arterial premature contraction
APE	Acute psychotic episode
APKD	Adult polycystic kidney disease
APTT	Activated thromboplastin time
aq dist	Distilled water
ARA-A	vidarabine
ara-C	Cytosine arabinoside
ARC	AIDS-related complex
ARD	Adult respiratory distress; acute respiratory disease
ARDS	Adult respiratory distress syndrome
ARF	Acute renal failure; acute rheumatic fever
AROM	Active range of motion
AS	Aortic stenosis; activated sleep; anal sphincter; left ear
ASA	Acetylsalicylic acid (aspirin); argininosuccinate

ASAP	As soon as possible	Bili	Bilirubin
ASAT	Aspartate transaminase (aspartate aminotransferase)	BK	Below knee
		BKA	Below knee amputation
ASCVD	Arteriosclerotic cardio-vascular disease	bkft	Breakfast
		BLE	Both lower extremities
ASD	Atrial septal defect	BLEO	Bleomycin sulfate
ASHD	Arteriosclerotic heart disease	BLS	Basic life support
AST	Aspartate transaminase (liver and heart enzyme), formerly SGOT	BM	Bowel movement; bone marrow; black male
		BMR	Basal metabolic rate
ATB	Antibiotic	B & O	Belladonna & opium
At Fib	trial fibrillation	BP	Blood pressure; benzoyl peroxide; British Pharmacopeia
ATN	Acute tubular necrosis		
ATP	Adenosine triphosphate		
ATPase	Adenosine triphosphatase	BPH	Benign prostatic hypertrophy
AU	Both ears; gold	BPM	Breaths per minute; beats per minute
AV	Arteriovenous; atrioventricular		
		BPRS	Brief psychiatric rating scale
AVR	Aortic valve replacement	BRP	Bathroom privileges
A & W	Alive and well	BS	Blood sugar; breath sounds; bowel sounds
A waves	Atrial contraction waves		
		BSA	Body surface area
		BSF	Busulfan
B	Bacillus; bands; black	BSO	Bilateral salpingooophorectomy
B_1	Thiamine HCl		
B_2	Riboflavin	BSP	Bromsulfophthalein
B_6	Pyridoxine HC1	BT	Breast tumor; brain tumor; bedtime
B_7	Biotin		
B_8	Adenosine phosphate	BUE	Both upper extremities
B_{12}	Cyanocobalamin	BUN	Blood urea nitrogen
Ba	Barium	BW	Body weight
BACOP	Bleomycin, adriamycin, cyclophosphamide, vincristine, prednisone	B	Phenobarbital
		BZ	Phenylbutazone
		Bx	Biopsy
BaE	Barium enema		
BAERs	Brainstem auditory-evoked responses		
		$\overline{c}$	With
baso	Basophil	C	Clubbing; cyanosis; carbohydrate; centigrade; ascorbic acid
BBB	Bundle branch block		
BBT	Basal body temperature		
B-cell	Large lymphocyte produced in the bone marrow	C_1	First cervical vertebra
		Ca	Calcium
BCG	Bacillus Calmette-Guérin vaccine	C & A	Clinitest and Acetest
		CA	Carcinoma; chronologic age
BCNU	Carmustine	CAB	Coronary artery bypass
BE	Barium enema; below elbow	CABG	Coronary artery bypass graft
BF	Black female	CAD	Coronary artery disease
BI	Bowel impaction; bladder irritation	CAL	Calories
		CAPD	Chronic ambulatory peritoneal dialysis
BID	Twice daily		

CARB	Carbohydrate	COAD	Chronic obstructive airway disease
CAT	Computed axial tomography; children's apperception test; cataract	COAP	Cyclophosphamide/vincristine/cytarabine/prednisone
cath.	Catheter; catheterization	COHB	Carboxyhemoglobin
CBC	Complete blood count; carbenicillin	COLD	Chronic obstructive lung disease
CBR	Complete bed rest	COP	Cyclophosphamide, vincristine, prednisone
CBS	Chronic brain syndrome		
CC	Chief complaint; cubic centimeter	COPD	Chronic obstructive pulmonary disease
CCMSU	Clean catch midstream urine	COPP	Cyclophosphamide/vincristine/procarbazine/prednisone
CCNU	Lomustine		
CCU	Coronary care unit		
CDC	Center for Disease Control; chenodexycholic acid	Cor	Coronary
CEA	Carcinoembryonic antigen	C.P., CP	Cerebral palsy; cleft palate; creatinine phosphokinase
CF	Cystic fibrosis; caucasian female; complement fixation; cardiac failure; cancer-free	CPA	Costophrenic angle
		CPAP	Continuous positive airway pressure
CGL	Chronic granulocytic anemia	CPD	Citrate-phosphate-dextrose
CGN	Chronic glomerulonephritis	CPK	Creatinine phosphokinase
CHD	Congential heart disease	CPKD	Childhood polycystic kidney
CHF	Congestive heart failure	CPP	Cerebral perfusion pressure
CHO	Carbohydrate	CPR	Cardiopulmonary resuscitation
CHOP	Cyclophosphamide/doxorubicin/vincristine/prednisone		
		CPZ	Chlorpromazine; Compazine
CI	Cardiac index	Cr	Creatinine
CIE	Counter immunoelectrophoresis	CrCl	Creatinine clearance
		CRF	Chronic renal failure
CK	Creatine kinase	Crit.	Hematocrit
Cl	Chloride	C & S	Culture and sensitivity
CLL	Chronic lymphocytic leukemia	C sect.	Cesarean section
		CSF	Cerebrospinal fluid; colony-stimulating factor
Cm,cm	Centimeter		
CM	Costal margin; capreomycin; continuous murmur; caucasian male; centimeter	CSR	Central supply room; Cheyne-Stokes respiration
		CT	Computed tomography; circulation time
CMF	Cyclophosphamide/fluorouracil/methotrexate		
		CTM	Chlortrimeton
CMI	Cell-mediated immunity	CTX	Cyclophosphamide
CMJ	Carpometacarpal joint	Cu	Copper
CML	Chronic myelogenous leukemia	CV	Cardiovascular; cell volume
		CVA	Cerebrovascular accident; costovertebral angle
CMV	Cytomegalovirus		
CN	Cranial nerve	CVAT	Costovertebral angle tenderness
CNS	Central nervous system		
C/O	Complaint of	CVP	Central venous pressure
CO_2	Carbon dioxide	C/W	Consistent with

Cx	Cervix	DNR	Do not resuscitate
CXR	Chest x-ray	D₅NS	5% dextrose in normal saline
DIC	Vincristine, adriamycin, dacarbazine	DO	Osteopathic physician
CZI	Crystalline zinc insulin	DOA	Dead on arrival; date of admission

		DOC	Drug of choice
		DOCA	Desoxycorticosterone acetate
		DOB	Date of birth
D	Diarrhea; cholecalciferol	DOE	Dyspnea on exertion
DA	Dopamine	DOSS	Docusate sodium (dioctyl sodium sulfosuccinate)
DACT	Dactinomycin		
db	Decibel	DP	Dorsalis pedic (pulse)
D & C	Dilation and curettage	DPH	Phenytoin; diphenhydramine
D/C, DC,	Discharge; discontinue;	DPT	Diphtheria, pertussis, tetanus
d/c	decrease	DRG	Diagnosis-related group
DC65	Darvon Compound 65 mg	DS	Double strength; disoriented
DCN	Darvocet-N	DSS	Docusate sodium
DCNU	Chlorozotocin	DT	Discharrge tomorrow; diphtheria tetanus; diphtheria toxoid
DD	Differential diagnosis		
DDAVP	Demopressin acetate		
DDD	Degenerative disc disease	DTIC	Dacarbazine
DDS	Dialysis disequilibrium syndrome; doctor of dental surgery	DTR	Deep tendon reflexes
		DTs	Delirium tremens
		DTT	Diphtheria, tetanus, toxoid
DDT	Chlorophenothane	DU	Duodenal ulcer
DES	Disequilibrium syndrome; diethylstilbestrol; diffuse esophageal spasm	DVT	Deep vein thrombosis
		D₅W	5% dextrose in water injection
dex.	Dexter (right)	DW	Dextrose in water; distilled water; deionized water
DHL	Diffuse histocytic lymphoma		
DI	Diabetes insipidus	5DW	5% dextrose in water
DIC	Disseminated intravascular coagulation; dacarbazine	Dx	Diagnosis
DIFF	Differential blood count		
Dig	Digoxin		
dis	Dislocation	e	Without
DJD	Degenerative joint disease	E → A	Say E.E.E. comes out as A.A.A. upon auscultation of lung showing consolidation
DK, DKA	Diabetic ketoacidosis		
DL, dl	Deciliter		
D5LR	Dextrose 5% in lactated Ringer's solution	EACA	Aminocaproic acid
		EBV	Epstein-Barr virus
DM	Diabetes mellitus; diastolic murmur; dextromethorphan	EC	Enteric coated
		ECF	Extracellular fluid
DMKA	Diabetes mellitus ketoacidosis	ECG	Electrocardiogram
		ECHO	Etoposide, cyclophosphamide, adriamycin, vincristine; echocardiogram
DMOOC	Diabetes mellitus out of control		
DMSO	Dimethyl sulfoxide		
DNA	Deoxyribosenucleic acid	ECT	Electroconvulsive therapy
DNCB	Dinitrochlorobenzene	ED	Emergency department

EDC	Estimated date of confinement; estimated date of conception	FRC	Functional residual capacity
		FROM	Full range of movement
		FSH	Follicle-stimulating hormone
EDTA	Ethylenediaminetetra acetate	FTA	Fluorescent titer antibody; fluoresecent treponemal antibody
EEG	Electroencephalogram		
EENT	Eyes, ears, nose, throat		
EFAD	Essential fatty acid deficiency	FTI	Free thyroid index
EGA	Estimated gestational age	FTND	Full-term normal delivery
EKG	Electrocardiogram	FTSG	Full-thickness skin graft
EMB	Ethambutol	FTT	Failure to thrive
EMG	Electromyograph	F & U	Flanks and upper quadrants
ENDO	Endotracheal	F/U	Follow-up
ENT	Eyes, nose, throat	5–FU	Fluorouracil
EOM	Extraocular movement	FUO	Fever of undetermined origin
EOMI	Extraocular muscles intact	Fx	Fracture
eos.	Eosinophil	Fx-dis	Fracture-dislocation
EPI	Epinephrine	Fxn	Function
epith.	Epithelial		
ER	Emergency room; estrogen receptors		
ERCP	Endoscopic retrograde cholangiopancreatography	G	Gauge; gravida; gram; gallop
		G 1/4	grade 1/4
ESR	Erythrocyte sedimentation rate	GA	Gastric analysis; glucose/acetone; general appearance
ESRD	End-stage renal disease	GABA	γ-aminobutyric acid
EST	Electroshock therapy	GB	Gallbladder
ETH	Elixir terpin hydrate	GBM	Glomerular basement membrane
ETH c̄ C	Elixir terpin hydrate with codeine		
		GBS	Gallbladder series
ETOH	Alcohol; alcoholic	GC	Gonococci (gonorrhea)
ext.	Extract; external	G and D	Growth and development
		GENT	Gentamicin
		GFR	Glomerular filtration rate
F	Fahrenheit; female	GG	γ-globulin; guaifenesin
FA	Folic acid	GH	Growth hormone
FBS	Fasting blood sugar	GI	Gastrointestinal
FC	Foley catheter	GIT	Gastrointestinal tract
5–FC	Flucytosine	GN	Graduate nurse; glomerulonephritis
F. cath	Foley catheter		
FDP	Fibrin-degradation products	GOT	Glutamic-oxaloacetic transaminase; aspartate aminotransferase
Fe, fe	Iron; female		
FEV_1	Forced expiratory volume in 1 sec		
		G6PD	Glucose-6–phosphate dehydrogenase
FFA	Free fatty acid		
FH	Family history	GPT	Glutamic pyruvic transaminase
FHR	Fetal heart rate		
FHT	Fatal heart tone	Grav.	Gravid (pregnancy)
FLK	Funny-looking kid	$GR_1P_0AB_1$	One pregnancy, no births, one abortion
FOB	Foot of bed; fiberoptic bronchoscope		
		GSW	Gunshot wound

GTT	Glucose tolerance test; drop	HS	Bedtime; Hartman's solution (lactated Ringer's); hereditary spherocytosis
GU	Genitourinary		
Gyn	Gynecology		
		HSV	Herpes simplex virus
		HT	Hypertension; hypodermic tablet
H	Hypodermic	5–HT	5–hydroxytryptamine
HA	Headache; hyperalimentation	HTN	Hypertension
HAA	Hepatitis-associated antigen	5–HTP	5–hydroxytryptophan
HAF	Hyperalimentation fluid	HU	Hydroxyurea
HB	Hemoglobin		
HBA$_g$	Hepatitis B antigen		
HBIG	Hepatitis B immune globulin		
HBP	High blood pressure	I	Iodine, impression
HBV	Hepatitis B virus; hepatitis B vaccine	IABP	Intraaortic balloon pump
		IADH	Inappropriate antidiuretic hormone
HC	Hydrocortisone; home care		
HCG	Human chorionic gonadotropin	IBC	Iron-binding capacity
		IBI	Intermittent bladder irrigation
HCl	Hydrochloric acid;		
HCO$_3$	Bicarbonate	ICF	Intracellular fluid
ˋHCT,	Hematocrit	ICM	Intracostal margin
✔ Hct		ICP	Intracranial pressure
HCTZ	Hydrochlorothiazide	ICN	Intensive care nursery
HCVD	Hypertensive cardiovascularr disease	ICU	Intensive care unit
		ID	Intradermal; initial dose; infectious disease
HD	Hearing distance; Hodgkin's disease		
		I & D	Incision and drainage
HDCV	Human diploid cell vaccine	IDDM	Insulin-dependent diabetes mellitus
HDL	High-density lipoprotein		
HEENT	Head, eyes, ears, nose, throat	IF	Intrinsic factor; interferon; interstitial
hemi	Hemiplegia		
Hgb	Hemoglobin	IFA	Indirect fluorescent antibody test
H & H	Hematocrit and hemoglobin		
5–HIAA	5 hydroxyindolacetic acid	IgA	Immunoglobulin A
Histo	Histoplasmin skin test	IgD	Immunoglobulin D
HJR	Hepatojugular reflux	IgE	Immunoglobulin E
HL	Hairline; heparin lock	IgG	Immunoglobulin G
HLA	Human lymphocyte antigen	IgM	Immunoglobulin M
H & N	Head and neck	IHD	Ischemic heart disease
HO, H/O	History officer	IHSS	Idiopathic hypertrophic subaortic stenosis
H$_2$O	Water		
H$_2$O$_2$	Hydrogen peroxide	IM	Intramuscular; infectious mononucleosis
HOB	Head of bed		
H & P	History and physical	IMP	Impression
HPF	High-power field	IMV	Intermittent mandatory ventilation
HPI	History of present illness		
HPN	Home parenteral nutrition	INH	Isoniazid
HR	Heart rate; hour	I & O	Intake and output

IOP	Intraocular pressure		KUB	Kidney, ureter, bladder
IP	Intraperitoneal		KVO	Keep vein open
IPD	Immediate pigment darkening; intermittent peritoneal dialysis		L	Left; liter
IPPB	Intermittent positive pressure breathing		L_2	Second lumbar vertebra
IPV	Inactivated polio vaccine		LA	Left atrium
ICS	Intercostal space		L & A	Light and accommodation
ISG	Immune serum globulin		lac.	Laceration
ISW	Interstitial water		LAD	Left anterior descending
IT	Intrathecal; inhalation therapy		LAG	Lymphangiogram
IU	International unit		LAP	laparotomy; leucine amino peptidase; left arterial pressure
IUD	Intrauterine device		LAT	Lateral
IV	Intravenous; four		LB	Low back
IVC	Intravenous cholangiogram, inferior vena cava		LBBB	Left bundle branch block
IVF	In vitro fertilization		LBP	Low back pain
IVH	Intravenous hyperalimentation		LBW	Low birth weight
IVP	Intravenous pyelogram; intravenous push		LCD	Coal tar solution (liquor carbonis detergens)
IVPB	Intravenous piggyback		LCM	Left costal margin; lymphocytic choriomeningitis
IVSS	Intravenous soluset		LD	Lethal dose; liver disease; lactic dehydrogenase; loading dose
IWMI	Inferior wall myocardial infarct		LDH	Lactic dehydrogenase
			LDL	Low-density lipoprotein
			LE	Lupus erythematosus; lower extremities
JODM	Juvenile onset diabetes mellitus		LES	Lower esophagheal sphincter
JRA	Juvenile rheumatoid arthritis		LFT	Liver function tests
JVD	Jugular venous distention		LGA	Large for gestational age
JVP	Jugular venous pulse		LH	Luteinizing hormone
			LHF	Left heart failure
			Li	Lithium
			LIH	Left inguinal hernia
K	Potassium; vitamin K		LKS	Liver, kidneys, spleen
K_1	Phytonadione		LLE	Left lower extremity
kcal	Kilocalorie		LLL	Left lower lobe; left lower lid
KCl	Potassium chloride		LLQ	Left lower quadrant
KDA	Known drug allergies		LMD	Local medical doctor; low molecular weight dextran
KF	Kidney function		LMP	Last menstrual period
Kg	Kilogram		LNMP	Last normal menstrual period
KI	Potassium iodide		LOC	Loss of consciousness; laxative of choice; level of consciousness
KJ	Knee jerk			
$KMnO_2$	Potassium permanganate			
KO	Keep open			

LOS	Length of stay	MDR	Minimum daily requirement
LP	Lumbar puncture; light perception	mEq	Milliequivalent
lpf	Low-power field	MF	Myocardial fibrosis; mycosis fungoides
LPN	Licensed practical nurse	MG	Myasthenia gravis; milligram; magnesium
LSB	Left sternal border		
L-Spar	Elspar (asparaginase)	MH	Marital history; menstrual history; mental health
LT	Light; left		
LTCF	Long-term care facility	MH/MR	Mental health & mental retardation
LUE	Left upper extremity		
LUL	Left upper lobe (lung)	MI	Myocardial infarction; mitral insufficiency
LUQ	Left upper quadrant		
LV	Left ventricle	MIC	Minimum inhibitory concentration
LVEDP	Left ventricular end diastolic pressure		
		MICU	Medical intensive care unit
LVEDV	Left ventricular end diastolic volume	MKAB	May keep at bedside
		ML	Midline; milliliter
LVH	Left ventricular hypertrophy	Mm, mm	Millimeter; mucous membrane
LVP	left ventricular pressure		
L & W	Living and well	M & M	Milk and molasses; morbidity and mortality
lytes	Electrolytes (Na$^+$, K$^+$, Cl$^-$, etc.)		
		mmole	Millimole
		MMPI	Minnesota Multiphasic Personality Inventory
M	Murmur; monocytes; male; molar		
		MMR	Measles, mumps, rubella
M$_1$	First mitral sound	MN	Midnight; manganese
M$_2$	Square meters (body surface)	MO	Mineral oil
MA	Mental age	MOM	Milk of magnesia
MAC	Maximal allowable concentration	mono	Monocyte; infectious mononucleosis
MAL	Midaxillary line	MOPP	Mechlorethamine/vicristine/ procarbazine/ prednisone
MAOI	Monoamine oxidase inhibitor		
MAP	Mean arterial pressure	mOsmole	Milliosmole
MBC	Maximum breathing capacity; minimal bacteriocidal concentration	MP	Metacarpophalangeal joint
		6–MP	Mercaptopurine
		MR	Mental retardation; may repeat
MBD	Minimal brain damage		
mcg, μg	Microgram	MR × 1	May repeat times one
MCH	Mean corpuscular hemoglobin	MS	Morphine sulfate; multiple sclerosis; mitral stenosis; musculoskeletal
MCHC	Mean corpuscular hemoglobin concentration		
		MSW	Multiple stab wounds
MCL	Midclavicular line; midcostal line	MTD	Monro tidal drainage
		MTX	Methotrexate
MCP	Metacarpophalangeal joint	MU	Million units
MCT	Medium chain triglyceride	MUGA	Multiple-gated acquisition
MCV	Mean corpuscular volume	MVA	Motor vehicle accident
MD	Mental deficiency; muscular dystrophy; medical doctor	MVI	Trade name parenteral multivitamin

MVI 12	Trade name parenteral multivitamin		NSR	Normal sinus rhythm
MVP	Mitral valve prolapse		NSS	Sodium chloride 0.9% (normal saline solution)
MVR	Mitral valve replacement		1/2 NSS	Sodium chloride 0.45% (1/2 normal saline solution)
			N & T	Nose and throat
			NTG	Nitroglycerin
N	Normal		NTP	Nitroprusside
NAD	No acute distress; no apparent distress		NV	Neurovascular
			N & V	Nausea and vomiting
NAS	No added salt		NVD	Neck vein distention; nausea, vomiting, and diarrhea; no venereal disease
NBS	Normal bowel sound			
NC	Neurologic check; no complaints; not completed; nasal cannula			
NCB	No code blue			
NE	Norepinephrine		O	Oxygen; objective findings; eye; oral
NET	Nasoendotracheal tube			
NG	Nasogastric		Ob	Obstetrics
NGU	Nongonococcal urethritis		OB	Occult blood
NHL	Non-Hodgkin's lymphomas; nodular histiocytic lymphoma		Ob-Gyn	Obstetrics and gynecology
			OBS	Organic brain syndrome
			OC	Oral contraceptive
NICU	Neurosurgical intensive care unit; neonatal intensive care unit		OCG	Oral cholecystogram
			OD	Right eye; overdose; doctor of optometry
NIDD	Noninsulin-dependent diabetes		OFC	Occipitofrontal circumference
NIDDM	Noninsulin-dependent diabetes mellitus		OH	Occupational history
			OHD	Organic heart disease; hydroxy vitamin D
NKA	No known allergies			
NKDA	No known drug allergies		OJ	Orange juice
NL	Normal; normal limits		OOB	Out of bed
NMT	No more than		OOBBRP	Out of bed with bathroom privileges
no.	Number			
NOR-EPI	Norepinephrine		OOC	Out of control
NPH	Normal pressure hydrocephalus; a type of insulin (Isophane)		OOR	Out of room
			OP	Outpatient
			O & P	Ova and parasites
NPN	Nonprotein nitrogen		OPV	Oral polio vaccine
NPO	Nothing by mouth		OR	Operating room
NREM	Nonrapid eye movement		OS	Left eye; opening snap
NREMS	Nonrapid eye movement sleep		OT	Occupational therapy
			OU	Both eyes
NS	Normal saline solution; nephrotic syndrome; nuclear sclerosis			
NSA	Normal serum albumin		P	Plan; protein
NSAID	Nonsteroidal anti-inflammatory drug		$\bar{p}$	After, post
			p_2	Pulmonic second heart sound

PA	Posteroanterior; pulmonary artery; pernicious anemia; physician's assistant	PFR	Peak flow rate; parotid flow rate
P & A	Percussion and ausculation	PFT	Pulmonary function test
PAC	Premature atrial contraction	PG	Pregnant; paregoric
PAH	Para-aminohippurate	pH	Hydrogen ion concentration
Pap	Papanicolaou smear	PH	Past history
PAR	Postanesthetic recovery	PHA	Peripheral hyperalimentation; passive hemagglutinating; phytohemagglutinin
PARA	Number of pregnancies		
PAS or PASA	Para-aminosalicylic acid	pHa	Arterial blood pH
		PHT	Phenytoin
PAT	Paroxysmal atrial tachycardia; preadmission testing	PI	Present illness
		PIAT	Peabody Individual Achievement Test
Path.	Pathology		
Pb	Lead; phenobarbital	PICU	Pediatric intensive care unit
P & B	Phenobarbital & belladonna	PID	Pelvic inflammatory disease
PBI	Protein-bound iodine	PIP	Proximal interphalangeal joint
PBN	Polymyxin B sulfate, bacitracin, and neomycin		
		Pit	Pitocin; pitressin
PBZ	Pyribenzamine; phenylbutazone; phenoxybenzamine	PKU	Phenylketonuria
		plts	Platelets
		PM	Postmortem, evening; pretibial myxedema
BZ	Phenylbutazone		
pc	After meal	PMC	Pseudomembranous colitis
PCU	Progressive care unit	PMH	Past medical history
PCN	Penicillin	PMI	Point of maximal impulse
PCO_2	Carbon dioxide pressure or tension	PMN	Polymorphonucleocytes
		PMP	Previous menstrual period
PCP	Phencyclidine; pneumocystitis; *Pneumocystis carinii* pneumonia	PMS	Premenstrual syndrome
		PMT	Premenstrual tension
		PND	Paroxysmal nocturnal dyspnea; postnasal drip
PCV	Packed cell volume	PNS	Peripheral nervous system
PCWP	Pulmonary capillary wedge pressure	Pnx	Partial nonprogressing stroke
		Pnx	Pneumothorax
PCZ	Prochlorperazine	PO	By mouth
PD	Peritoneal dialysis; Parkinson's disease	POD 1	Postoperative day 1
		POLY	Polymorphonucleocytes
PE	Physical examination; pulmonary embolism; pulmonary edema	POMP	Prednisone, vincristine, methotrexate, mercaptopurine
Peds.	Pediatrics	POMR	Problem-oriented medical record
PEEP	Positive end-expiratory pressure		
		POp	Postoperative
PEG	Pneumoencephalogram; polyethylene glycol	post op	Postoperative
		PP	Postpartum; postprandial; paradoxical
PEP	Protein electrophoresis		
perf.	Perforation	PP	Pulse; pin prick
PERRLA	Pupils, equal, round, reactive to light and accommodation	PPBS	Postprandial blood sugar
		PPBG	Postprandial blood glucose

PPD	Purified protein derivative; packs per day; postpartum day		Px	Physical exam; pneumothorax
P & PD	Percussion and postural drainage		PZA	Pyrazinamide
PPF	Plasma protein fraction		PZI	Protamine zinc insulin
PPI	Patient package insert			
PPM	Parts per million		q, Q	Every
PPVT	Peabody Picture Vocabulary test		qd	Every day
			q4h	Every four hours
PR	Per rectum; pulse rate		qh	Every hour
P & R	Pulse and respiration		qhs	Every night
PRBC	Packed red blood cells		qid	Four times daily
Pred	Prednisone		qod	Every other day
pre-op	Before surgery		quad	Quadriplegic
prep	Prepare for surgery			
PRN, prn	As needed (pro re nata)			
PRO	Protein			
PROCTO	Proctoscopic; proctology		R	Respiration; right; rectum
prog.	Prognosis		RA	Rheumatoid arthritis; right atrium; right auricle
PROM	Passive range of motion; premature rupture of membrane		RAI	Radioactive iodine
			RAIU	Radioactive iodine uptake
PS	Pulmonary stenosis; paradoxic sleep; pathologic stage		RBBB	Right bundle branch block
			RBC	Red blood cell
			RBP	Retinol-binding protein
PT	Physical therapy; patient; prothrombin time; pine tar		RCM	Right costal margin
			RD	Renal disease
PTA	Prior to admission; plasma thromboplastin antecedent		RDA	Recommended daily allowance
PTCA	Percutaneous transluminal coronary angioplasty		RDS	Respiratory distress syndrome
PTH	Post-transfusion hepatitis; parathyroid hormone		RE	Reticuloendothelial
			Rehab	Rehabilitation
PTS	Prior to surgery		REM	Rapid eye movement
PTT	Partial thromboplastin time		REMS	Rapid eye movement sleep
PTU	Propylthiouracil		RES	Reticuloendothelial system
PUD	Peptic ulcer disease		Resp	Respiratory; respirations
pul.	Pulmonary		RF	Rheumatoid factor; renal failure; rheumatic fever
P & V	Pyloroplasty and vagotomy			
PVC	Premature ventricular contraction; pulmonary venous congestion		Rh	Rhesus factor in blood
			RHD	Rheumatic heart disease
			RHF	Right heart failure
PVD	Patient very disturbed; peripheral vascular disease		RIA	Radioimmunoassay
			RICU	Respiratory intensive care unit
PVP	Peripheral venous pressure; polyvinyl pyrolidone		RIG	Rabies immune globulin
			RIH	Right inguinal hernia
PVT	Paroxysmal ventricular tachycardia		RLE	Right lower extremity
PWP	Pulmonary wedge pressure		RLL	Right lower lobe

RLQ	Right lower quadrant	segs	Segmented neutrophils
RML	Right middle lobe (lung)	SEM	Systolic ejection murmur
RNA	Ribonucleic acid	SENS	Sensorium
R/O	Rule out	S.G.	Specific gravity
ROM	Range of motion	SGOT	Serum glutamic-oxaloacetic transaminase (also AST)
ROS	Review of systems		
RPGN	Rapidly progressive glomerulonephritis	SGPT	Serum glutamic-pyruvic transaminase (also ALT)
RPR	Rapid plasma reagin	SH	Social history; serum hepatitis
RQ	Respiratory quotient		
RR	Recovery room; respiratory rate	S & H	Speech and hearing
		SHEENT	Skin, head, eyes, ears, nose, throat
RRE	Round, regular, and equal (pupils)	SIADH	Syndrome of inappropriate antidiuretic hormone secretion
RRR	Regular rhythm and rate		
RSR	Regular sinus rhythm		
RT	Right; radiation therapy	sibs	Siblings
RTA	Renal tubular acidosis	SICU	Surgical intensive care unit
RTC	Return to clinic	SIDS	Sudden infant death syndrome
RUE	Right upper extremity		
RUL	Right upper lobe	SIT	Slossen Intelligence Test
rupt	Ruptured	SL	Sublingual
RUQ	Right upper quadrant	SLE	Systemic lupus erythematosus
RV	Right ventricle; residual volume; rectovaginal		
		SMA	Sequential multiple analyzer, simultaneous multichannel autoanalyzer
RVH	Right ventricular hypertrophy		
RXN	Reaction	SMX/TMP	Sulfamethoxazole/trimethoprim
		S-O	Salpingooophorectomy
s̄	Without	SOAP	Subjective, objective, assessment, and plans
S	Subjective findings		
S₁	First heart sound	SOB	Shortness of breath
S₂	Second heart sound	SOP	Standard operating procedure
SA	Sinoatrial; salicylic acid	SOS	May be repeated once if urgently required
S/A	Sugar and acetone		
S-A node	Sinoatrial node	S/P	Status post
SAH	Subarachnoid hemorrhage	SPA	Albumin human (formerly known as salt-poor albumin)
SBE	Subacute bacterial endocarditis		
		SPEC	Specimen
SB-LM	Stanford Binet Intelligence Test-Form LM	SPF	Sun protective factor
		sp fl	Spinal fluid
SBO	Small bowel obstruction	SQ	Subcutaneous
SC	Subcutaneous; subclavial; sickle cell; Snellen's chart; subclavian	SR	Sedimentation rate
		SrCr	Serum creatinine
		SRS-A	Slow-reacting substance of anaphylaxis
SDH	Subdural hematoma		
sed	Sedimentation	SS	Saline solution; sickle cell half
sed rt	Sedimentation rate		

S & S,	Signs and symptoms; support	TEN	Toxic epidermal necrolysis
S & Sx	& stimulation	TF	Tube feeding
SSE	Saline solution enema;	6–TG	Thioguanine
	soapsuds enema	THC	Transhepatic cholangiogram;
SSKI	Saturated solution potassium		tetrahydrocannabinol
	iodide	THP	Total hip replacement;
SSS	Sick-sinus syndrome		trihexphenidyl
ST	Speech therapist	TIA	Transient ischemic attack
staph	*Staphylococcus aureus*	TIBC	Total iron-binding
stat	Immediately		capacity
STD	Sexually transmitted diseases	TIG	Tetanus immune globulin
STD TF	Standard tube feeding	TL	Tubal ligation; team leader,
STG	Short-term goals		trial leave
strep	*Streptococcus* ; streptomycin	TLC	Tender loving care; total lung
STS	Serologic test for syphilis		capacity
sub q	Subcutaneous	TM	Tympanic membrane
SULF-	Trimethoprim and	TMP	Trimethoprim
PRIM	sulfamethoxazole	TMP/	Trimethoprim/
SVC	Superior vena cava	SMX	sulfamethoxazole
SVT	Supraventricular tachycardia	TMTC	Too many to count
SW	Social worker	TMX	Tamoxifen
SWI	Sterile water for injection	TNTC	Too numerous to count
Sx	Signs, symptom	TOPV	Trivalent oral polio
SZ	Seizure		vaccine
		TP	Total protein
T	Temperature	TPPE	Time, person, place, and
$T_{1/2}$	Half-life		event
T_1	Tricuspid; first sound; first	TPN	Total parenteral nutrition
	thoracic vertebra	TPR	Temperature, pulse, and
T_3	Liothyronine (3,5,3'-		respiration; total peripheral
	triiodithyronine)		resistance
T_4	Free thyroxine factor	trach.	Tracheal; tracheostomy
T & A	Tonsillectomy and	TRH	Thyrotropin-releasing
	adenoidectomy		hormone
TAH	Total abdominal	TRIG	Triglycerides
	hysterectomy	TRM-	Trimethoprim-
TAM	Tamoxifen	SMX	sulfamethaxazole
TB	Tuberculosis	TSH	Thyroid-stimulating hormone
TBG	Thyroxine-binding globulin	TSS	Toxic shock syndrome
TBI	Total body irradiation	TT	Transtrachael; thrombin time;
TBW	Total body water		tetanus toxoid
T & C	Type and crossmatch	TTP	Thrombotic
TCAD	Tricyclic antidepressant		thrombocytopenic purpura
T cell	Small lymphocyte	TU	Tuberculin units
TCN	Tetracycline	TUR	Transurethral resection
TD	Transverse diameter; tardive	TURP	Transurethral resection of
	dyskinesia		prostate
Td	Adult tetanus-diphtheria	TVP	Transvenous pacemaker
	toxoid	Tx	Treatment; therapy

U	Units		VT	Ventricular tachycardia
UA	Uric acid; urinalysis; unauthorized absence		VZIG	*Varicella-zoster* immune globulin
UE	Upper extremity			
UGI	Upper gastrointestinal series			
UK	Unknown			
UR	Utilization review		WAIS	Wechsler Adult Intelligence Scale
URI	Upper respiratory infection			
urol	Urology		WAIS-R	Wechsler Adult Intelligence Scale-Revised
USP	United States Pharmacopeia			
UTI	Urinary tract infection		WB	Whole blood
UV	Ultraviolet		WBC	White blood cell
			WDL	Well-differentiated lymphocytic
			WDWNBM	Well-developed, well-nourished black male
V	Vomiting; vein; five			
VA	Visual acuity; valproic acid		WDWNWF	Well-developed, well-nourished white female
VAC	Vincristine, adriamycin, cyclophosphamide		WF	White female
VAG HYST	Vaginal hysterectomy		WFI	Water for injection
			WHO	World Health Organization
Vas.	Vascular		WM	White male
VBI	Vinblastine		WNL	Within normal limits
VC	Vital capacity; vena cava		W/O	Without
VCR	Vincristine sulfate		WR	Wassermann reaction
VD	Venereal disease		W/U	Workup
Vd	Volume of distribution			
VDRL	Venereal Disease Research Laboratory (test for syphilis)			
vent.	Ventricular; ventral		×	Times; ten
VER	Visual-evoked responses		X-mat.	Cross match (blood)
VF	Vision field; ventricular fibrillation		XRT	X-ray therapy
V.Fib	Ventricular fibrillation			
VLDL	Very low density lipoprotein			
VMA	Vanillylmandelic acid		YO, Y/O	Year-old
VNA	Visiting nurse's association			
VO	Verbal order			
V/P, V/Q	Ventilation and perfusion			
VPC	Ventricular premature contractions		Z-ERS	Zeta erythrocyte sedimentation rate
VS	Vital signs		ZIZ	*Zoster* serum immune globulin
VSD	Ventricular septal defect			
VSS	Vital signs stable		ZIP	*Zoster* immune plasma

Miscellaneous—Examples of how some laboratory test values may be written in the medical chart

140	101	17
3.4	25	1.0

— 140

$Na = 140$, $Cl = 101$
$BUN = 17$
glucose $= 140$
$K = 3.4$, $CO_2 = 25$,
$SrCr = 1.0$

Na	Cl	BUN
K	CO_2	SrCr

— Gluc.

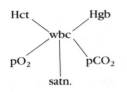

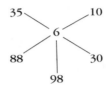

Hct	=	35
Hgb	=	10
wbc	=	6
pO_2	=	88
satn.	=	98
pCO_2	=	30

Glossary of Common Medical Terms (6–11)

Acholia	Suppressed secretion of bile
Adenopathy	Swelling of the lymph nodes
Akathisia	Inability to keep still, irresistible urge to be in motion
Akinesia	Absence or loss of voluntary motion
Amyloidosis	Deposits of amyloid in various organs or tissues
Aneurysm	Circumscribed dilation of an artery or vein wall forming a sac that is filled with blood
Anisocytosis	Red blood cell size variation
Anorexia	Loss of appetite
Aphonia	Loss of speech
Apnea	Without breath or respiration
Arrhythmia	Irregularity, loss of rhythm
Ascites	Collection of fluid in the abdomen
Atheroma	Fatty degeneration and infiltration of the walls of the arteries by lipids
Azotemia	Uremia
Babinski's reflex	Extension instead of flexion of the great toe, sometimes with plantar flexion of the other toes following stroking of the sole

Bleb	Collection of fluid beneath the skin
Bradycardia	Slowness of the heart beat
Bradykinesia	Extreme slowness of movement
Bronchioecstasis	Dilation of a bronchus or of the bronchial tubes
Bronchopleural fistula	A pathologic sinus or abnormal passage leading from the abscess cavity to the outside of the bronchial tree

Cardiomegaly	Enlargement of the heart
Cheyne-Stokes	Pattern of breathing with gradual increase in depth respiration and sometimes in rate to maximum—followed by a decrease resulting in apnea—30- to 60-sec cycles
Cholelithiasis	Calculi in the gallbladder or bile ducts
Cytotoxic	Destructive to cells

Dacryocystitis	Inflammation of the lacrimal sac
Digitalization	Administration of digitalis until sufficient amounts are present in the body to produce desired therapeutic effects
Diverticulitis	Inflammation of small pockets in the colon (symptomatic)
Diverticulosis	Asymptomatic small pockets in the colon
Dysarthria	Disorder of articulation due to sensory-neural abnormalities
Dyspnea	Difficult breathing, frequently rapid

Ecchymosis	A purplish patch caused by extravasation of blood into the skin
Edema	A perceptible accumulation of excessive clear, watery fluid in the tissue
Edentulous	Toothless
Empyema	Pus in a body cavity; when used without qualification, pus in the pleural cavity
Endarteritis	Inflammation of the inner coat of the artery
Epigastrium	Pit of the stomach
Epistaxis	Hemorrhage, nosebleed
Exacerbation	Increase in speed of course that a disease takes; increases in severity
Extrapyramidal	Indicating descending nerve tracts that do not enter into the formation of the pyramids of the medulla
Extravasation	Act of escaping from a vessel into the tissues, said of blood, lymph, or serum

Febrile	Relating to fever, pyretic
Fibroplasia	Production of fibrous tissue
Fibropurulent pleuritis	Pus containing fibrin located in the pleura

Glaucoma	Disease of the eye characterized by increased intraocular pressure due to restricted outflow of the aqueous through the aqueous veins and Schlemm's canal
Glomerulonephritis	Renal disease with an inflammatory change in the glomerulus
Gynecomastia	Excessive development of the mammary glands

Hectic	Relating to the daily rise in temperature in active TB
Hectic malar flush	Localized hectic flush of the malar eminences, often occurring in TB
Hemosiderin	Hydrated ferrous oxide in combination with protein
Hemosiderosis	Deposition of iron in the tissue
Hepatomegaly	Enlargement of the liver
Holosystolic	Throughout systole
Hyalin	A clear homogeneous substance occurring in amyloid, colloid, or hyaloid degeneration
Hypercapnia	Presence of an abnormally large amount of carbon dioxide in circulating blood; increased carbon dioxide tension resulting in extra stimulation of the respiratory center
Hypertrophy	General increase in bulk, overgrowth
Hyperplasia	Increased size by increasing the actual amount of tissue
Hypochromia	Percentage of hemoglobin in red blood cells is less than normal
Hypokalemic	Abnormally small amount of potassium in the circulating blood
Hypophonia	Abnormally weak voice due to incoordination of the muscles concerned in vocalization
Hypoxia	Decreased amount of oxygen in organs and tissues, less than the physiologically normal amount

Infarct	Death of tissue resulting from arrest of circulation in the artery supplying the body part
Insidious	Denoting a disease that progresses with few or no symptoms to indicate its gravity
Intumescent	Enlarging, swelling
Ipsilateral	On the same side

| Kyphosis | Curvature of the spine, humpback |

| Lordotic position | Erect "military attention"; somewhat swaybacked (lordosis) |

Melena	Black vomit; the passage of dark, tarry stools due to the presence of blood
Metabolism	Tissue change, the sum of the chemical changes whereby the function of nutrition is affected
Metamyelocyte	Immature granulocyte
Metastasis	The shifting of a disease, or its local manifestations, from one part of the body to another
Microcyte	A hollow nonnucleated red blood cell
Myelocyte	A young cell of the granulocyte series occurring normally in the bone marrow
Myeloid metaplasia	Enlargement of the spleen
Myerson's sign	Lack of facial expression
Nevus flammeus	Any congenital lesion
Oliguria	Scanty urination
Oophorectomy	Removal of an ovary
Orthopnea	Discomfort on breathing in any but the erect, sitting, or standing position (i.e., number of pillows used to prop up)
Palliative	Mitigating, reducing severity of
Pancytopenic	Pronounced reduction of erythrocytes, all white blood cells, and platelets in the circulating blood
Papilledema	Inflamed optic nerve head, edema, with redness due to congestion
Percutaneous	Through unbroken skin
Pericarditis	Inflammation of the pericardium
Petechiae	Minute hemorrhage spots
Plaque	A patch or small differentiated area on the skin or mucous membrane
Pneumatocele	Thin-walled cavity
Poikilocytosis	Red blood cell of irregular shape present in peripheral blood
Polychromatophilia	Presence in the blood of polychromatophils
Polycythemia	Increased red blood cells
Polydipsia	Excessive thirst
Polyphagia	Excessive hunger
Polyuria	Excessive urination
Proprioception	Receiving stimuli originating in muscles, tendons, or internal tissue
Pyelography	Radiography of the ureter and pelvis of the kidney
Pyemia	Pus in the blood, a type of septicemia
Retinopathy	Noninflammatory degenerative disease of the retina

Sarcoma	A tumor, usually highly malignant; a malignant connective tissue neoplasm
Scoliosis	Lateral deviation of the spine
Sclerotic	Hardening
Splenomegaly	Enlargement of the spleen
Spirometer	Pneumatometer, an instrument used for measurement of respired air
Sublaxated	Incompletely dislocated
Sulfhemoglobinemia	Persistent cyanotic condition due to sulfhemoglobin in the blood

Thrombocytopenia	Abnormally small number of platelets in the blood
Thromboembolism	Embolism from a thrombus dislodged from a vein
Thrombophlebitis	Inflammation of a vein with secondary thrombus formation
Torticollis	Wry-neck, stiff neck
Trabecular meshwork	Supporting fibers traversing the substances of a structure (bone)

Common Medical Prefixes

A-(AN-),	without, deficiency. Amentia, subnormal mental development.
AB-,	from, away from. Abduction, withdrawal of a part from the axis of the body.
ABORTO-,	miscarry. Aborticide, killing an unborn fetus.
ACANTHO-,	thorny, spiny. Acanthoid, resembling a spine.
ACARO-,	mites or itch. Acarodermatitis, skin inflammation.
ACRO-,	extremities. Acrohypothermy, abnormal coldness of the extremities.
ACTINO-,	ray or radiated structure. Actinogen, substance producing radiation.
AD-,	adherence, increase, near, toward. Adduction, movement of a part toward the median of the body.
ADENO-,	gland, glandular. Adenopathy, glandular disease.
ADIPO-,	fat or fatty tissue. Adiposis, excessive accumulation of fat in the body.
AERO-(AER-),	air or gas. Aerogram, an x-ray film of an organ inflated with air.
ALGIO-,	pain. Algiogenesis, the source or origin of pain.
ALLO-,	differentiation from normal, reversal. Allochezia, passage of feces from the body through an abnormal opening.
ALVEO-,	hollow. Alveolus, air cell of the lung.

AMBI-,　　both. Ambilateral, affecting both sides.

AMBLY-,　　dulled, faint. Amblyopia, dimness of vision.

AMPHI-,　　both, about or on both sides. Amphibious, capable of living both on land and in water.

AMYLO-,　　starch. Amylodyspepsia, inability to digest starchy foods.

ANA-,　　on, up, back, or through. Anasarca, literally, throughout the flesh. A generalized edema.

ANDRO-,　　man. Androphobia, morbid dislike of men or the male sex.

ANEURISMO-,　　a widening. Aneurysm, areterial dilatation due to pressure of blood on weakened tissue forming sac of clotted blood.

ANGIO-,　　blood vessel. Angiorrhexis, rupture of a blood vessel.

ANISO-,　　unequal or dissimilar, Anisocytosis, inequality in the size of red blood cells.

ANKYLO-,　　crooked or a growing together of parts. Ankylosis, stiffness or fixation of a joint.

ANO-,　　anus or anal. Anoscope, an instrument for examining the rectum.

ANTE-,　　before or in front of. Anteaural, in front of the ear.

ANTERO-,　　anterior or front. Anteroinferior, situated in front and below.

ANTHRACO-,　　coal or carbuncle. Anthracosis, black pigmentation of the lungs due to the accumulation of carbon dust.

ANTI-,　　against. Antiemetic, an agent relieving or preventing nausea and vomiting.

ANTRO-,　　cavern or cavity. Antrum, a cavity or hollow space in a bone.

AORTO-,　　aorta. Aortitis, inflammation of the aorta.

APO-,　　away from or separated. Apositia, aversion to or loathing of food.

ARCH-,　　first or original. Archetype, basic model or prototype.

ARCTO-,　　contract or compress. Arctation, stricture of any canal opening.

ARGYRO-,　　silver. Argyria, bluish opening, discoloration of skin due to prolonged administration of silver preparations.

ARRHENO-,　　male. Arrhenogenic, producing only male offspring.

ARTERIO-,　　artery. Arteriosclerosis, hardening of the arteries.

ARTHRO-(ARTH-),　　joint. Arthropathy, any joint disease.

ASTRO-,　　star. Astrocyte, stellate cells of the neuroglia found in the brain and spinal cord.

ATELO-,　　imperfect development. Ateloglossia, congenital defect in the tongue.

ATHERO-,　　porridge. Atheroma, a sebaceous cyst.

ATRETO-,　　not perforated. Atretocystia, imperforation of the bladder.

AUDIO-,　　hearing. Audiology, science of hearing.

AURI-,　　ear or gold. Aurist, specialist in diseases of the ear.

AUTO-,　　self. Autolysis, self-digestion of tissues within the living body.

AUXO-,　　increase. Auxometer, device for measuring magnifying power of lenses.

AXO-,　　axis or axis cylinder. Axon, the efferent process or a nerve cell.

BARO-,	weight or difficult. Barometer, instrument measuring atmospheric pressure.
BASI-,	base. Basicranial, relating to the base of the skull.
BI-,	two. Bilateral, relating to both sides.
BILI-,	bile or biliary system. Biliuria, presence of bile salts in the urine.
BIO-,	life. Biopsy, excision, during life, of tissue for microscopic examination and diagnosis.
BLASTO-,	germ. Blastomycosis, disease produced by budding yeastlike agents.
BLENNO-,	mucous. Blennorrhea, excessive mucous discharge.
BLEPHARO- (BLEPHAR-),	eyelid. Blepharoptosis, drooping of the upper eyelid.
BRACHIO- (BRACHI-),	arm. Brachiotomy, surgical cutting or removal of an arm.
BRACHY-,	short. Brachyglossal, having a short tongue.
BRADY-,	slow. Bradycardia, slowness of the heart.
BREVI-,	short. Brevicollis, having a short neck.
BROMO-,	bad smell, bromine. Bromhidrosis, excretion of sweat with an unpleasant odor.
BRONCHO-,	bronchus. Bronchostenosis, narrowing of the lumen of the bronchi.
BUBO-,	groin. Buboadenitis, inflammation of an inguinal lymph node.
BUCCO- (BUCCA-),	cheek. Buccolabial, pertaining to the cheek and the lip.

CACO-,	bad, deformed. Cacophony, an abnormally discordant voice.
CAPITO-,	head. Capitulum, a small rounded articular end of a bone.
CARBO-,	carbon. Carboluria, presence of carbolic acid in the urine.
CARCINO-,	cancer. Carcinogen, any cancer-producing substance.
CARDIO-,	heart. Cardioplegia, paralysis of the heart.
CATA-,	downward, against. Catabolism, destructive phase of metabolism.
CAUDO-,	tail. Caudocephalad, in the direction from the tail toward the head.
CELIO-,	abdomen. Celiotomy, opening of the abdominal cavity.
CENTRO-,	center. Centrifugal, receding from the center to the periphery.
CEPHALO- (CEPHAL-),	head. Cephalocentesis, surgical puncture of the cranium.
CEREBRO- (CEREBA-),	brain. Cerebrospinal, pertaining to the brain and spinal cord.
CERO- (CERA-),	wax. Cerosis, condition of a membrane where it seems to consist of waxlike scales.
CERVICO- (CERV-),	neck. Cervicodynic, cramp or pain of the neck.
CHEILO- (CHEIL-),	lips. Cheilosis, disorder of the lips due to avitaminosis.
CHEMO-,	chemistry. Chemotaxis, response of organisms to chemical stimuli.
CHIRO- (CHIR-),	hand. Chiromegaly, enlargement of one or both hands.
CHLORO-,	green. Chlorophidrosis, a condition characterized by greenish perspiration.
CHOLE- (CHOL-),	bile. Cholecystitis, inflammation of the gallbladder.
CHONDRO- (CHONDR-),	cartilage. Chondromalacia, softening of a cartilage.

CHRONO-,	time. Chronograph, instrument recording small intervals of time.
CHYLO-,	emulsion of fat globules in lymph. Chylemia, presence of chyle in the blood.
CILIO-,	eyelid, cilia. Cillosis, trembling of the eyelid.
CIRCUM-,	around. Circumoral, surrounding the mouth.
CLEIDO-,	clavicle. Cleidocostal, pertaining to the ribs and clavicle.
CO-, (COM-,CON-),	with, together. Coarctation, compression of the walls of a vessel or canal.
COLEO-,	sheath. Coleocele, vaginal tumor or hernia.
COLO-,	colon. Colostomy, formulation of an artificial anus in the abdominal wall.
COLPO-,	vagina. Colposcope, instrument for visual examination of the vagina.
CON-,	with, together. Congenital, born with or existing at birth.
CONDYLO-,	knuckle, joint. Condyle, any rounded eminence such as occurs in the joints of many bones.
CONTRA-,	against, in opposition. Contralateral, on the opposite side.
COPRO-,	feces. Coprolith, hard mass of fecal matter in the bowels.
CORE-,	pupil. Corestenoma, narrowing of the pupil.
CORPUS-,	body. Corpuscle, a small round body.
CORTICO-,	cortex. Corticospinal, pertaining to the brain cortex and the spinal cord.
COSTO- (COST-),	rib. Costochondral, pertaining to the ribs and their cartilages.
COUNTER-,	against. Countertraction, traction which offsets another, as in reducing fractures.
CRANIO- (CRANI-),	skull. Craniocleidodysostosis, congenital defect of the clavicle associated with imperfect ossification of the bones of the skull.
CRYPTO-,	hidden. Cryptorchism, defect where the testes fail to descend and remain within the abdomen or inguinal canal.
CUTI-,	skin. Cuticolor, simulating the color of skin.
CYANO-,	blue. Cyanosis, bluish discoloration of the skin and mucous membranes due to a lack of oxygen.
CYCLO-,	circular, a cycle. Cyclothymia, disposition marked by alternations of mood between elation and depression.
CYRTO-,	curved. Cyrtoid, resembling a hump or swelling.
CYSTO- (CYST-),	bladder, cyst. Cystorrhaphy, suture of the bladder.
CYTO-,	cell. Cytosome, the body of a cell apart from its nucleus.
DACRYO-,	tear. Dacryorrhea, excessive flow of tears.
DACTYLO- (DACTYL-),	finger or toe. Dactylogram, a fingerprint.
DE-,	away from, separation. Decapitation, removal of the head.
DENTI-, (DENTO-),	tooth. Dentiform, tooth-shaped.
DERMATO-, (DERM-DERMO-),	skin. Dermatitis, inflammation of the skin.
DESMO-,	bond, ligament. Desmotomy, incision of a ligament.
DEXTRO-,	right. Dextrocardia, transposition of the heart to the right side of the thorax.

DI-,	two. Dichromic, marked by two colors.
DIA-,	across, through. Diapedesis, passage of blood cells through the unruptured vessel walls into tissues.
DIPLO-,	double. Diplopia, double vision, one object being seen as two.
DIPSO-,	thirst. Dipsophobia, morbid fear of drinking.
DIS-,	reversal, separation. Discrete, not running together, separate.
DOLICHO-,	long, narrow. Dolichomorphic, marked by a long or narrow form.
DORSO-,	back. Dorsoventral, pertaining to the dorsal and ventral regions.
DUODENO-,	duodenum. Duodenoplasty, reparative operation of the duodenus.
DYS-,	painful, difficult. Dysmenorrhea, painful menstruation.

E-, (ED-),	out of, out from. Eccentric, situated away from the center.
ECTO-,	without, on the outer side. Ectoplasm, outer layer of cytoplasm of a cell.
ELECTRO-,	electricity. Electrocoma, coma produced by electroshock therapy.
EMETO-,	vomiting. Emetatrophia, atrophy due to persistent vomiting.
EN- (EM-),	in, into. Encapsulation, surrounding of a part with a capsule.
ENCEPHALO- (ENCEPHAL-),	brain. Encephalonarcosis, stupor from some brain lesion.
ENDO-,	within. Endocarditis, inflammation of the living membrane of the heart.
ENTERO- (ENTER-),	intestine. Enterotome, an instrument of cutting open the intestine.
ENTO-,	within. Entocele, internal hernia.
EPI-,	on, upon. Epicystitis, inflammation of the tissues above the bladder.
EPISIO-,	vulva. Episiotomy, incision of the vulva during childbirth.
EQUI-,	equally. Equiaxial, having equal axes.
ERGO-,	work. Ergophobia, morbid dread of work.
ERO-,	love. Erotism, sexual excitment or desire.
ERYTHRO-,	red. Erythrocyte, red blood cells.
ESO-,	within. Estotropia, strabismus with one eye fixing on an object and the other deviates inward.
EU-,	well, well-being. Euphoria, an exaggerated sense of well-being.
EX-, (EXO-),	out away from, over. Exanthema, an eruption upon the skin.
EXTRA-,	outside of. Extracellular, external to the cells of an organism.

FIBRO-,	fiber. Fibroplasia, the growth of fibrous tissue.
FISTULO-,	pipe or tube. Fistuloenterostomy, anastomosis between a biliary fistula and the duodenum.
FLAVO-,	yellow. Flavedo, yellowness of the skin.

| FORE-, | before, in front. Forefinger, index finger. |
| FRONTO-, | anterior position, forehead. Frontad, toward the frontal aspect. |

GALACTO-,	milk. Galactagogue, agent increasing the secretion of milk.
GAMO-,	marriage. Gamomania, insane desire for marriage.
GASTRO- (GASTR-),	stomach. Gastroenteritis, inflammation of stomach and intestine.
GENITO-,	genital. Genitourinary, relating to the genitalia and the urinary organs or functions.
GERO-,	old. Gerontology, study of old age.
GLAUCO-,	gray-green. Glaucoma, disease of the eye due to high intraocular pressure with a lessening of vision.
GLIO-,	glue. Glioma, tumor of the supporting tissue of the central nervous system.
GLOSSO-,	tongue. Glossitis, inflammation of the tongue.
GLUCO-,	glucose. Gluconeogenesis, formation of glucose from noncarbohydrate sources.
GLYCO- (GLYC-),	sweet. Glycosuria, presence of sugar in the urine.
GONADO-,	ovary or testis. Gonadotrophic, gonad-stimulating.
GONO-,	seed. Gonocyte, a germ cell.
GRAPHO-,	writing. Graphology, study of handwriting.
GYNO- (GYNE-),	woman, female reproductive organ. Gynecology, science of diseases of women, especially those affecting the sexual organs.

HELICO-,	spiral. Helicoid, spiral, coiled like a snail shell.
HELIO-,	sun. Heliotherapy, treatment of disease by exposure to sunlight.
HEMI-,	half. Hemisection, act of division into two lateral halves.
HEM- (HEMO-, HEMAT-, HEMATO-),	blood. Hemolysia, destruction of red blood cells.
HEPATO- (HEPAT-),	liver. Hepatomegaly, enlargement of the liver.
HERNIO-,	hernia. Herniotomy, operation for relief of irreducible hernia.
HETERO-,	other, different. Heterogenous, of a different species.
HIDRO-,	sweat. Hidrosis, formation and excretion of sweat.
HISTO- (HISTIO-),	tissue, web. Histology, study of microscopic anatomy of tissues.
HOLO-,	whole, complete. Holoacrania, complete absence of the cranial vault.
HOMEO- (HOMO-),	like, similar. Homeostasis, maintenance of a constant, unchanging internal environment.
HYALO-,	glass, hyalin. Hyaloid, transparent, glasslike.
HYDRO-,	water. Hydronephrosis, a collection of urine in the distended pelvis of the kidney.

HYPER-,	above, excessive, beyond. Hypertrophy, increase in the size of an organ.
HYPNO-,	sleep. Hypnotic, agent which induces sleep.
HYPO-,	beneath, below, deficient. Hypodermic, pertaining to the region under the skin.
HYSTERO- (HYSTER-),	uterus or hysteria. Hysterectomy, surgical removal of the uterus.

ICTERO-,	jaundice. Icterogenic, causing icterus.
IDEO-,	idea. Ideology, the science of ideas.
IDIO-,	self-produced. Idiosyncrasy, a peculiar situation in which an individual will react differently from most persons to drugs or treatments.
ILEO-,	ileum. Ileitis, inflammation of the ileum.
ILIO- (ILI-),	flank, iliac. Iliopagus, twins united in the iliac region.
IMMUNO-,	immune. Immunologist, a specialist in the science of immunity.
IN-,	not, within, on. Inanimate, dead, without life.
INFRA-,	below. Infrared, beyond the red end of the spectrum.
INTER-,	between. Interlobular, between lobules.
INTRA- (INTRO-),	within, into. Intravenous, within, or into, the veins.
IRIDO-,	iris. Iridectomy, cutting out a part of the iris.
ISCHO-,	suppression. Ischomenia, suppression of the menstrual flow.
ISO-,	equal. Isopia, equal acuteness of vision in the two eyes.

JEJUNO-,	jejunum. Jejunostomy, making an artificial opening through the abdominal wall in the jejunum.
JUXTA-,	nearness. Juxtaposition, situated adjacent to another.

KARYO-,	nucleus of a cell. Karyolysis, dissolution of the nucleus of a cell.
KERA- (KERATO-),	horn, horny tissue, or cornea. Keratinization, development of a horny quality in a tissue. Keratitis, inflammation of the cornea.
KINESI-,	movement, motion. Kinesia, any form of motion sickness.
KONIO-,	dust. Koniology, science of dust and its effects.
KYMO-,	wave. Kymograph, instrument for recording physiologic cycles or actions.
KYPHO-,	humped. Kyphosis, hunchbacked.

LABIO-,	lip. Labiogingival, pertaining to the lips and gums.
LACRI-,	tear. Lacrimation, secretion of tears.

LACTO-,	milk. Lactation, the formation or secretion of milk.
LAPARO-,	abdomen. Laparotomy, incision through the abdominal wall.
LARYNGO-,	larynx. Laryngoscopy, examination of the interior of the larynx with the laryngoscope.
LATERO-,	side. Laterotorsion, twisting to one side.
LEIO-,	smooth. Leiodermia, abnormal smoothness of the skin.
LEPIDO-	scale, scaly. Lepidoptera, an order of insects distinguished by featherlike scales.
LEPTO-,	thin, small, weak. Leptocephalis, abnormal smallness of the skull.
LEUCO- (LEUKO-),	white. Leukemia, a disease of the blood-forming organs characterized by uncontrolled proliferation of the leukocytes.
LEVO-,	left. Levophobia, morbid fear of objects on the left side of the body.
LIENO-,	spleen. Lienopathy, any disorder of the spleen.
LIPO- (LIP-),	fat. Lipomatosis, a general deposition of fat; obesity.
LITHO- (LITH-),	stone. Lithotomy, removal of a calculus, usually urinary, through an operative incision.
LOBO-,	lobe. Lobotomy, section of brain tissue.
LUMBO-,	loin or lumbar. Lumbosacral, pertaining to the lumbar vertebrae and to the sacrum.
LUTEO-,	yellow. Luteotrophin, hormone of the anterior pituitary which maintains the corpus luteum.
LYMPHO-,	lymph, water. Lymphocytosis, excess of lymphocytes in the blood.
LYO-,	dissolve, loose. Lyophilization, process of rapidly freezing a substance and then dehydrating it in a vacuum.

MACRO-,	large. Macroscopic, large enough to be seen by the naked eye.
MACULO-,	spot. Maculopapular, having the characteristics of a macule and a papule.
MAL-,	ill, bad. Malaise, general feeling of illness.
MAMMO- (MAMM-),	breast. Mammectomy, excision or amputation of the breast.
MAMMILLO-,	nipple. Mammilliform, nipple-shaped.
MASTO- (MAST-),	breast or mastoid. Mastitis, inflammation of the breast.
MEDIO-,	middle. Mediofrontal, pertaining to the middle of the forehead.
MEGA- (MEGALO-),	large, great. Megacolon, hypertrophic dilatation of the colon.
MELANO- (MELAN-),	Dark-colored or melanin. Melanoma, tumor which originates in a pigmented nevus.
MENINGO- (MENING-),	membrane. Meningitis, inflammation of the membranes of the brain or cord.
MENO-,	month, relation to the menses. Menopause, physiologic cessation of menstruation.
MERO-,	part. Merosmia, partial loss of the sense of smell.
MESO-,	middle, mesentery, partial. Mesocolon, mesentery connecting the colon with the posterior abdominal wall.

META-,	over, after, change, beyond. Metacarpus, part of the hand between the carpus and the phalanges.
METRO- (METR-),	uterus. Metrophlebitis, inflammation of the veins of the uterus.
MICRO-,	small. Microcyte, a small red blood cell.
MID-,	middle. Midaxilla, the center of the armpit.
MIO-,	less or smaller. Miosis, constriction of the pupil.
MISO-,	hatred. Misogyny, hatred of women.
MITO-,	thread. Mitosis, indirect nuclear division.
MOGI-,	painful or difficult. Mogiphonia, difficulty in speaking.
MONO-,	single. Monoplegia, paralysis of a single limb or a single muscle.
MORBI-,	disease. Morbidity, state of being diseased.
MORPHO-,	form. Morphometry, measurement of the forms of organisms.
MUCO-,	mucus. Mucopurulent, containing mucus mingled with pus.
MULTI-,	many. Multigravida, a pregnant woman who has had two or more previous pregnancies.
MUSCULO-,	muscle. Musculocutaneous, pertaining to or supplying the muscles and skin.
MYCO-,	fungus. Mycology, the science of fungi.
MYELO- (MYEL-),	bone marrow or spinal cord. Myelopore, opening in the spinal cord.
MYO-,	muscle. Myoneural, pertaining to both muscle and nerve.
MYRINGO-,	eardrum. Myringoscope, instrument for examining the tympanic membrane.
MYXO-,	mucus, mucus tissue. Myxoma, a connective-tissue tumor.

NARCO-,	narcosis, stupor. Narcohypnosis, state of deep sleep induced by hypnosis.
NASO-,	nose. Nasolabial, pertaining to the nose and lip.
NECRO-,	dead. Necroscopy, the examination of a dead body; autopsy.
NEO-,	new. Neonatal, newborn.
NEPHRO- (NEPHR-),	kidney. Nephrotoxic, destructive to the kidney cells.
NEURO-,	nerve. Neurospasm, nervous twitching of a muscle.
NON-,	not. Nonmalignant, lacking any features of malignant disease, usually referring to tumors.
NOSO-,	disease. Nosology, science of classification of disease.
NUCLEO-,	nucleus. Nucleoprotein, a protein constituent of cell nuclei.
NYCTO-,	night. Nyctalopia, night blindness.

OCULO-,	eye. Oculomotor, pertaining to the movement of the eye.
ODONTO-,	tooth. Odontologist, dental surgeon.
OLIGO-,	few. Oliguria, decrease in the quantity of urine excreted.
OM-, (OMO-),	shoulder. Omodynia, pain of the shoulder.
OMPHALO-,	umbilicus. Omphalotomy, cutting of the umbilical cord.

ONCO-,	bulk, tumor. Oncometer, instrument for measuring variations of the volume of an organ.
ONYCHO-,	nail or claw. Onychomalacia, abnormally soft nails.
OO-,	egg. Oogenesis, origin, growth and formation of the ovum.
OOPHORO-,	ovary, ovarian. Oophoropathy, disease of the ovary.
OPHTHALMO- (OPHTHALM-),	eye. Ophthalmoptosis, protrusion of the eyeball.
OPISTHO-,	behind. Opisthotonos, tetanic spasm of the muscles of the back, where the head and lower limbs bend backward and the trunk arches forward.
OPTO-,	sight, vision. Optometry, measurement of visual powers.
ORCHIO-,	Testes. Orchitis, inflammation of the testes.
ORGANO-,	organ. Organotrophic, relating to the nutrition of living organs.
ORO-,	mouth, oral. Orohorrhea, a colorless discharge.
ORTHO-,	straight or normal. Orthodontics, branch of dentistry concerned with the treatment of malocclusion.
OS-,	mouth or bone. Osculum, a small aperture. Ossicle, a small bone.
OSCILLO-,	swing. Oscillometry, measurement of oscillations.
OSMO-,	smell, odor, or osmosis. Osmometer, instrument for testing the sense of smell.
OSTEO-,	bone. Osteomyelitis, inflammation of the marrow of bone.
OTO-,	ear. Otitis, inflammation of the ear.
OVARIO-,	ovary. Ovariocele, tumor or hernia of an ovary.
OVI- (OVO-),	egg. Oviduct, duct which transports the ovum from the ovary to the exterior, i.e., Fallopian tube.
OXY-,	sharp, acute or oxygen. Oxyesthesia, condition of increased acuity of sensation.

PACHY-,	thick. Pachydermia, abnormal thickening of the skin.
PALATO-,	roof of mouth or palate. Palatomaxillary, pertaining to the palate and the jaw.
PALEO-,	old, ancient. Paleontology, science which is based on the study of fossil remains from past geologic periods.
PAN-,	all, general. Pandemic, epidemic over a wide geographic area.
PAPILLO-,	pustule or pimple. Papilliform, shaped like a papilla.
PAPULO-,	small elevation of the skin. Papulosquamous, characterized by both papules and scales.
PARA-,	beyond, near, around, abnormal. Parahepatic, about or near the liver.
PATHO-,	disease. Pathogenicity, capacity to produce disease.
PEDO- (PED-),	child. Pedology, science regarding childhood diseases, hygiene, etc.
PERI-,	around, near. Pericardium, the membranous sac enveloping the heart.
PHACO-,	lens or lens or the eye. Phacoid, lens-shaped.

PHAGO- (PHAGIA), devour, eat, swallow. Phagocyte, a cell which can engulf and digest particles or cells harmful to the body.

PHARMACO-, drug. Pharmacology, science of the nature, properties and actions of drugs.

PHARYNGO-, pharynx. Pharyngospasm, spasmodic contraction of the pharynx.

PHLEBO- (PHLEB-), vein. Phlebitis, inflammation of a vein.

PHONO-, sound, voice. Phonetics, the science dealing with the mode of production of sounds.

PHOTO-, light. Photophobia, intolerance or morbid fear of light.

PHRENO-, diaphragm. Phrenicectomy, resection of a section of the phrenic nerve.

PHYTO-, plant. Phytopharmacology, branch of pharmacology concerned with effect of drugs on plant growth.

PILO-, hair. Pilomotor, causing movement of the hair.

PLANO-, flat or wandering. Planoconvex, flat on one side and rounded on the other.

PLASMO-, plasma. Plasmolysis, shrinkage of a cell due to withdrawal of water by osmosis.

PLATY-, broad, flat. Platyhelminth, flatworm.

PLEO-, more. Pleocytosis, increase of cells in the cerebrospinal fluid.

PLURI-, more or several. Plurigravida, a gravid woman who has had two or more pregnancies.

PLEURO-, membrane enveloping the lung. Pleurisy, inflammation of the pleura.

PNEUMATO-, air, breath. Pneumatosis, air or gas in abnormal situations in the body.

PNEUMONO- (PNEUMA-), lung, air. Pneumonectomy, excision of an entire lung.

POLIO-, grey. Poliomyelitis, inflammation of the grey matter of the spinal cord.

POLY-, many. Polyuria, passage of an excessive quantity of urine.

POST-, behind. Postoperative, occurring after an operation.

PRE-, before. Preganglionic, situated in front of a ganglion.

PRESBY-, old. Presbyopia, condition of vision in the aged.

PRIMO-, first. Primipara, a woman bearing her first child.

PRO-, before. Prootic, in front of the ear.

PROCTO-, rectum. Proctoscope, instrument for inspecting the rectum.

PROTO-, first. Protocol, the original notes or records of an experiment, etc.

PSEUDO-, false. Pseudoanemia, pallor and appearance of anemia without blood changes to support the diagnosis.

PSORO-, itching. Psoriasis, inflammatory skin disease.

PTYALO-, saliva. Ptyalism, excessive secretion of saliva.

PULMO-, lung. Pulmonary, pertaining to or affecting the lungs.

PURI-, pus. Purohepatitis, purulent inflammation of the liver.

PYELO- (PYEL-), pelvis of kidney. Pyelitis, inflammation of the kidney pelvis.

PYLORO-, pyloris, opening of the stomach into the duodenum. Pylorospasm, spasm of the pylorus.

PYO-, pus. Pyogenesis, formation of pus.

PYRO-, fire or fever. Pyromania, a monomania for incendiarism.

QUADRI-, four. Quadriplegia, paralysis affecting the four extremeties of the body.

QUINTI-, five. Quintipara, a woman who has had five children.

RACHIO-, spine. Rachioplegia, spinal paralysis.

RADIO- (RADI-), ray. Radioactive, emitting radiant energy.

RE-, back, again. Reflected, turned back upon itself.

RECTO-, rectum. Rectovaginal, pertaining to the rectum and vagina.

RENI- (RENO-), kidney. Renotrophic, to produce hypertrophy of the kidney.

RETRO-, backward. Retroflexion, state of being bent backward.

RHEO-, current. Rheostat, instrument for altering the intensity of an electric current.

RHINO-, nose. Rhinitis, inflammation of the nasal mucous membrane.

SACRO-, sacrum. Sacroiliac, pertaining to the sacrum and the ilium.

SALPINGO-, trumpet or auditory or uterine tube. Salpingotomy, operation of cutting into a uterine tube.

SANGUI-, blood. Sanguirenal, pertains to blood supply of the kidneys.

SAPRO-, rotten, decaying organic matter. Saprophyte, organism living on dead organic matter.

SARCO-, flesh. Sarcolemma, sheath enveloping a muscle fiber.

SCAPULO-, shoulder or scapula. Scapulopexy, fixation of the scapula to the ribs.

SCHISTO- (SCHIZO-), split, cleft. Schizonychia, disease of the nails characterized by irregular splitting.

SCLERO-, hard. Sclerosis, hardening of a part by overgrowth of fibrous tissue.

SCOLIO-, curved or crooked. Scoliosis, lateral curvature of the spine.

SCOTO-, darkness. Scotoma, a dark spot in the visual field.

SEBO-, grease or tallow. Sebolith, an inorganic mass formed in a sebaceous gland.

SEMI-, half. Semilunar, resembling a half moon in shape.

SEMINO-, seed or semen. Seminoma, tumor of the testes.

SEPTI-, putrefaction. Septimetritis, pathogenic infection of the uterus.

SERO-, serum. Seromucous, having the nature of or containing both serum and mucous.

SIALO-, saliva. Sialoadenotomy, incision of a salivary gland.

SIDERO-, iron. Siderosis, chronic inflammation of the lungs due to prolonged inhalation of dust containing iron salts.

SINO-, sinus. Sinusitis, inflammation of a sinus.

SKIA-, shadow. Skiametry, measurement of x-ray intensity.

SOMATO-, body. Somesthesia, sensibility to bodily sensations.

SOMNO- (SOMA-), sleep. Somnambulism, condition in which the individual walks during sleep.

SPASMO-,	sudden muscular contraction. Spasmophilia, morbid tendency to convulsions.
SPERMATO-,	seed, germ. Spermatogenesis, production of mature male germ cells.
SPHENO-,	wedge or sphenoid bone. Sphenoid, wedge-shape.
SPHYGMO-,	pulse. Sphygmomanometer, an instrument for measuring arterial blood pressure.
SPIRO-,	spiral or respiration. Spirometer, instrument for measuring vital capacity.
SPLANCHNO-,	viscera. Splanchnic, pertaining to or supplying the viscera.
SPLENO-,	spleen. Splenectomize, excise the spleen.
SPONDYLO- (SPONDYL-),	vertebra. Spondylopathy, any disease of the vertebrae.
SPORO-,	spore, seed. Sporicide, agent which destroys spores.
STAPHYLO-,	grape cluster or uvula. Staphyledema, swelling of the uvula.
STEATO-,	fat. Steatorrhea, passage of stools having an excessive amount of fat intermixed.
STENO-,	narrow, constricted. Stenothorax, an unusually narrow chest.
STEREO-,	solid. Stereoanesthesia, inability to ascertain the form or shape of objects by feeling them.
STERNO-,	breast or sternum. Sternodynia, pain in the sternum.
STETHO-,	breast or chest. Stethoscope, instrument for detection and study of sounds arising within the chest.
STOMATO-,	mouth. Stomatitis, inflammation of the soft tissues of the mouth.
STREPTO-,	twisted, curved. *Streptobacillus*, bacillus which remains attached end to end, forming chains.
STRIC-,	closure or narrowing. Stricture, the abnormal narrowing of a canal, duct or passage.
SUB-,	under, below. Substernal, beneath the sternum.
SUDO-,	sweat. Sudorific, an agent inducing sweating.
SUPER- (SUPRA-, SUPRE-),	above, excessive. Supraliminal, lying above the threshold.
SYN- (SYM-),	union, with, together, beside. Syndactylism, adhesion of fingers or toes; webbed fingers; webbed toes.
SYPHILO-,	syphilis. Syphiloma, tumor due to syphilis.
SYRINGO-,	tube, pipe. Syringobulbia, presence of cavities in the medulla oblongata.
TACHO- (TACHY-),	swift. Tachycardia, excessive rapidity of the heart's action.
TELE-,	far off, end. Telepathy, action of one mind upon another when the two persons are separated by a considerable distance.
TENO-,	tendon. Tenosynovitis, inflammation of the tendon and its sheath.
TETANO-,	tetanus. Tetanism, a form of continuous muscular hypertonicity.
TETRA-,	four. Tetrotus, having four ears.
THANATO-,	death. Thanatoid, resembling death.
THERMO-,	heat. Thermohyperalgesia, condition where the application of heat causes excessive pain.

THORACO- (THORAC-),	thorax. Thoracentesis, the aspiration of the chest cavity for the removal of fluid.
THROMBO-,	clot of blood within the heart of blood vessels. Thromboangitis, thrombosis with inflammation of the intima of a vessel.
THYRO-,	thyroid. Thyrotoxicosis, hyperthyroidism of any type.
TOCO-,	childbirth or labor. Tocology, science of obstetrics.
TOPO-,	place or localized. Topography, study of the regions of the body or its parts.
TOXICO-,	poison. Toxicology, science of the nature and effects of poisons, and their detection and treatment.
TRACHELO-, TRACHEO- (TRACHEL-),	neck. Trachelodynia, pain in the neck.
TRANS-,	through, across. Translucent, permitting a partial transmission of light; somewhat transparent.
TRAUMATO-,	injury or wound. Traumatology, science of wounds and their care.
TRI-,	three. Tribrachius, having three arms.
TRICHO-,	hair. Trichoglossia, hairy tongue, thickening of the papillae causing a hairy appearance.
TROPHO-,	nutrition. Trophodynamics, the study of the laws governing nutrition.
TUBER- (Tubercel-),	swelling. Tubercle, a small nodule; rounded prominence on a bone.
TUBO-,	tube. Tuboovarian, pertaining to the uterine tube and the ovary.
TYMPANO-,	drug or middle ear. Tympanitis, inflammation of the tympanum; otitis media.

ULTRA-,	excess, beyond. Ultrasonic, relating to energy waves similar to those of sound but of higher frequencies.
UNI-,	one. Unilateral, pertaining to or affecting but one side.
URETERO-,	ureter. Ureteronephrectomy, removal of the kidney and its ureter.
URETHRO-,	urethra. Urethrogram, a roentgenographic visualization of the urethra.
URINO- (URA-, URO-),	urine. Urolithiasis, presence of urinary calculi.
UTERO-, uterus.	Uteroplacental, pertaining to the uterus and placenta.

VAGINO-,	vagina. Vaginitis, inflammation of the vagina.
VAGO-,	vagus nerve. Vagotomy, division of the vagus nerve.
VARICO-,	a dilated vein. Varicotomy, excision of a varicose vein.
VASO- (VAS-),	vessel. Vasomotor, regulating the contraction and expansion of blood vessels.
VENTRO-,	abdomen or anterior of body. Ventromedian, middle of the ventral surface.

VERMI-,　　　worm. Vermifuge, agent that kills or expels intestinal worms.
VERTEBRO-,　　vertebra. Vertebrocostal, pertaining to the vertebra and ribs.
VESICO-,　　　bladder. Vesicotomy, incision of the bladder.
VISCERO- (VICER-),　viscera or organs. Viscerosensory, relating to sensation in the viscera.
VITA-,　　　　life. Vitagen, nutrient needed for body-building material or energy.
VIVI-,　　　　living. Vivisection, surgical preparation of anesthetized animals for study of functions or derangements.

XANTHO-,　　yellow. Xanthopsia, yellow vision, condition in which objects look yellow.
Xeno-,　　　foreign or strange. Xenodiagnosis, procedure of using a suitable arthropod to transfer a disease from a patient to a susceptible laboratory animal.
XERO-,　　　dry. Xerostomia, dry mouth, caused by insufficient secretion of saliva.

ZOO-,　　　animal. Zoology, the study of animals.
ZYMO-,　　fermentation. Zymogen, inactive precursor of an enzyme.

Common Medical Suffices

-ABLE (-IBLE).　capable of. Palpable, capable of being touched.
-ACEAE.　　of the nature of. Bacteriaceae, of the nature of the genus *Bacterium*.
-AGRA.　　gout, a seizure of pain. Podagra, gout, especially of the foot or toe.
-AL.　　　belonging to, pertaining to. Neural, pertaining to nerves.
-ALGIA.　　pain. Myalgia, pain in the muscles.
-APHIA.　　touch. Amblyaphia, dullness of the sense of touch.
-ASE.　　denotes an enzyme. Amylase, an enzyme hydrolyzing starch to sugar.
-ASTHENIA.　weakness. Myasthenia, muscular weakness or excessive fatigue.
-ATE.　　having the shape or nature of. Stellate, star-shaped.

-BLAST.　　a formative cell or germ layer. Normoblast, a nucleated red blood cell of normal size.

-CELE (-OCELE). hernia or swelling. Hydrocele, accumulation of fluid in the testes.

-CENOSIS. discharge, surgical removal. Lithocenosis, removal of crushed calculi from the bladder.

-CENTESIS. puncture. Paracentesis, puncture of the wall of a cavity to draw off the contained fluid.

-CIDE. destroy. kill. Bactericide, destructive to bacteria.

-CLASIA (-CLAST). breaking. Hemoclasia, destruction of the erythrocytes.

-CLE. small. Corpuscle, a small rounded body.

-CLEISIS. closure. Enterocleisis, closure of a wound in the intestines.

-CYESIS. pregnancy. Pseudocyesis, false pregnancy.

-CYTE. cell. Spermatocyte, a cell which divides to form male germ cells.

-CYTOMA. a neoplasm made up of cells. Leukocytoma, tumorlike mass composed of leukocytes.

-DEMA. swelling. Edema, the presence of abnormally large amounts of fluid in the intercellular tissue spaces.

-DERMA. skin or skin disease. Scleroderma, disease characterized by induration of the skin.

-DESIS. binding fixation. Cirsodesis, ligation of varicose veins.

-DYNIA. pain. Pleurodynia, a sharp pain in the intercostal muscles.

-ECTASIA (-ECTASIS). distension or stretching. Bronchiectasis, dilatation of bronchi due to an inflammatory process.

-ECTOMY. surgical removal of. Hysterectomy, removal of the uterus.

-EMBOLUS. a plug. Aeroembolus, presence of nitrogen bubbles in the blood.

-EMIA (-CEMIA). blood. Septicemia, systemic disease caused by bacteria in the bloodstream.

-ERGY (-URGY). work. Energy, capacity for doing work.

-ESTHESIA. sensation. Anesthesia, loss of sensation.

-FEROUS. to bear; produce. Ossiferous, containing or producing bone.

-FICATION. making; causing. Calcification, formation of calcium.

-FORM. form or shape. Pustuliform, resembling a pustule.

-FUGE. to flee. Taeniafuge, an agent that destroys tapeworms.

-GEN (-GENESIS). producing. Spermatogenesis, formation of spermatozoa.

-GENIC. origin.

-GLOSSAL. tongue. Hypoglossal, situated under the tongue.

-GOGUE. to make flow. Sialagogue, producing a flow of saliva.

-GONY. Knee. Gonyocele, swelling of the knee.

-GRAM. a tracing. Cardiogram, a record of the heart's pulsation.

-GRAPH (-GRAPHIA). to write. Myograph, instrument for recording muscular contraction.

-GRAVIDA. pregnant. Multigavida, a woman who has borne two or more children.

-IASIS. disease. Trichomoniasis, disease caused by the presence of *Trichomonas*.

-INE (-IN). denotes a drug preparation. Narcotine, an alkaloid from opium.

-ISM. condition. Narcissism, condition of self-love.

-ITIS. inflammatory disease. Arthritis, inflammation of a joint.

-IZE. to treat by special method. Cauterize, to destroy tissue by heat, etc.

-LEMMA. sheath or envelope. Neurilemma, the sheath encasing a nerve fiber.

-LITH. stone. Cholelith, gallstone.

-LITHOTOMY. incision for removal of stones.

-LOGY. science or study of. Histology, study of microscopic anatomy.

-LYSIS (-LYTIC). dissolving or reduction. Hemolysis, destruction of red blood cells.

-MALACIA. softening. Adenomalacia, abnormal softening of a gland.

-MANIA. insanity. Monomania, mental disorder where the thoughts and action are dominated by one subject or idea.

-MEGALY. large, enlargement. Cardiomegaly, enlarged heart.

-MENTIA. mind. Dementia, loss of the mental faculties.

-MERE. part. Blastomere, segmentation cell.

-METRY. measure. Thermometry, measuring temperature with the thermometer.

-MYCIN. fungus. Neomycin, literally new fungus.

-NOMY. law. Taxonomy, science of the classification of organisms.

-NOSIS. disease. Diagnosis, the art of determining the nature of a disease.

-ODONT. tooth. Orthodontics, branch of dentistry concerned with treating malocclusion.

-ODYNIA.   state of pain. Neurodynia, severe pain along the course of a nerve.
-OID.   like or resembling. Sigmoid, shaped like the letter *S*.
-OLE.   small. Bronchiole, small subdivision of the bronchi.
-OMA.   tumor. Lipoma, a fatty tumor.
-OPIA.   sight or defect of the eye. Myopia, nearsightedness.
-OPSIA.   condition of vision. Xanthopsia, condition where objects look yellow.
-OREXIA.   appetite. Anorexia, loss of appetite.
-OSE.   sugar or carbohydrate. Fructose, fruit sugar.
-OSIS.   a condition or disease. Necrosis, pathologic death of cells in contact with living cells.
-OSTOMY.   to furnish with a mouth. Gastrostomy, establishing an opening into the stomach.
-OTOMY.   a cutting. Hysterotomy, incision of the uterus.
-OUS (-OBE).   full of or made of. Squamous, of the shape of a scale.

-PAROUS.   to bear. Primipara, woman giving birth to, or having had, first child.
-PATHY.   disease. Adenopathy, any glandular disease, especially of the lymph nodes.
-PENIA.   lack or deficiency. Granulocytopenia, deficiency of granulocytes in the blood.
-PEXIA (-PEXY).   fixation. Pneumonopexy, fixation of lung tissue to chest wall.
-PHAGE.   eating. Aerophagia, swallowing of air.
-PHOBIA.   fear. Photophobia, morbid fear of light.
-PHONY.   voice. Cacophony, abnormally harsh or discordant voice.
-PHYLAXIS.   protection. Anaphylaxis, state of hypersensitivity.
-PHYMA.   swelling or growth. Arthrophyma, swelling of a joint.
-PHYTE.   plant. Hematophyte, a vegetable organism living in the blood.
-PLAST (-PLASTY).   formation or molded. Myoplasty, plastic surgery on muscle.
-PLEGIA.   stroke, paralysis. Hemiplegia, paralysis of one side of the body.
-PNEA.   breathing. Dyspnea, difficult breathing.
-POESIS (-POIETIC).   making or producing. Hematopoiesis, formation of blood.
-POD (-PODY).   foot. Polypod, individual having an additional foot.
-PTOSIS.   a falling. Blepharoptosis, dropping of the upper eyelid.

-RRHAGIA.   abnormal or excessive discharge. Menorrhagia, excessive menstruation.
-RRHAPY.   suturing or stitching. Angiorrhaphy, suture of a blood vessel.
-RRHEA.   flow. Diarrhea, increased frequency and fluid consistency of the stools.
-RRHEXIS.   rupture. Plasmorrhexis, the rupture of a cell with the loss of protoplasm.
-RHYTHMIA.   rhythm. Arrythmia, absence of rhythm.

-SCOPE (-SCOPY).	to view. Laryngoscopy, examination of interior of larynx with the laryngoscope.
-SOMA.	body. Asoma, a fetal monster with only a rudimentary body.
-SPASM.	involuntary contraction. Bronchospasm, spasmodic contractions of the walls of the bronchi.
-STALSIS.	constriction. Peristalsis, wave of contraction seen in tubes.
-STAT.	stoppage. Hemostat, agent or instrument which arrests flow of blood.
-STOMY.	creation of a more or less permanent opening.

-TAXIA (-TAXY).	arrangement. Ataxia, incoordination of muscular action.
-THANASIA.	death. Euthanasia, an easy or calm death.
-THERAPY.	treatment. Pneumotherapy, treatment of lung disease.
-THYMIA.	condition of the mind. Agriothymia, insanity characterized by violence.
-TOMY.	incision into. Celiotomy, an incision made through the abdominal wall.
-TRIPSY.	crushing, rubbing. Lithotripsy, crushing calculi in the bladder.
-TROPHY.	nourishment. Atrophy, a reduction in size of an organ or cell.
-TROPE (-TROPIC).	a turning. Phototropic, tendency of a plant to turn toward light.

-URIA.	urine. Glycosuria, sugar in the urine.
-ULE.	small. Venule, a small vein.
-VOROUS.	eat. Herbivorous, living on vegetable food.

■ References

1. Tyrrell WB. *Medical Terminology for Medical Students*, Charles C Thomas, Springfield, IL, 1979, pp. 3–15.
2. Frenay AC. *Understanding Medical Terminology*, 4th ed, The Catholic Hospital Association, St. Louis, MO, 1969, pp. 1–16.
3. Caldwell E, Hegner BR, *Foundation for Medical Communication*, Reston Publishing Company, Inc, Reston, VA, 1978, pp. 51–68.
4. Sugar O. How the sacrum got its name. *JAMA* 1987; 257:2061–2063.
5. Chabner D. *The Language of Medicine*, 3rd ed, WB Sanders, Philadelphia, 1985.
6. Thomas J. Medical terminology. *Aust J Pharmacol* 1972; 53:357.
7. Collin MA. *Medical Terminology and the Body Systems*. Harper & Row, Hagerstown, MD, 1974, pp. 9–11.
8. Davies PM. *Medical Terminology in Hospital Practice*, 2nd ed, William Heinemann Medical Books, London, 1974, pp. 338–345.
9. Young CG, Barger JD. *Learning Medical Terminology Step By Step*, 3rd ed, CV Mosby, St. Louis, MO, 1975, pp. 8–14.
10. Bergman HD. Medical terminology, *US Pharm* 1980; 1:42–48.
11. Davis NM. 1700 medical abreviations: convenience at the expense of communications and safety. *Hosp Pharm* 1983; 18:175–211.

Chapter 7
Drug Dosage Forms That Should Not Be Crushed

It is not uncommon for a patient, nurse, or physician to ask a pharmacist if a drug product may be crushed or chewed to help ease drug administration. In many hospitals and long-term care facilities, it is a common practice to crush tablets or open capsules and mix the contents with water, juice, or certain foods. This practice generally helps improve a patient's compliance with his or her drug regimen. However, all medication dosage forms cannot be handled in this manner. There are many different types of oral medications available that have been specially formulated to release the drug over a prolonged period of time or at a predetermined time following administration. Examples of these special drug dosage forms include: extended release, enteric-coated, encapsulated beads, wax-matrix, and sublingual products. Altering the manufacturer's formulation design of products by crushing, chewing, or breaking may: (*a*) radically affect the drug's rate of absorption and distribution; (*b*) increase the risk of adverse and/or toxic side effects; or (*c*) seriously affect pharmacologic activity. Since all drug dosage form types are not readily identifiable from the drug name or from the package, the pharmacist must exercise a great deal of professional judgment when questioned on the matter. The problem of decreased patient compliance may be greatly improved by crushing drug products, but, in the process, the patient may be at a much higher risk of having adverse and/or toxic side effects from the drug (1).

■ Extended-release Drug Dosage Forms

Extended-release or controlled release drug dosage forms were developed to provide a mechanism that would allow medication to be released slowly from the tablet or capsule. An extended-release dosage form is defined as "one that allows at least a twofold reduction in dosing frequency as compared to that drug presented as a conventional dosage form" (1). In most instances, extended-release drug products enable patients to take fewer tablets or capsules each day without losing therapeutic efficiency and helps patients avoid adverse side effects from the drug. Both of these advantages could help improve patient compliance. Many drug delivery systems prolong the therapeutic action of a drug by prolonging its release from the core of the tablet. As the drug dosage form passes through the gastrointestinal (GI) tract, the outermost layer of the tablet/particles comes into contact with the fluid contents of the GI tract and the drug is released. This process might be best described as a shedding or dissolving of multiple layers of dosage forms over a period of time. As each layer is dissolved, a proportion of the medication is released and absorbed, ultimately producing a pharmacologic effect in the patient.

Although in a tablet dosage form, wax-matrix tablets are manufactured to provide the same extended-release of the drug, but by a different release mechanism. These tablets are based on the concept that liquid medication embedded in the wax will be released slowly as the wax matrix passes through the GI tract and melts or passes on in the feces.

Other drug dosage forms utilize a special semipermeable membrane that helps regulate the amount of fluid that enters the core of a tablet/particle in the GI tract. This process produces a slow, extended release or controlled release of the drug by affecting the dissolution rate and/or ion exchange properties of the drug. Drug dosage forms that may utilize this process include: tablets, capsules with beads, and some suspensions.

As a general rule, drug dosage forms manufactured as tablets or capsules with extended release properties should never be crushed or chewed by the patient. However, capsules that contain many small beads often may be opened and the capsule's contents mixed with a liquid or food product and consumed without chewing the beads.

■ Enteric-coated Drug Dosage Forms

Enteric-coated drug dosage forms are formulated to allow the medication to pass from the stomach into the intestine before releasing the active drug. The coating process is used for two primary reasons: to prevent stomach irritation and to avoid denaturation of the drug in the stomach (1).

Since some drugs, such as aspirin, are particularly irritating to the delicate lining of the stomach, some manufacturers produce these types of drugs with an enteric coating to prevent the stomach from becoming irritated. The coating helps prevent the medication from coming into contact with the stomach lining, but allows it to pass into the less acidic portion of the intestine where it is absorbed. Coating a tablet also protects the product against destruction of the active ingredient by the gastric juices of the stomach.

In general, crushing or chewing enteric-coated tablets is likely to produce undesirable side effects and possibly cause inactivation of the active ingredient.

■ Sublingual Drug Dosage Forms

Sublingual and buccal tablets are formulated to dissolve completely in the mouth when placed under the tongue or in the buccal cavity and to allow the drug to be quickly absorbed and have a rapid onset of action. The proximity of blood vessels and the relatively large blood supply in the buccal area enable the active ingredient to be absorbed and avoid possible destruction by gastric acids or rapid hepatic metabolism. Sublingual tablets are usually less effective or in-effective when taken orally by swallowing.

In general, crushing sublingual tablets is unnecessary and makes it very dif-ficult to place the powder properly under the tongue. Crushing the sublingual tablet may also render a major portion of the drug unusable and/or ineffective.

■ Alternatives to Crushing

For patients who cannot swallow whole tablets or capsules, the most logical approach is to replace the drug product with an oral liquid or suspension, a rectal suppository, a subcutaneous, intradermal, or intramuscular injection; or an intra-venous dosage form of the same medication. The pharmacist must always keep in mind that when changing a drug from an oral solid dosage form to a liquid, suspension suppository, or parenteral dosage form, it may be necessary to make an adjustment in drug dosage due to the drug's altered (increased or decreased) bioavailability in a different dosage form. The following table and product infor-mation code sheet may be used as a guide for selected drug products that generally should not be crushed. The product information code may be utilized to help determine a product's dosage form and to show how altering some dosage forms may not be detrimental to the drug or to the patient.

■ References

1. United States Pharmacopeia Convention, 21st ed, Mack Printing, Easton, PA, 1984.
2. Kastrup EK, Boyd JR, eds. *Facts and Comparisons*. JB Lippincott, Philadelphia, 1989.
3. McEvoy GK. *American Hospital Formulary Service*, American Society of Hospital Pharmacists, Bethesda, MD, 1989.
4. Mitchell JF. Oral dosage forms that should not be crushed: 1985 revision. *Hosp Pharm* 1985; 20:309–319.
5. Drug Information for the Health Care Provider, vol 1, *USP-DI*, 7th ed, 1989, United States Pharmacopeial Convention, Inc., Mack Printing, Easton, PA, 1989.
6. Hufford B, Voegele C, Harrison L. *Drugs That Should Not Be Chewed or Crushed*, Healthcare Prescription Services, Inc, Indianapolis, IN, 1985.

TABLE 7.1. ORAL DRUG DOSAGE FORMS THAT SHOULD NOT BE CHEWED OR CRUSHED (2–6)

Drug Product	Dosage Form	Drug Category	Product Information Code[a]
Accutane	Liquid-filled capsule	Vitamin	1b
Aerolate SR, JR, III	Controlled-release capsule	Bronchodilator	2
Afrinol Repetabs	Controlled-release tablet	Antihistamine/decongestant	3a
Aminodur Dura-Tabs	Controlled-release tablet	Bronchodilator	3e
Ammonium chloride tablets	Enteric-coated tablet	Urinary acidifier	1b
Artane Sequels	Controlled-release capsule	Antiparkinson	2
Arthritis Bayer Timed-Release	Controlled-release capsule	Analgesic	2
A.S.A. Enseals	Enteric-coated tablet	Analgesic	1b
Asbron G Inlay	Multiple compressed layered tablet	Bronchodilator	3c
Avazyme, Avazyme-100	Enteric-coated tablet	Digestive enzyme	1a
Azulfidine EN-tabs	Enteric-coated tablet	Antibiotic/antibacterial	1c
Belladenal-S	Controlled-release tablet	Antispasmodic	3b
Bellergal-S	Controlled-release tablet	Antispasmodic	3b
Bisacodyl	Enteric-coated tablet	Laxative	1b
Bontril-SR	Controlled-release capsule	Anorexiant	2
Breonesin	Liquid filled capsule	Expectorant	4a
Bronchobid Duracaps	Controlled-release capsule	Bronchodilator	2
Bronkodyl S-R	Controlled-release capsule	Bronchodilator	2
Butibel-Zyme	Controlled-release capsule	Digestive enzyme	3a
Calan SR Caplets	Controlled-release tablet	Antihypertensive	3b
Cama Arthritis Pain Reliever	Multiple compressed layered tablet	Analgesic	3c
Cardizem-SR	Controlled-release tablet	Antiarrhythmia	2
Carter's Little Pills	Enteric-coated tablet	Diuretic/analgesic	1b
Centrax	Controlled-release tablet	Antianxiety	3b
Chlorpheniramine Maleate T-D	Controlled-release capsule	Antihistamine	2
Chlor-Trimeton Repetabs	Controlled-release tablet	Antihistamine	3a
Chlor-Trimeton Decongestant Repetabs	Controlled-release tablet	Antihistamine/decongestant	3a
Choledyl SA	Controlled-release tablet	Bronchodilator	3e
Chymoral	Coated tablet	Enzyme	1a
Clistin R-A	Controlled-release tablet	Antihistamine	3a
Codimal-L.A. Cenules	Controlled-release capsule	Antihistamine/decongestant	2
Combist L.A.	Controlled-release capsule	Antihistamine/decongestant	2
Compazine Spansule	Controlled-release capsule	Antiemetic	2
Congress SR, JR	Controlled-release capsule	Antitussive/decongestant	2

Drug	Dosage Form	Category	Code
Constant-T	Controlled-release tablet	Bronchodilator	3
Contac	Controlled-release capsule	Antihistamine/decongestant	2
Cotazym-S Capsules	Enteric-coated microspheres (beads)	Digestive enzyme	1a
Cystospaz-M Capsules	Controlled-release capsule	Antispasmodic	2
Deconamine-SR	Controlled-release capsule	Antihistamine/decongestant	2
Demazin Repetabs	Controlled-release tablet	Antihistamine/decongestant	3a
Depakene	Controlled-release tablet	Anticonvulsant	4a
Desoxyn Gradumet	Controlled-release tablet	CNS stimulant	3a
Dexamyl Spansules	Controlled-release capsule	Anticonvulsant	2
Dexedrine Spansules	Controlled-release capsule	Anticonvulsant	2
Diamox Sequels	Controlled-release capsule	For glaucoma	2
Diatac	Controlled-release capsule	Anorexiant	2
Diethylstilbestrol Enseals	Enteric-coated tablet	Hormone	1b
Dilatrate-SR Capsules	Controlled-release capsule	Coronary vasodilator	2
Dimetane Extentabs	Controlled-release tablet	Antihistamine	3a
Dimetapp Extentabs	Controlled-release tablet	Antihistamine/decongestant	3a
Disophrol Chronotabs	Controlled-release tablet	Antihistamine/decongestant	3a
Donnatal Extentabs	Controlled-release tablet	Antispasmodic	3a
Donnazyme	Enteric-coated tablet	Digestive enzyme	3a
Dristan Capsules	Controlled-release capsule	Antihistamine/decongestant	2
Drixoral Repetabs	Controlled-release tablet	Antihistamine/decongestant	3a
Dulcolax	Enteric-coated tablet	Laxative	1b
Duotrate	Controlled-release capsule	Coronary vasodilator	2
Easprin	Enteric-coated tablet	Analgesic	2b
Ecotrin	Enteric-coated tablet	Analgesic	1b
E.E.S. Tablets	Enteric-coated tablet	Antibiotic/antibacterial	1a
Elixophyllin SR	Controlled-release capsule	Bronchodilator	2
E-Mycin	Enteric-coated tablet	Antibiotic/antibacterial	1a
Entozyme	Enteric-coated tablet	Digestive enzyme	3a
Equanil	Compressed tablet	Muscle relaxant	4a
Ergomar	Sublingual Tablet	Migraine	5
ERYC	Enteric-coated capsule	Antibiotic/antibacterial	2
ERY-Tab	Enteric-coated tablet	Antibiotic/antibacterial	1a
Eskabarb Spansule	Controlled-release capsule	Sedative	2
Eskalith CR	Controlled-release tablet	Antimanic	3a
Extendryl JR, SR	Controlled-release capsule	Antihistamine	2
Extex LA	Controlled-release tablet	Expectorant/decongestant	3
Fedahist	Controlled-release capsule	Antihistamine	2

TABLE 7.1. *Continued*

Drug Product	Dosage Form	Drug Category	Product Information Code[a]
Feldene	Gelatin capsule	Anti-inflammatory/analgesic	4a
Feosol	Enteric-coated tablet	Iron supplement	1b
Feosol Spansule Capsules	Controlled-release capsule	Iron supplement	2
Fergon	Controlled-release capsule	Iron supplement	1b
Fero-Grad 500 mg	Controlled-release tablet	Iron supplement	3d
Fero-Gradumet	Controlled-release tablet	Iron supplement	3d
Ferro-Sequels	Controlled-release capsule	Iron supplement	2
Ferrous Sulfate Enseals	Enteric-coated tablet	Iron supplement	1b
Festal, Festal II	Enteric-coated tablet	Digestive enzyme	1a
Fiogesic	Multiple compressed layered tablet	Analgesic	1b
Histabid	Controlled-release capsule	Antihistamine	2
Hydergine Sublingual	Sublingual tablet	Dementia	5
Iberet Filmtab	Controlled-release tablet	Vitamin/mineral	3d
Iberet-500 Filmtab	Controlled-release tablet	Vitamin/mineral	3d
Ilotycin	Enteric-coated tablet	Antibiotic/antibacterial	1a
Inderal-LA Capsule	Controlled-release capsule	β-blocker	2
Indocin SR	Controlled-release capsule	Anti-inflammatory/analgesic	2
Isoclor Timesule Capsules	Controlled-release capsule	Antihistamine	2
Isoptin SR Tablet	Controlled-release tablet	Antihypertensive	3b
Isordil Sublingual	Sublingual tablet	Coronary vasodilator	5
Isordil Tembids Tablets	Controlled-release tablet	Coronary vasodilator	3
Isordil Tembids Capsules	Controlled-release capsule	Coronary vasodilator	2
Isuprel Glossets	Sublingual tablet	Bronchodilator	5
K-Lyte	Effervescent tablet	Potassium supplement	4h, 1b
K-Tab	Controlled-release tablet	Potassium supplement	3e, 1b
Kaon-Cl 10	Controlled-release tablet	Potassium supplement	3e, 1b
Kaon-Cl 6.7 mEq	Controlled-release tablet	Potassium supplement	3e, 1b
K-Dur Tablets	Controlled-release tablet	Potassium supplement	3b, 1b
KEFF	Effervescent tablet	Potassium supplement	4g, 1b
Klor-Con Tablets	Controlled-release tablet	Potassium supplement	3e, 1b
Klorvess	Effervescent tablet	Potassium supplement	4g, 1b
Klotrix	Controlled-release tablet	Potassium supplement	3b, 1b
K-Ten Tablets	Controlled-release tablet	Potassium supplement	3b, 1b
Lithobid	Controlled-release tablet	Antimanic	3b

Mandelamine	Enteric-coated tablet	Urinary antiseptic	1b
Measurin	Controlled-release tablet	Analgesic	1b
Meprospan	Controlled-release capsule	Muscle relaxant	2
Mestinon Timespan Tablets	Controlled-release tablet	For myasthenia gravis	3a
Metandren Linguets	Sublingual tablet	Hormone	5
Mi-Cebrin	Coated tablet	Vitamin/mineral	4a
Mi-Cebrin T	Enteric-coated tablet	Vitamin/mineral	4a
Micro-K	Controlled-release capsule	Potassium supplement	2
Modane Soft	Liquid-filled capsule	Fecal softener	4a
Mol-Iron Chronsules	Controlled-release capsule	Iron supplement	2
Motrin	Coated tablet	Anti-inflammatory/analgesic	4a
MS Contin	Controlled-release tablet	Analgesic	3
MSC Triaminic	Enteric-coated tablet	Antihistamine/decongestant	3a
Multicebrin	Coated tablet	Vitamin/mineral	4a
Myobid Capsules	Controlled-release capsule	Vasodilator	2
Naldecon	Controlled-release tablet	Antihistamine/decongestant	3a
Napril	Timed-release capsule	Antihistamine/decongestant	2
Nico-400 Plateau-Caps	Controlled-release capsule	Vasodilator	2
Nicobid	Controlled-release capsule	Vasodilator	2
Nico-Span	Controlled-release capsule	Vasodilator	2
Niferex-150 Capsules	Controlled-release capsule	Iron supplement	2
Nitro-Bid	Controlled-release capsule	Coronary vasodilator	2
Nitrogard Buccal Tablets	Buccal tablet	Coronary vasodilator	5
Nitroglycerin T-D	Controlled-release capsule	Coronary vasodilator	2
Nitroglyn	Controlled-release tablet	Coronary vasodilator	3
Nitrostat Sublingual	Sublingual tablet	Coronary vasodilator	5
Nitrostat SR	Controlled-release capsule	Coronary vasodilator	2
Noctec	Liquid-filled capsule	Hypnotic	4a
Nolamine	Controlled-release tablet	Antihistamine/decongestant	3a
Norflex	Controlled-release tablet	Muscle relaxant	4a
Norpace CR Capsules	Controlled-release capsule	Antiarrhythmic	2
Novafed	Controlled-release capsule	Antihistamine/decongestant	2
Novafed A	Controlled-release capsule	Antihistamine/decongestant	2
Novahistine LP	Controlled-release tablet	Antihistamine/decongestant	1c
Nu'Leven	Enteric-coated tablet	Digestive enzyme	1a
Obestat	Controlled-release capsule	Anorexiant	2
Oragrafin	Liquid-filled capsule	Radiopaque	4a
Ornade Spansule Capsules	Controlled-release capsule	Antihistamine	2

TABLE 7.1. *Continued*

Drug Product	Dosage Form	Drug Category	Product Information Code[a]
Pabalate	Enteric-coated tablet	Analgesic	1b
Pabalate SF	Enteric-coated tablet	Analgesic	1b
Pabirin Buffered	Multiple compressed layered tablet	Analgesic	4a
Pancrease	Enteric-coated microspheres (beads)	Digestive enzyme	2
Panmycin	Gelatin capsule	Antibiotic/antibacterial	4a
Papaverine HCl T-R	Controlled-release capsule	Vasodilator	2
Pathilon Sequels	Controlled-release capsule	Anticholinergic	2
Pavabid Plateau-Caps	Controlled-release capsule	Vasodilator	2
PBZ-SR	Controlled-release tablet	Antihistamine	3a
PCE Tablet	Enteric-coated tablet	Antibiotic/antibacterial	1a
Penritol Timesules	Controlled-release capsule	Coronary vasodilator	2
Perdiem	Wax-coated granules	Laxative	4f
Peritrate SA	Controlled-release tablet	Coronary vasodilator	3c
Permitil Chronotabs	Controlled-release tablet	Neuroleptic	3a
Phazyme	Controlled-release tablet	Digestive enzyme	1a
Phazyme 95	Controlled-release tablet	Digestive enzyme	1a
Phazyme PB	Controlled-release tablet	Digestive enzyme	1a
Phenergan	Compressed tablet	Antihistamine	4a
Polaramine Repetabs	Controlled-release tablet	Antihistamine	3a
Povan Filmseals Tablets	Coated tablet	Antihelminthic	4b
Prelu-2	Controlled-release capsule	CNS stimulant	2
Preludin Endurets	Controlled-release tablet	CNS stimulant	3b
Procan SR	Controlled-release tablet	Antiarrhythmic	3d
Procardia	Gelatin capsule	Antiarrhythmic/antiangina	4d
Pronestyl-SR	Controlled-release tablet	Antiarrhythmic	3e
Quibron-T,SR	Controlled-release tablet	Bronchodilator	3a
Quinaglute Dura-Tabs	Controlled-release tablet	Antiarrhythmic	3e
Quinidex Extentabs	Controlled-release tablet	Antiarrhythmic	3a
Resbid	Controlled-release tablet	Bronchodilator	2
Ritalin-SR	Controlled-release tablet	CNS stimulant	3a
Robimycin Robitabs	Enteric-coated tablet	Antibiotic/antibacterial	1a
Roniacol Timespan	Timed-release tablet	Vasodilator	3a
Roxanol-Sr	Controlled-release tablet	Analgesic	3a
Seldane	Controlled-release tablet	Antihistamine	3a

Drug	Dosage form	Category	Code
Singlet	Controlled-release tablet	Antihistamine/decongestant	3a
SK-Bisacodyl	Enteric-coated tablet	Laxative	1b
SK-Erythromycin	Enteric-coated tablet	Antibiotic/antibacterial	1a
Slo-Bid Gyrocaps	Timed-release capsule	Bronchodilator	2
Slo-Phyllin-CRT	Controlled-release capsule	Bronchodilator	2
Slo-Phyllin GG	Controlled-release capsule	Bronchodilator	2
Slo-Phyllin Gyrocaps	Timed-release capsule	Bronchodilator	2
Slow-FE	Controlled-release tablet	Iron supplement	3a
Slow-K	Controlled-release tablet	Potassium supplement	3e
Sodium Salicylate Enseal	Enteric-coated tablet	Anti-inflammatory/analgesic	1b
Sodium Chloride Enseal	Enteric-coated tablet	NaCl supplement	1b
Somophyllin-CRT	Timed-release capsule	Bronchodilator	2
Sorbitrate S.A.	Controlled-release tablet	Coronary vasodilator	3a
S-P-T	Liquid-filled capsule	Thyroid supplement	4a
Sudafed S.A.	Controlled-release capsule	Decongestant	2
Sustaire	Controlled-release tablet	Bronchodilator	3a
Symmetrel	Controlled-release capsule	Antiviral	2
Tavist-D	Controlled-release tablet	Antihistamine/decongestant	3a
Tedral SA	Controlled-release tablet	Bronchodilator	3a
Teldrin Spansules	Controlled-release capsule	Antihistamine	2
Temaril Spansules	Controlled-release capsule	Antihistamine	2
Tenuate Dospan	Controlled-release tablet	Anorexiant	3e
Tepanil Ten-tab	Controlled-release tablet	Anorexiant	3e
Tessalon Perle	Capsule	Antitussive	4e
Theo-24 Capsules	Controlled-release capsule	Bronchodilator	2
Theobid	Controlled-release capsule	Bronchodilator	2
Theobid Jr.	Controlled-release capsule	Bronchodilator	2
Theo-Dur	Controlled-release tablet	Bronchodilator	3b
Theo-Dur Sprinkles	Controlled-release capsule	Bronchodilator	2
Theolair-SR	Controlled-release tablet	Bronchodilator	3b
Theophyl SR	Controlled-release capsule	Bronchodilator	2
Theospan Capsules	Controlled-release capsule	Bronchodilator	2
Theovent	Controlled-release capsule	Bronchodilator	2
Thorazine Spansules	Controlled-release capsule	Neuroleptic	2
Trental	Controlled-release tablet	Hemorrheologic agent	3a
Triaminic	Enteric-coated tablet	Antihistamine/decongestant	3a
Triaminic-12	Controlled-release tablet	Antihistamine/decongestant	3a
Triaminic TR	Multiple compressed layers	Antihistamine/decongestant	3c

TABLE 7.1. *Continued*

Drug Product	Dosage Form	Drug Category	Product Information Code[a]
Triaminic Juvelets	Controlled-release tablet	Antihistamine/decongestant	3a
Trilafon Repetabs	Controlled-release tablet	Neuroleptic	3a
Trinalin Repetabs	Controlled-release tablet	Antihistamine	3a
Tussagesic	Enteric-coated tablet	Decongestant/analgesic	1b
Tuss-Ornade Spansules	Controlled-release capsule	Antitussive/antihistamine	2
Ursinus Inlay	Multiple compressed layered tablet	Bronchodilator	3c
Valrelease	Controlled-release capsule	Antianxiety	2
Wyamycin-S	Controlled-release tablet	Antibiotic/antibacterial	1a
Zorprin	Controlled-release tablet	Anti-inflammatory/analgesic	3b

[a] **Product Information Code**

1. **Enteric-coated tablet**
   Designed to pass through the stomach whole and then dissolve in the intestines. Reasons for this type of formulation include:
   a. To prevent the destruction of the drug by stomach acid
   b. To prevent irritation to the stomach
   c. To achieve a prolonged action

2. **Timed-release capsules**
   Designed to release medication over a period of 8–12 hr. The beads within the capsules are designed to dissolve at different times. It should not hurt the medication to open the capsule and administer the contents, but **do not** crush or chew the contents. The beads may be carefully mixed with soft foods, e.g., apple sauce, pudding.

3. **Timed-release tablets**
   Designed to give medication release over a period of 8–12 hr. Some formulations are designed to reduce gastric irritation. Specific types include:
   a. Slow release core—outer coating may dissolve to give initial dose of medication followed by the slow dissolving of the core to give a prolonged release of medication
   b. Mixed release granules—formulated with regular and slow release granules to give immediate and also prolonged medication release
   c. Multilayer tablets—usually two or three layers with one layer designed to dissolve fast to give a loading dose of the medication; the remaining layers dissolve at a slow rate to maintain constant blood levels of the medication
   d. Porous inert carriers—a small plastic pellet with thousands of small passages filled with the medication, medication slowly releases into the gastric fluids
   e. Soluble matrix—a wax matrix that allows a slow release of a drug into the gastric fluids, prevents a large concentration of drug in a local area, thus preventing gastric upset

4. **Miscellaneous**
   a. Taste—extremely unpleasant
   b. Stains mouth red
   c. Burning sensation of oral mucosa due to irritation
   d. Delays absorption, but capsule may be opened
   e. Causes anesthesia to oral mucosa
   f. Wax-coated granules
   g. Tablet must be dissolved in water or juice

5. **Sublingual and buccal tablets**
   Designed to dissolve in the oral fluids and be rapidly absorbed in the mouth. Swallowing, chewing, or crushing may prevent the drugs from reaching the bloodstream, thus making them ineffective. Some medications are destroyed by gastric juices. Some medications are available in both oral and sublingual forms but are formulated differently.

Answers for Review Questions

■ Chapter 1

1. Any five of the following:

   a. General information—age, date of birth, sex, race, religion, date of admission

   b. Attending physician(s)

   c. Admitting diagnosis(es)

   d. Patient allergies

   e. Physical assessment by nurse

   f. Physical therapy assessment

   g. Occupational therapy assessment

   h. Speech therapy assessment

   i. Social worker's assessment and discharge plan

2. Any five of the following:

   a. Current chief complaint of the patient

   b. History of patient's present illness

   c. Patient's past medical history

   d. Allergies/drug sensitivities

   e. Patient's family and social history

   f. Patient's physical examination

    g. Physician's impressions of what is wrong with the patient and his or her admitting diagnosis

3. Any five of the following:

    a. Routine medication orders

    b. Medication orders (prn)

    c. Vital signs, fluid intake and/or urine output

    d. Treatments

    e. Therapies (physical, occupational, speech)

    f. Laboratory tests

    g. Diet (e.g., 1500 kcal, low-sodium diet, American Diabetes Association)

    h. Approved bedside medication or health items

4. Any five of the following:

    a. Patient's subjective complaints of acute problems

    b. Patient's subjective complaints of chronic problems

    c. Physician's objective evaluation of patient's status

    d. Laboratory tests

    e. Vital signs of patient

    f. Physician's assessment of patient's status

    g. Physician's plans to help correct or improve the patient's status

5. Any five of the following:

    a. Vital signs (temperature, apical pulse, respirations, blood pressure)

    b. Adverse drug reactions

    c. Documentation of prn medication administered

    d. Assessment of the patient status on a daily basis

    e. Patient's refusal to take medications

    f. Current weight

    g. Social involvement with visitors, residents, and staff

    h. Documentation of the pharmacist's drug regimen review

i. Onset of acute medical conditions

j. Catheter changes, appearance of urine

k. Complaints of the patient

l. Notes from therapists (physical, occupational, and speech)

m. Notes from dietician

n. Notes from activities director

o. Response to drug therapy

6. Any five of the following:

a. Medication—strength, dose, dosage interval, and duration (oral, parenteral, external)

b. Record of medication administration times (routine and prn)

c. Record of medication refused by the patient

d. Daily initialed record of who administered the medication

e. Patient allergies/drug sensitivities

f. Whether medication should be crushed

g. Dates when medication was started and stopped or discontinued

h. Initials/names of all nurses administering medication during the month

i. Limitations or contraindications to medication as ordered (e.g., apical pulse less than 0, systolic blood pressure less than 100 mm Hg, respiration less than 12)

7. Answers:

a. Results of current laboratory tests (e.g., complete blood count, fasting blood sugar, chemistry profile, electrolytes, blood urea nitrogen, creatinine, urinalysis, culture and sensitivity report, prothrombin time, partial thromboplastin time)

b. Results of previous laboratory reports from another hospital or long-term care facility.

c. Serum drug levels (e.g., digoxin, phenytoin, theophylline, phenobarbital, Mysoline, aminoglycosides, procainamide)

d. X-rays, CAT scans, ECG/EKG, EEG and related tests

8. Answers:

   a. Vital signs (e.g., temperature, apical pulse, respirations, blood pressure)

   b. Body weight

   c. Eating habits

   d. Continence (e.g., bowel and bladder)

   e. Sleeping habits

9. False

10. True

■ Chapter 2

1. True

2. Answers:

   a. Admissions Record

   b. History and Physical Examination

3. Any two of the following:

   a. Clues to the patient's present condition

   b. Clues to past psychological and sociological problems

   c. Clues to genetic illness patterns

4. Any three of the following:

   a. Drug allergies/sensitivities

   b. Past and present medical problems

   c. Extent of recovery of past medical problems

   d. Previous laboratory tests

   e. Current physical and medical status of the patient

5. Answer:

   To help determine that all current drugs being taken are necessary and that all medical problems the patient has are being addressed or treated.

6. Any three of the following:

   a. Direct indicators of a patient's medical condition

   b. A guide for rapid and thorough understanding of a patient's medical condition

   c. A diagnostic tool in reviewing vital body systems of metabolism and excretion

   d. Degree of disease control

   e. An indication of present or impending complications for the patient

   f. Therapeutic or toxic serum level

7. True

8. True

9. Any four of the following:

   a. Clinical improvements in the patient's condition

   b. Clinical signs and/or symptoms of an acute medical problem

   c. Clinical signs and/or symptoms of a failure to reverse a disease process

   d. Clinical signs and/or symptoms of an improvement of a disease

   e. Clinical signs and/or symptoms of a lack of response to appropriate drug therapy

   f. Adverse and/or toxic side effects of drugs

   g. Clinical laboratory values

   h. Diagnostic tests

   i. Serum and/or urine drug levels

   j. Body or organ functions

10. True

11. True

12. True

13. True

14. Any four of the following:

   a. Alternative drug and nondrug therapies

   b. Discontinue drug(s)

   c. Modify drug dose

   d. Modify drug dosage interval

   e. Change route of administration

   f. Advise against taking drugs together

   g. Advise against taking drugs with or without food

   h. Request laboratory tests

   i. Change diet

   j. Suggest the patient learn more about his or her medication and/or disease

   k. Request vital signs be taken more often

   l. Continue to monitor unclear or problematic situations

   m. Continue present drug and nondrug therapies

15. False

Index

Page numbers followed by "t" denote tables.

Spectrobid. *See* Bacampicillin

Spironolactone
    drug-monitoring parameters for, 173
    lab tests for monitoring of, 235t, 243t

Spironolactone and hydrochlorothiazide, drug-monitoring parameters for, 173–174

Spironometer, definition of, 270

Splenomegaly, definition of, 270

SSKI. *See* Potassium iodide

Stadol. *See* Butorphanol

Staphcillin. *See* Methicillin

Stelazine. *See* Trifluoperazine

Stop-order policies, 67

Streptokinase, drug-monitoring parameters for, 155

Streptomycin, drug-monitoring parameters for, 135

Subluxated, definition of, 270

Sucralfate, drug-monitoring parameters for, 176

Sudafed. *See* Psuedoephedrine hydrochloride

Suffixes, 284–288

Sulbactam sodium and ampicillin sodium, drug-monitoring parameters for, 139

Sulfamethoxazole, drug-monitoring parameters for, 143–144

Sulfamethoxazole and trimethoprim, drug-monitoring parameters for, 143–144

Sulfhemoglobinemia, definition of, 270

Sulfinpyrazone
    drug-monitoring parameters for, 174–175
    lab tests for monitoring of, 243t

Sulfisoxazole, drug-monitoring parameters for, 143–144

Sulfonamides, drug-monitoring parameters for, 143–144

Sulindac
    drug-monitoring parameters for, 165–166
    lab tests for monitoring of, 239t, 243t

Sumycin. *See* Tetracycline hydrochloride

Sus-phrine. *See* Epinephrine

Symmetrel. *See* Amantadine hydrochloride

Sympathomimetic agents, drug-monitoring parameters for, 153

Synophylate. *See* Theophylline

Synthroid. *See* Levothyroxine sodium

Tagamet. *See* Cimetidine

Talwin. *See* Pentazocine

Tambocor. *See* Flecainide

Tamm-Horsfall mucoproteins, 226

Tamoxifen, drug-monitoring parameters for, 151

Tapazole. *See* Methimazole

Tavist. *See* Clemastine fumarate

Tazicef. *See* Ceftazidime

Tazidime. *See* Ceftazidime

Tegopen. *See* Cloxacillin

Tegretol. *See* Carbamazepine

Temazepam, drug-monitoring parameters for, 170

Tenex. *See* Guanfacine hydrochloride

Teniposide, drug-monitoring parameters for, 149

Ten-K. *See* Potassium chloride

Tenoretic. *See* Chlorthalidone and atenolol

Tenormin. *See* Atenolol

Terazosin, drug-monitoring parameters for, 162

Terbutaline, drug-monitoring parameters for, 181

Terfenadine, drug-monitoring parameters for, 134

Terminology, medical, 249–288. *See also* Medical terminology

Terramycin. *See* Oxytetracycline

Tes Tape, 225

Testosterone, lab tests for monitoring of, 244t

Tetracycline hydrochloride, drug-monitoring parameters for, 140

Theo–24. *See* Theophylline

Theo-Dur. *See* Theophylline

Theophylline, 64t
    drug-monitoring parameters for, 181
    lab tests for monitoring of, 244t

Theo-Sprinkles. *See* Theophylline

Thiazide diuretics, drug-monitoring parameters for, 173

Thioguanine, drug-monitoring parameters for, 152

Thioridazine, drug-monitoring parameters for, 170